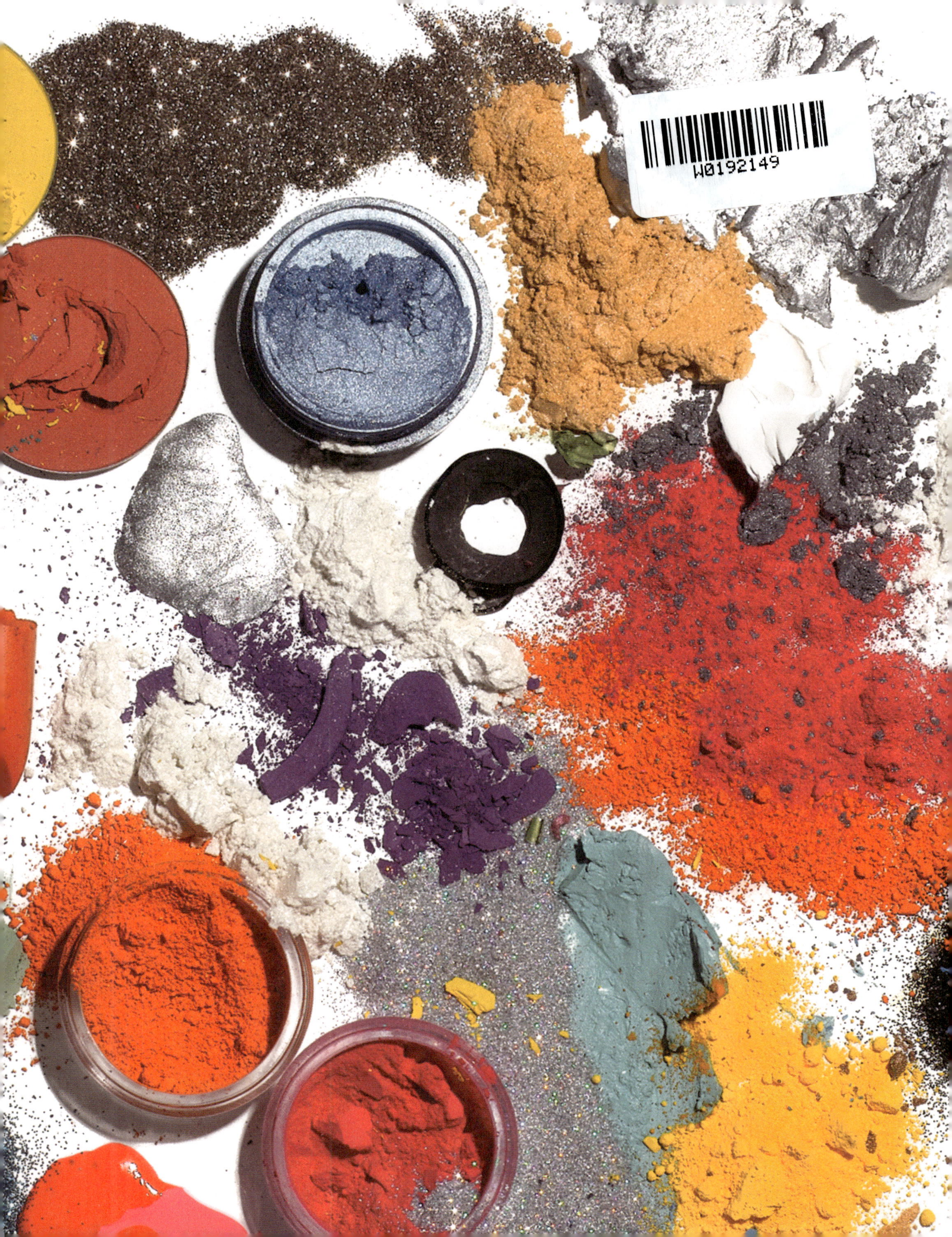

BOBBI BROWN MAKEUP MANUAL

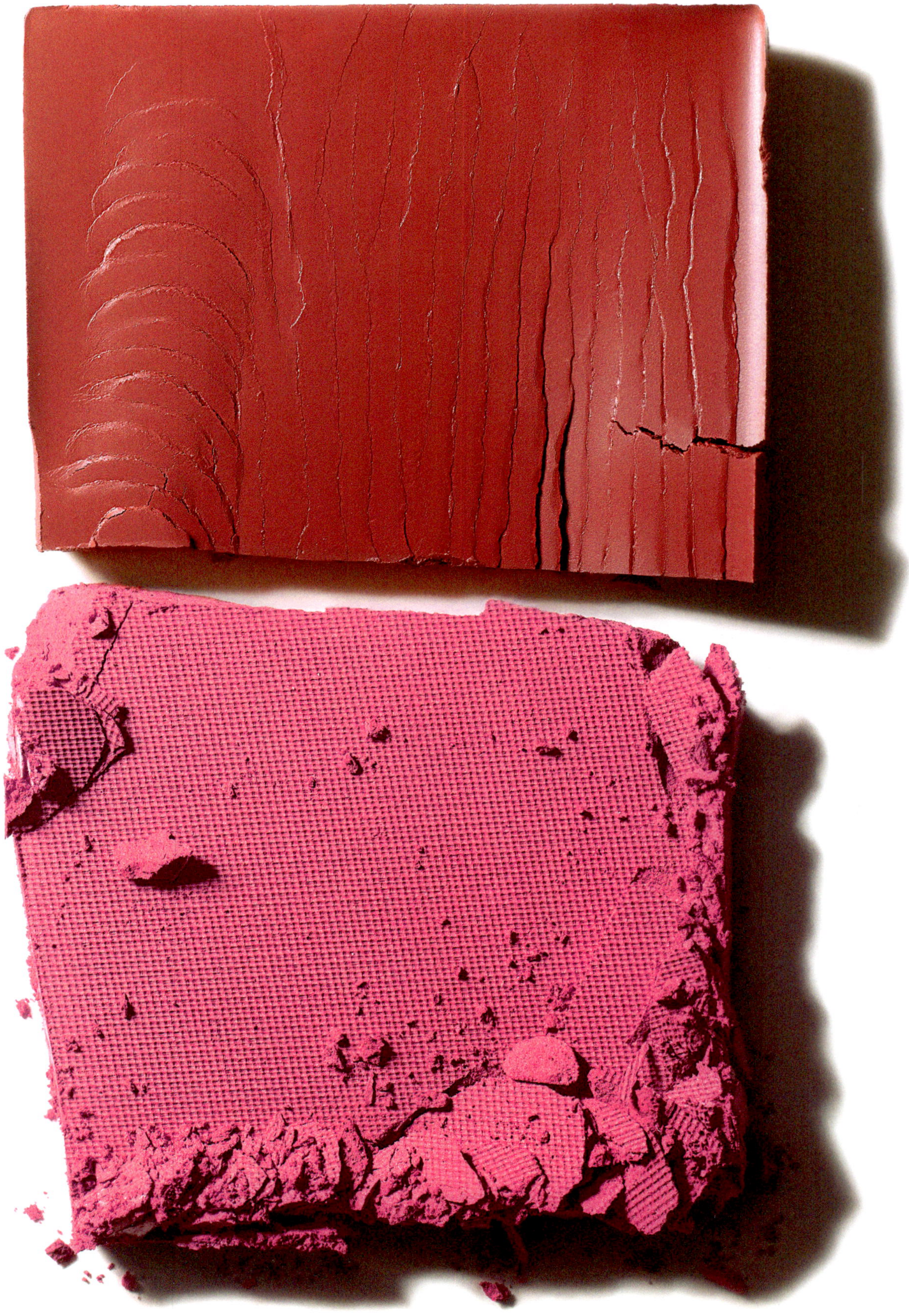

For Everyone from Beginner to Pro

BOBBI BROWN MAKEUP MANUAL

Bobbi Brown

with Debra Bergsma Otte and Sally Wadyka

with photographs by Henry Leutwyler

GRAND CENTRAL Life & Style

NEW YORK • BOSTON

Photography credits and permissions information on p. 221.

Grand Central Life & Style
Hachette Book Group
1290 Avenue of the Americas, New York, NY 10104
www.GrandCentralLifeandStyle.com

Grand Central Life & Style is an imprint of Grand Central Publishing. The Grand Central Life & Style name and logo are trademarks of Hachette Book Group, Inc.

First Edition: December 2008

Design by Ruba Abu-Nimah & Eleanor Rogers

Library of Congress Cataloging-in-Publication Data
Brown, Bobbi.
Bobbi Brown makeup manual: for everyone from beginner to pro / By Bobbi Brown.
p. cm.
ISBN: 978-0-446-58134-9
1. Cosmetics. 2. Beauty, Personal. 3. Women—Health and hygiene. I. Title.
RA778.B8786 2008
646.7'2—dc22
2008004307

10 9 8 7 6

Printed in the United States of America

This book is dedicated to makeup artists everywhere — from the ones that taught me to the ones that I now teach.

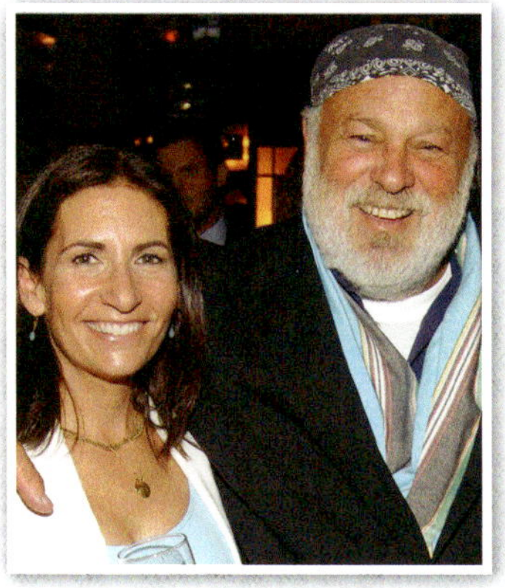

And to Bruce Weber, who taught me how to see the natural tones in people's faces — and that you can be both talented and famous, humble and nice.

And, always, to the boys/men in my life who make my heart sing.

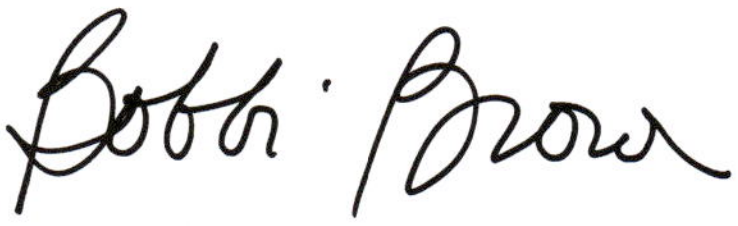

CONTENTS

I BASICS

II ARTISTRY

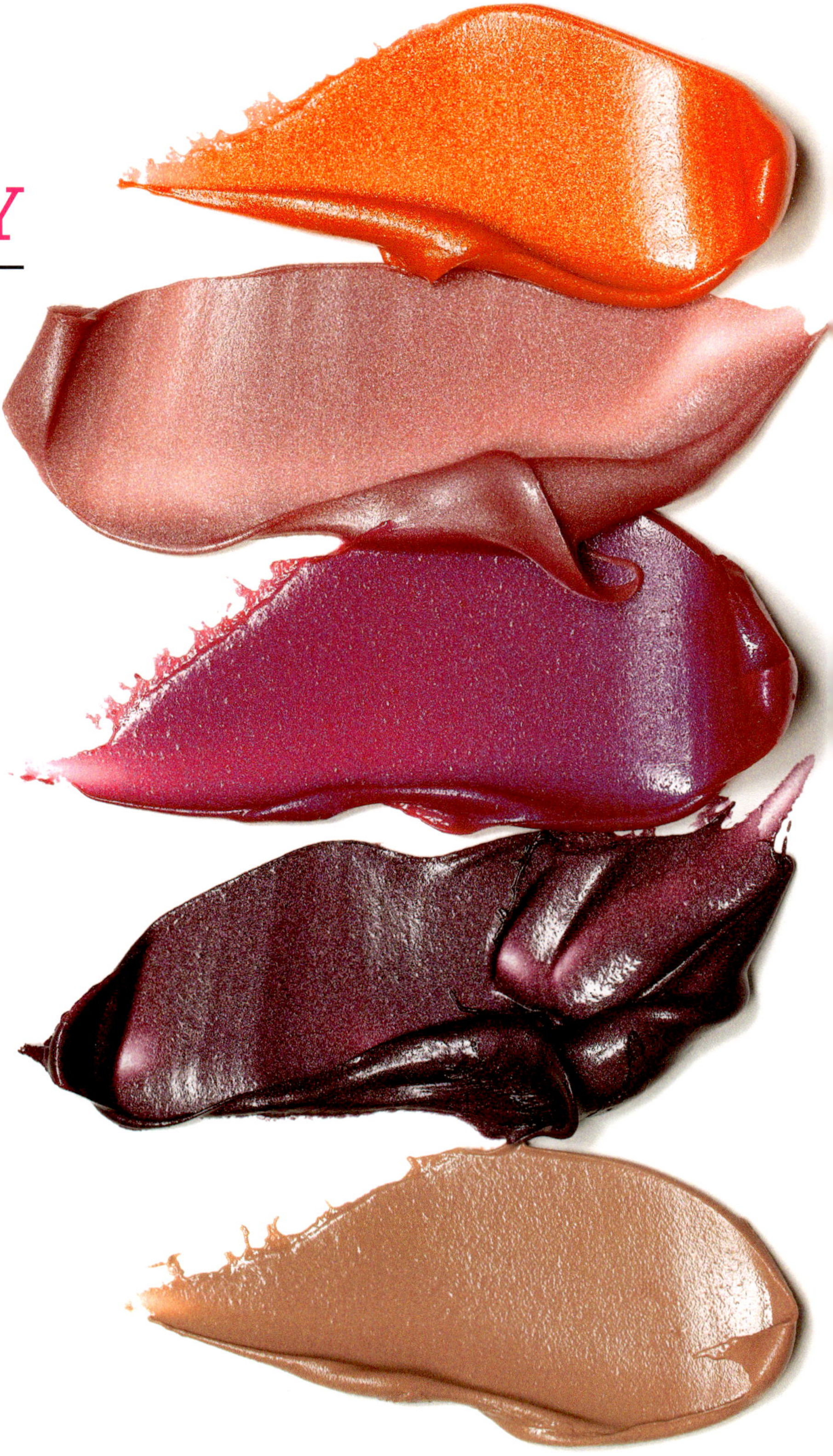

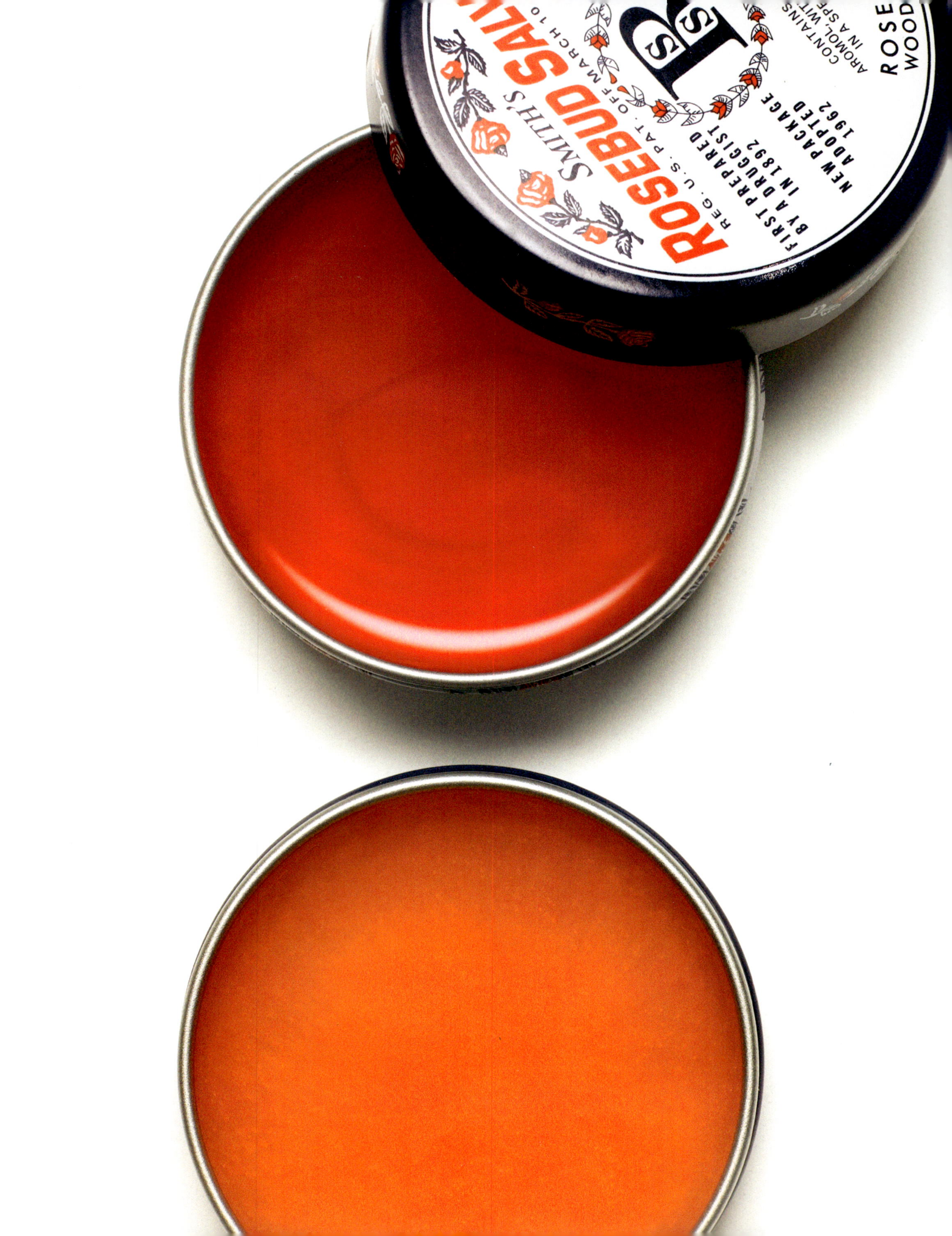
SMITH'S
ROSEBUD
FIRST PREPARED BY A DRUGGIST IN 1892
NEW PACKAGE ADOPTED 1962

PART I: BASICS

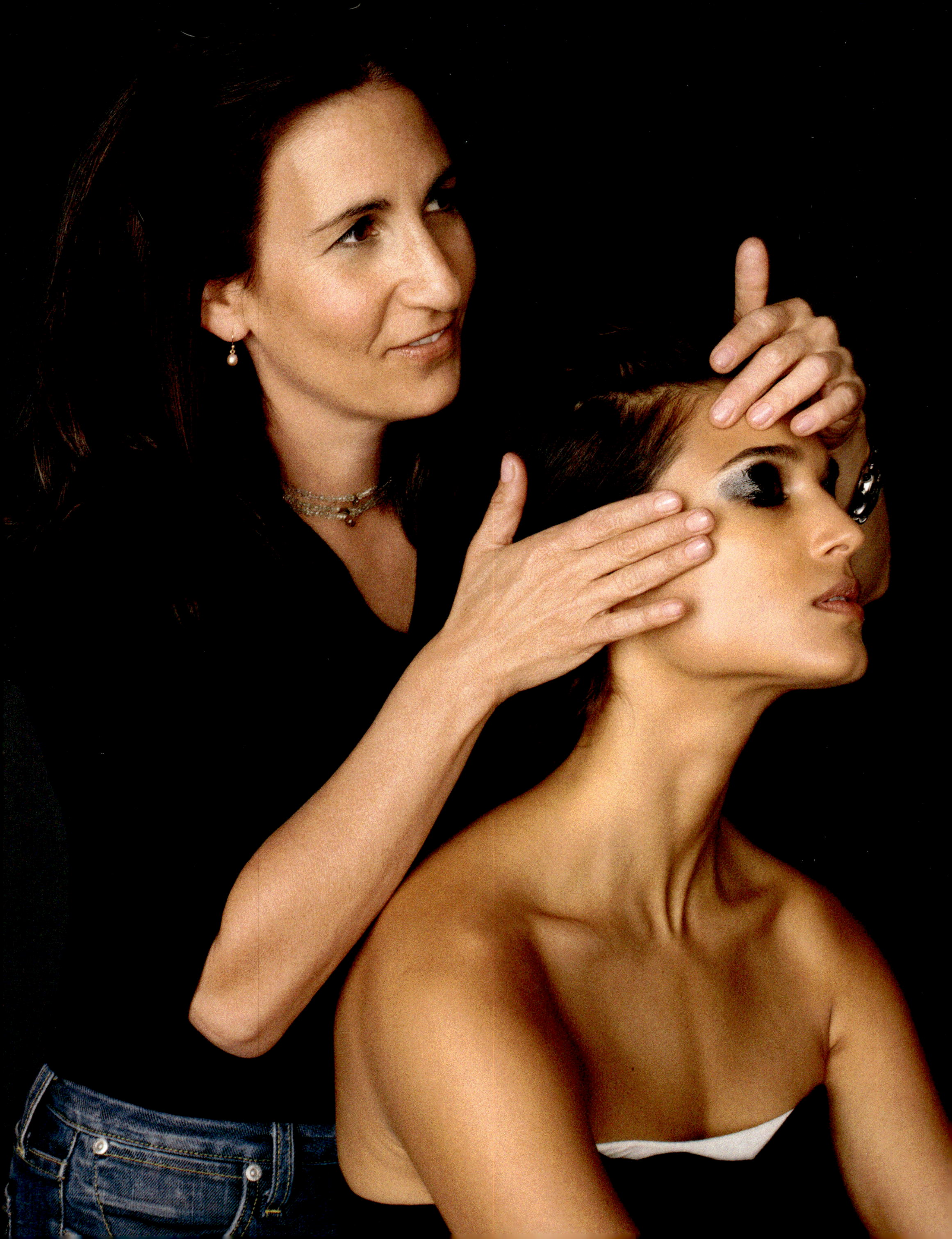

Chapter 1

MAKEUP ARTISTRY

I've set out to write the **simplest, most comprehensive makeup lesson you will ever have.** I've written this book for everyone: my artists, students, friends, and every woman who ever wanted to put on makeup like a professional.

When I first started working as a freelance makeup artist, it was almost impossible to find books dedicated to makeup artistry. This situation has improved over the years, but there is still a noticeable lack of good and accessible resources on makeup artistry. After scouring countless bookstores in search of the perfect makeup reference, I finally decided to write my own guide. My vision for this book is simple. I wanted it to be filled with complete step-by-step lessons, industry tips, and beautiful pictures. I wanted this book to serve as a complete reference guide for everyone who wants to know about beauty and makeup.

I have found that women are either intrigued with or mystified by cosmetics, but most are interested in learning more about makeup and how it can transform a face. All women really want the same thing: to look like themselves, only prettier and more confident. That desire is what actually inspired me, at twelve years old, to create the "natural look" for which I'm known. In seventh grade, the coolest thing was to hear how tan you were. So I used my mother's bronzer, put it on my cheeks, forehead, nose, and chin—until it looked like a real tan. I put on her lipstick and then rubbed it off. I wanted people to say I looked pretty—and not notice the makeup.

Years later, when I worked as a makeup artist, I learned from many of the leading professionals. My early work was a mixture of the natural look with risky bolts of color. I worked with George Newell, who did beautiful pale skin, very 80s red lips, bronze cheeks, and dark eyes. His style was not mine, but he was a great talent who taught me things I could not have learned elsewhere. I also studied under Linda Mason, the artist known for her abstract uses of color on the face. She taught me to go beyond my comfort zone and push myself to the unexpected. Then I met my mentor, Bonnie Maller. I first saw her work in a magazine profile. She did all the makeup for Bruce Weber and all the ads for Perry Ellis, Calvin Klein, and Ralph Lauren. Her style was outdoorsy, as you can imagine. She had the same aesthetic as I did, and perfected the look. It changed my life. Her makeup was most instrumental in helping my style emerge. It was clean, natural, and always beautiful.

In the early days, I was like a sponge, learning from others, and then experimenting to see what I liked. I now look back on this time as graduate school. I read and studied every fashion spread. I loved the way light hit the colors on the face, and tried to recreate the looks. I began assisting makeup artists and eventually, with that experience, started to lead my own team.

When you are hired to do a show, you meet with the designer, and sometimes the stylist, to discuss the desired look and to possibly try the makeup on a model. The makeup has to be beautiful and work with the clothes. I used to experiment with concealer on lips to make a pale lip color statement while doing Brigitte Bardot–inspired, dark, smoky eyes or the brightest red and pink lips with very little on the eyes. I also remember using brown eye pencil on lips, which started the whole brown lip look.

By the time I started Bobbi Brown Cosmetics, I already had a group of artists who helped me do fashion shows. Early in my career, I couldn't pay them much, so I hired the ones who were eager to do the work for the experience and training. I started by inviting them to assist me—even if they just held brushes or observed. I watched them do makeup. I watched them watch me do makeup.

I love working with people who soak up information. Everyone has potential. I've never met anyone who could not master the skills needed, but many who lacked the confidence. I do believe that there is always more to learn, and I love the process.

I also believe every woman would gain confidence if she understood more about applying her makeup, using the right tools, finding the colors that work for her and perfecting the basic techniques.

I've written this book for everyone: my artists, students, friends, and every woman who ever wanted professional instruction. I've gone into more detail than ever before and photographed hundreds of step-by-step photos to show you as much detail as possible. I've also put the entire "class" into the sequence that I believe works best. Understanding the skin is the best way to start, and then building from foundation and concealer to color, lips, eyes, and everything in between. I believe this will be the most comprehensive makeup lesson you will ever have.

For the makeup artist or those who aspire to be one, I've written a section for professionals in the second part of the book. In this section, you'll find important information from how to pack a professional makeup kit to how to work with photographers.

The best artists continually want to learn. Artists who think they know everything don't grow. Professional makeup artists must love makeup. They need to be obsessed with the art and the business and cannot be afraid of hard work. Artists have to be able to see, evaluate their work, and take criticism as an

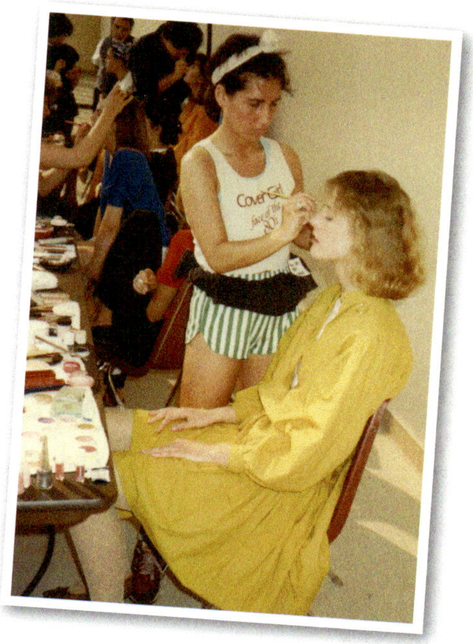

opportunity to grow. In makeup that means learning to recognize skin condition and texture, evaluate and effectively use color, and determine when formulation and application choices work and what to do when they don't.

This book is a true labor of love. It was written with the help of my team of makeup artists, friends, and customers—who have all contributed questions, concerns, and tips about makeup. Even though I've been in the makeup industry for over twenty years, I continue to learn.

The beauty industry is constantly changing, so it is important to stay open to new ideas, to acknowledge when techniques or styles don't work anymore, and to try new approaches and solutions. The goal is always to help women look and feel beautiful.

I expect that aspiring makeup artists will want to read every word of this book. Others may pick and choose to read those sections that apply to their concerns. Makeup artistry is incredibly gratifying. So be open, have fun, and never stop learning.

Bobbi Brown

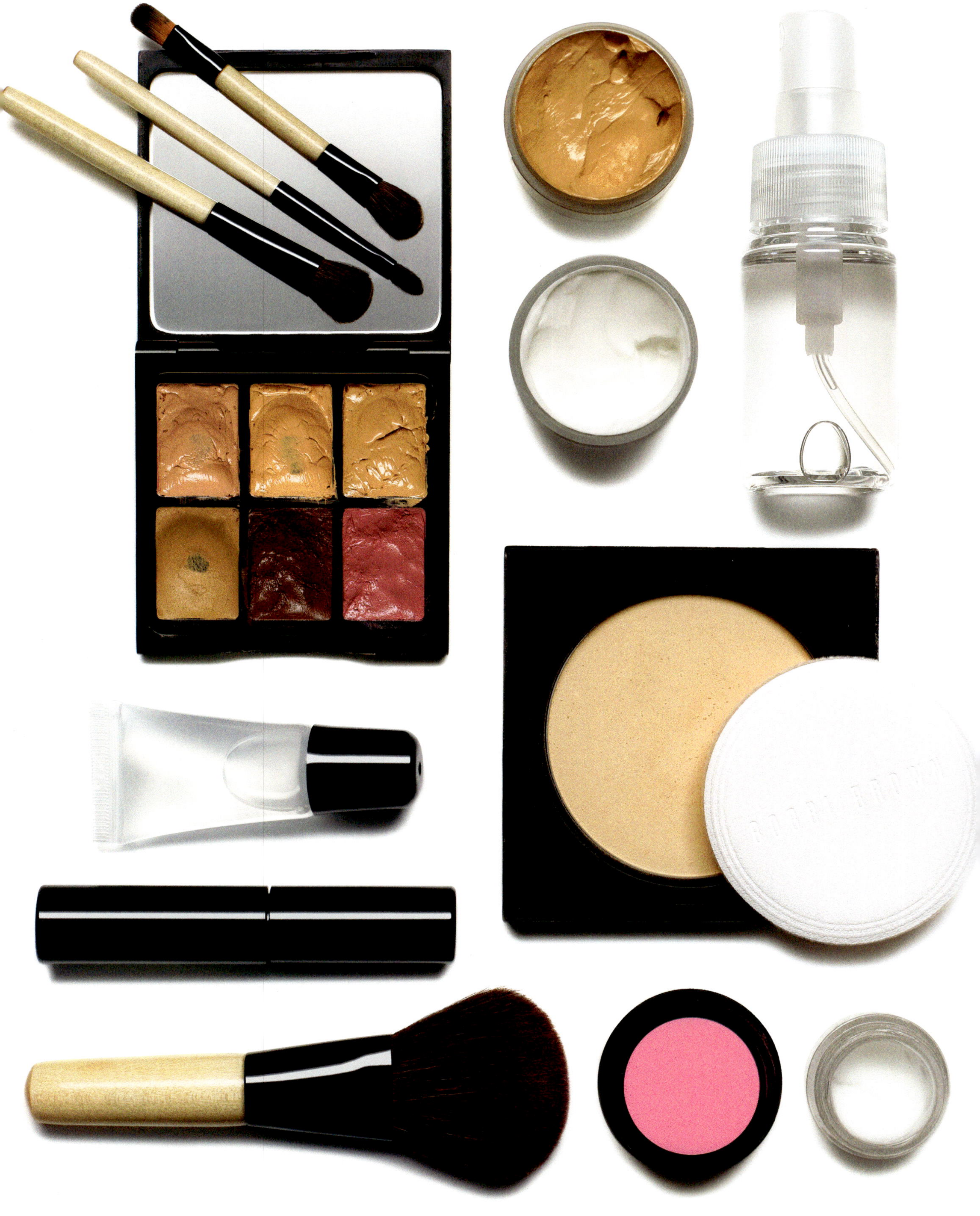

Chapter 2

EQUIPMENT

Being well organized is essential.

Whether you're a minimalist whose makeup kit rarely holds more than a lipstick and powder or a working makeup artist who routinely totes around a complete collection of cosmetics, it takes a plan.

MAKEUP KITS

Home Makeup

Organize your makeup either in your bathroom drawer, on top of the counter, or in a box. Keep basics and items used only occasionally separate. At least twice a year make sure your colors and formulas are working. Basics include:

Concealers and correctors

Foundation or tinted moisturizer

Powder (two colors)

Eye shadow (three to four basic colors)

Eyeliner (powder and gel)

Mascara

Blush (powder or cream)

Lipstick, gloss, lip pencil

Everyday Bag

Pack the following essentials in a small bag:

One or two palettes that contain your foundation, concealer, blush, and lip color

A compact of pressed powder with a mirror

A basic eye palette—the smaller the better

Mini mascara

Lip gloss

Mini brushes

Small sample sizes of face cream

Evening Bag

Tiny purses don't lend themselves to toting around lots of products, so you need to be selective. Pack the following items:

Lipstick or gloss

Lip pencil

A powder compact

Customizable face palette (containing concealer, foundation, blush)

Mini perfume

Breath mints

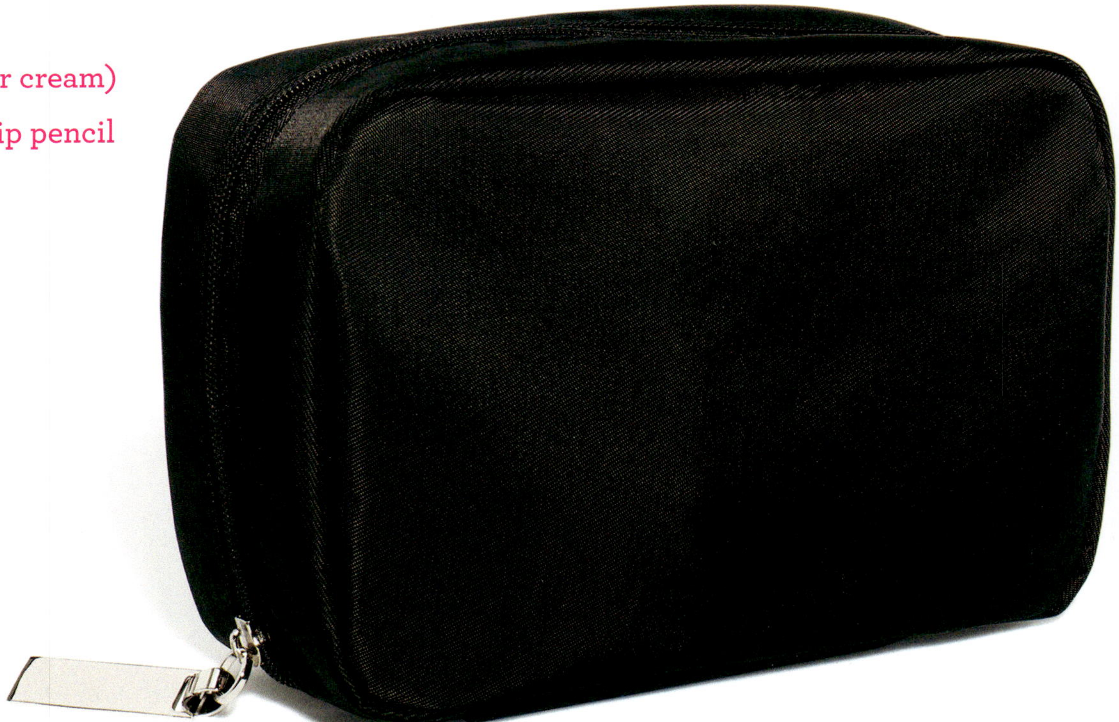

In Your Desk Drawer

It's worth investing in duplicates of your makeup to keep in your office to freshen up before a big meeting or for reapplying if you need to go straight out after work. These basics include the following items:

Concealer

Foundation

Pressed powder (with mirror)

Blush

Lip balm, lip color, and/or gloss

Black eyeliner and white or silver eye shadow to create an evening eye

Mini brushes

Travel toothbrush and toothpaste set

In Your Gym Bag

After a workout, you will want to clean your face and start your makeup from scratch. So be sure to bring the following items to the gym:

Face-cleansing cloths

Moisturizer

Customized face palette, or at least a tinted moisturizer, lip color or gloss, and mascara

For Travel

Keep your travel kit packed at all times so you never have to worry about arriving somewhere only to realize you've left something important in your bathroom cabinet. Invest in several small plastic bottles, label them, and fill them with your essentials. Purchase mini brushes, mascara, and a small eye palette. Include the following items:

Travel-size shampoo and conditioner

Body and facial moisturizers

Makeup palettes with all your basics

Mini mascara

Face powder, bronzer (great for the travel weary)

Self-tanner

Lipstick or gloss

A brush roll of travel-size brushes

Tweezers

Hairbrush and hair spray

Perfume in a mini or compact version

Perfumed body creams are also great

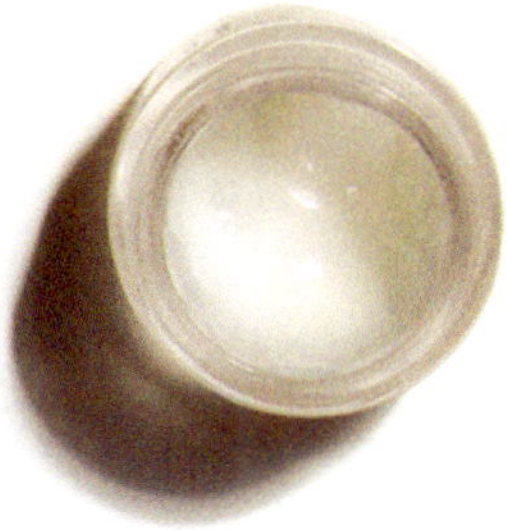

Tip

Collect deluxe samples from makeup counters—they are perfect for travel.

ESSENTIAL TOOLS

Brushes make all the difference in makeup application. Everyone from the most skilled makeup artist to the woman who wears only the basics can benefit from using the right tools. Consider investing in at least a few key brushes. High-quality blush, eye shadow, eyebrow, and eyeliner brushes are basic. Good brushes are not hard to find. Look at those made by makeup artists' lines as well as less expensive versions available at beauty and art supply stores. To find out which brushes you need and which ones are good quality, familiarize yourself with a variety of styles, shapes, and bristle types.

Assessing Brush Quality

Before purchasing brushes, you have to know what you are looking for and which brushes are worthwhile investments. Assess the quality of a brush by testing the way the bristles feel against the skin and by running your fingers through the bristles to make sure that they don't shed. It's important to test how a brush feels when you hold it in your hand. It needs to feel comfortable and easy to maneuver.

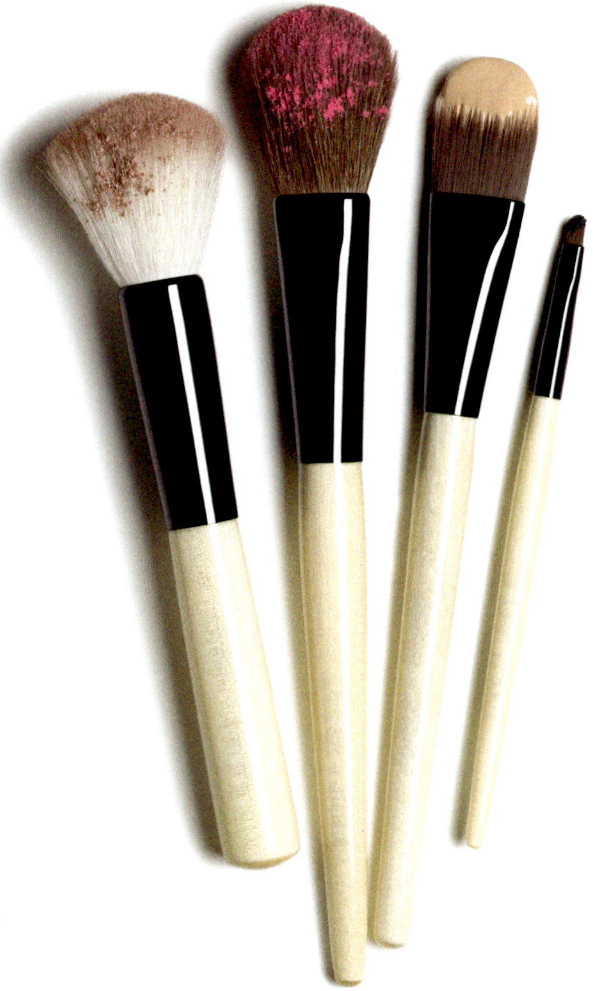

Tips

Brush Size
The brushes that come with most makeup compacts are too small and narrow for proper blush application. Toss them and use a brush designed specifically for that purpose instead.

Natural Bristles
Natural bristles (such as squirrel, goat, pony, or sable) are very soft and offer a more blended, natural application. They're best for working with powder-based products—blush, powder, and eye shadow.

Synthetic Bristles
Synthetic bristles are the best choice for brushes that will be used with creamy products, such as concealer, gel liners, and lip colors. They are generally stiffer than natural hair, so they give you greater control and a more precise application.

Tool Guide

This alphabetized glossary describes the different types of brushes as well as other tools you might want to keep in your kit. It will help you decide what brushes work best for a specific need or technique.

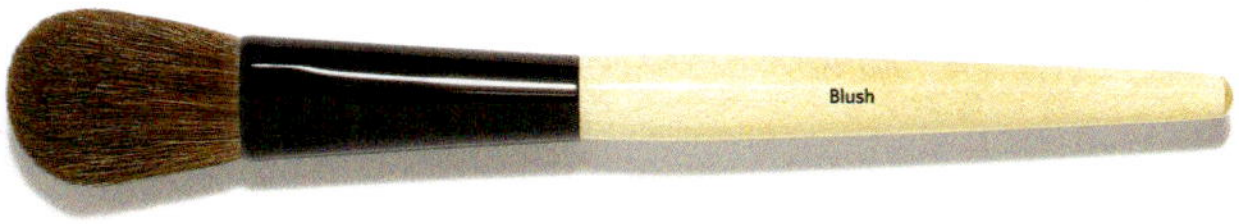

BLUSH BRUSH
This needs to be wide enough to cover the apple of the cheek. The bristles should be soft, natural hair with beveled and curved edges.

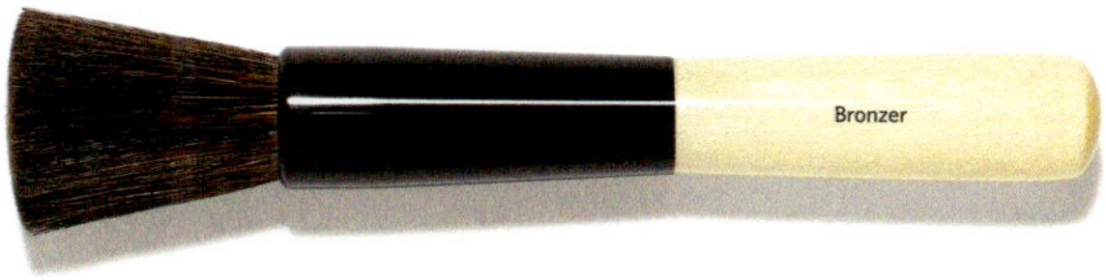

BRONZER BRUSH
This is thicker and fuller than a blush brush and has a flat profile. It is designed for sweeping and pressing bronzer over cheeks, forehead, nose, and chin to provide natural-looking warmth to the skin.

BROW BRUSH
A brush with stiff, short bristles cut on an angle. Designed for applying shadow to the brows. Look for a synthetic/natural blend of bristles, as the 100 percent synthetic brushes are too stiff and don't deposit color as effectively.

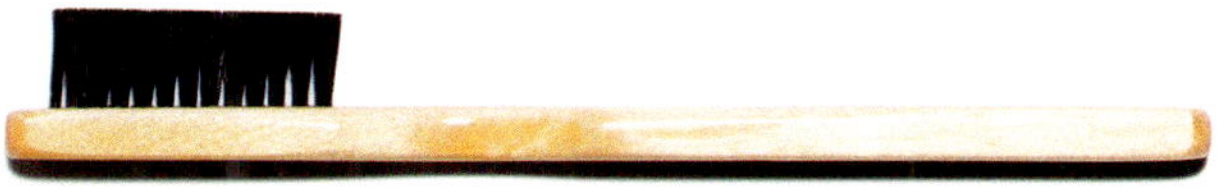

BROW GROOMING BRUSH
This is for brushing brows into place. It has stiff bristles cut straight across, like a toothbrush.

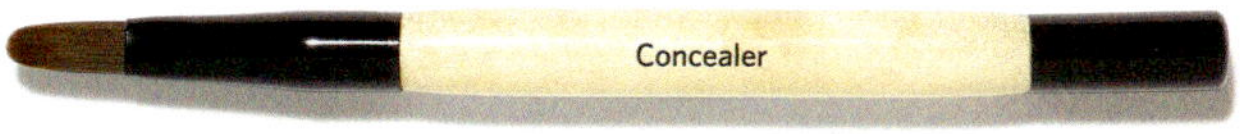

CONCEALER BRUSH
This should have firm but soft bristles that aren't too hard or scratchy, since the brush will be used on the delicate skin under the eyes. Look for a brush with glossy synthetic hairs, as these slip along the skin. The ends of the bristles should be tapered to help you place concealer in hard-to-reach spots, such as the inner corners of the eyes, and apply stick foundation to cover any redness around the nose.

EYE BLENDER BRUSH
A soft, fluffy, natural-hair brush with long bristles designed to blend eye shadow and eliminate lines of demarcation on the lids after applying multiple shades. It is also great for applying powder to set corrector, concealer, or foundation around the eyes or over blemish cover.

EYE CONTOUR BRUSH
A round, flat-head, natural-hair brush. Short, dense bristles apply a greater amount of shadow in the crease to contour the eye.

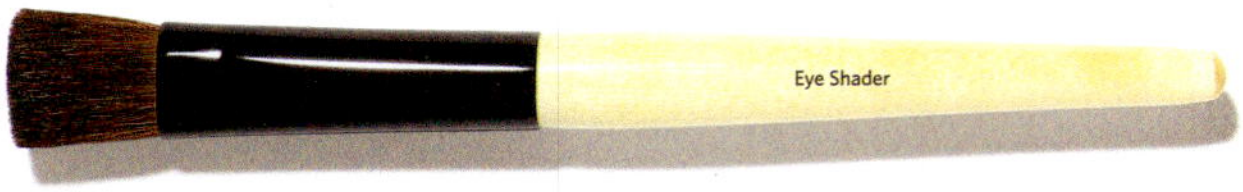

EYE SHADER BRUSH
A wide, flat-head brush that can gently sweep eye shadow color over the entire lid, from the lash line to the brow bone.

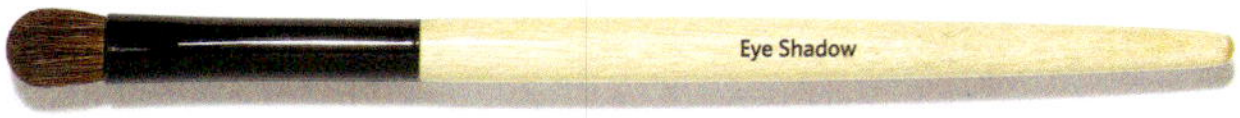

EYE SHADOW BRUSH
Wide enough to cover about half the eyelid. This brush has natural, soft, rounded bristles with beveled edges that deposit a sweep of shadow across the lower lid without leaving any harsh lines.

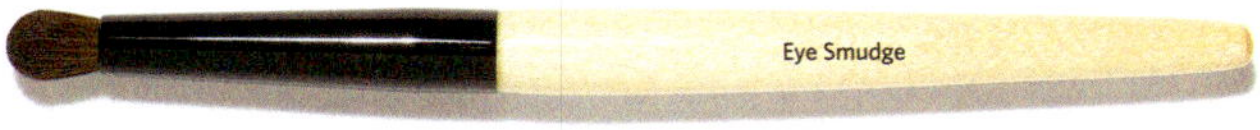

EYE SMUDGE BRUSH
A small-head brush with a slightly rounded point. This brush has soft, flexible bristles that help smudge liner to create a smoky look.

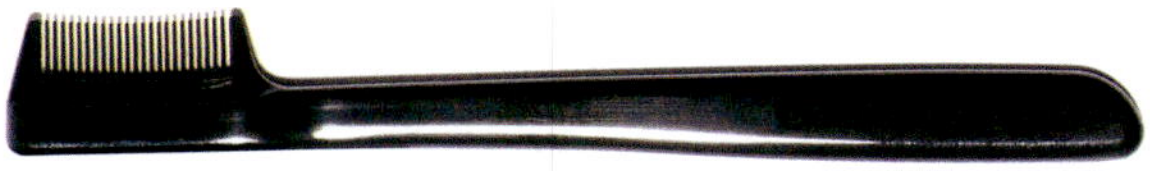

EYELASH COMB
This has straight, stiff (often plastic), fine teeth and is designed to separate lashes immediately after applying mascara (while the lashes are still wet). Mascara wands work just as well and are more convenient.

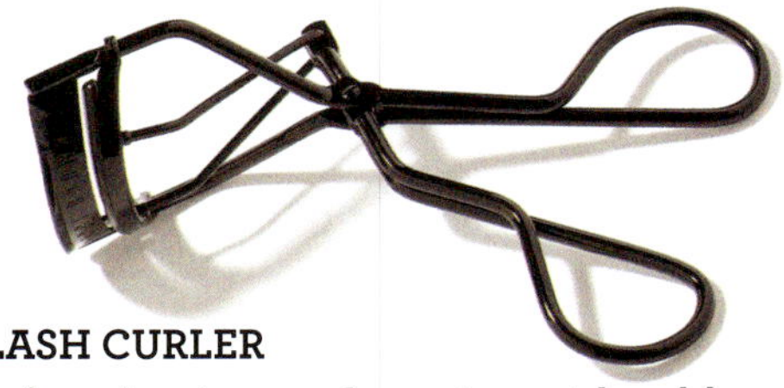

EYELASH CURLER
Look for a basic metal version with rubber pads. An eyelash curler shapes lashes into a natural-looking curl. Replace pads regularly. To avoid breakage, always curl the lashes before applying mascara.

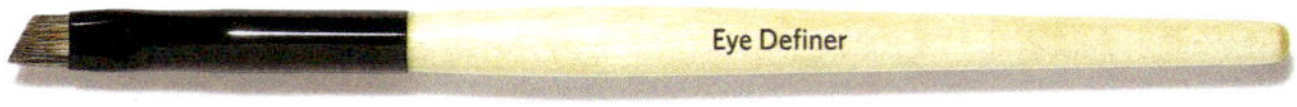

EYELINER BRUSH (ANGLED)/ EYE DEFINER BRUSH
This small brush has very short, dense bristles cut on an angle. It is designed to use with shadow to strengthen thin brows or as an alternative to an eyeliner brush.

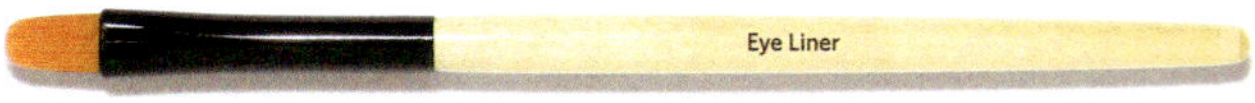

EYELINER BRUSH (FLAT)
With flat, dense, synthetic bristles that are slightly rounded at tip, this brush can be used wet or dry to apply a precise line at the lash line.

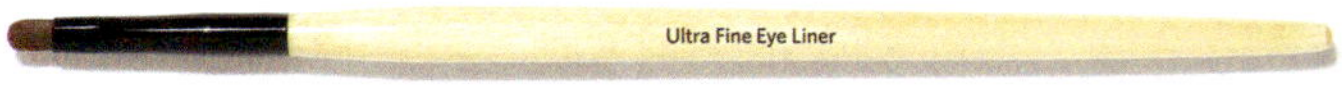

EYELINER BRUSH (ULTRA FINE)
The bristles on this small brush are synthetic, dense, and curve to a point. Perfect for the precise application of liquid or gel eyeliner.

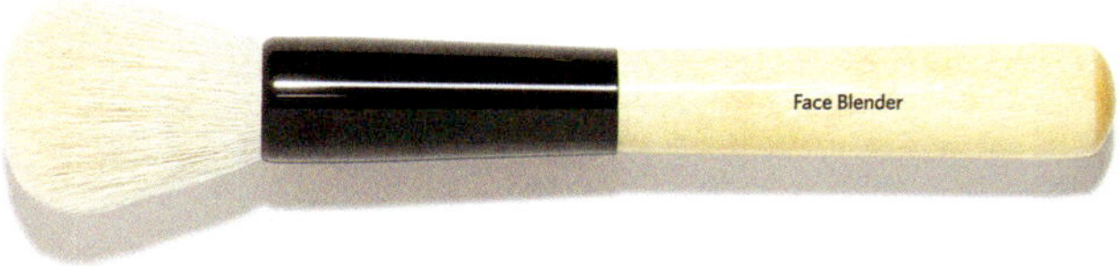

FACE BLENDER BRUSH
A natural or synthetic brush used to deposit shimmer, bronzer, powder, or blush.

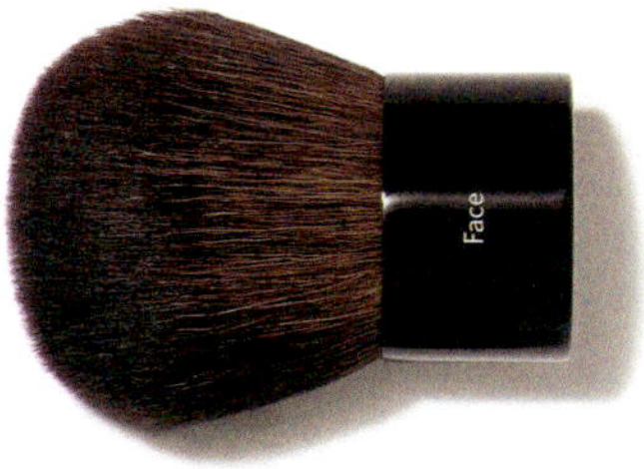

FACE BRUSH
A natural or synthetic fluffy, curved brush that can be used to apply bronzer, blush, or powder.

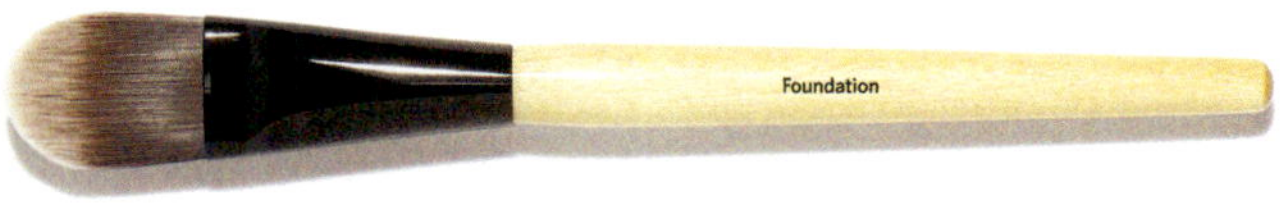

FOUNDATION BRUSH

Synthetic bristles in this full, flat-edged brush deposit just the right amount of foundation onto the skin.

LIP BRUSH

Firm, long bristles come to a slightly pointed tip. This brush allows for the precise placement of lip color. Bristles can be either synthetic or natural.

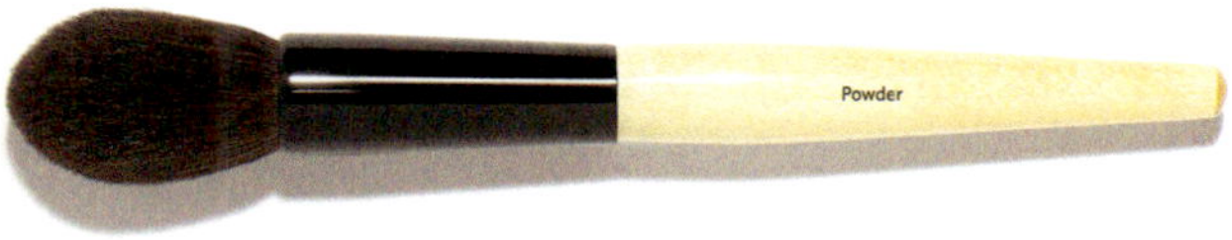

POWDER BRUSH

A natural-hair, large, fluffy brush with soft bristles that bevel to a slight point (for navigating around the nose and under the eyes). Designed for use with both loose and pressed powders.

Tip

Using Your Fingers

Nothing beats the warmth of the fingers to blend makeup into the skin. Lipstick can be blotted onto the lips to create a stain effect. Face cream, balm, or oil rubbed between both palms and then gently pressed onto cheeks adds moisture and a youthful glow to the face. I use my hands to warm concealers, blend foundation, and mix lip shades together. I also use my hands to work makeup into the face so that the makeup feels like a part of the skin and not like a mask.

POWDER PUFF

A velour puff that's about the size of your palm. Designed to press powder onto the face to lock foundation in place. Can be hand washed or tossed in the dishwasher (at least once a week).

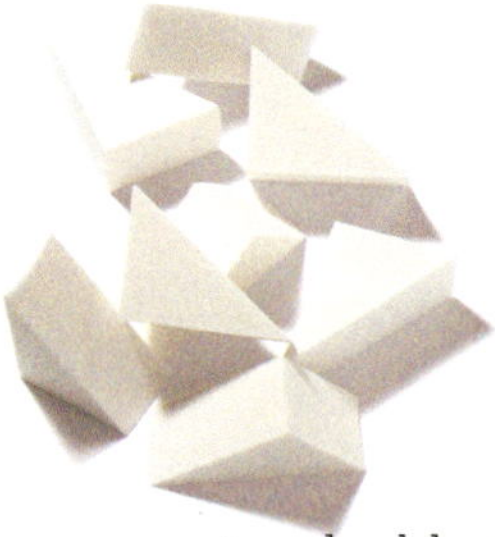

SPONGES

Disposable sponges are invaluable. Wedge-shaped ones are great for applying foundation around the nose and other hard-to-reach places, as well as for blending. Don't bother washing them—toss dirty ones, and take a new one. Higher-quality sponges can be washed and reused many times.

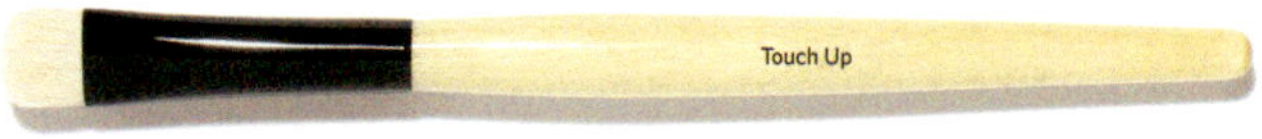

TOUCH UP BRUSH

Short, firm, natural-bristled brush used with foundation for spot touch-ups and for hard-to-reach areas around the nose and mouth. This brush can also be used to touch up concealer and apply eye shadow.

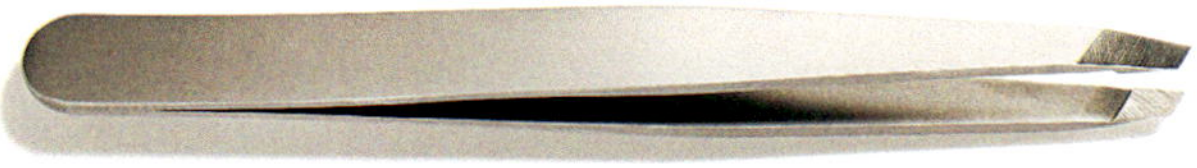

TWEEZERS

It's well worth investing in a good pair. Look at the Tweezerman or Rubis brands. Tweezers that are angled at the tip are easier to control than those that come to a sharp point. Always cover tweezers' tips with the included rubber cap when they are not in use.

SHOPPING FOR SUPPLIES

Whether you are starting your first professional makeup kit, replacing a few personal items, or looking for something new, shopping is a time to experiment, test cosmetics, and research trends. One of the best and easiest ways to stay current is to test the latest products on the cosmetics floor of any large department store. The makeup artist at the counter will show you new items and techniques. You can try the cosmetics and get information, all without any cost. Magazines and the Internet are great for research and information, but when you are ready for a purchase, it is important to touch and feel the products so you know the quality you are getting.

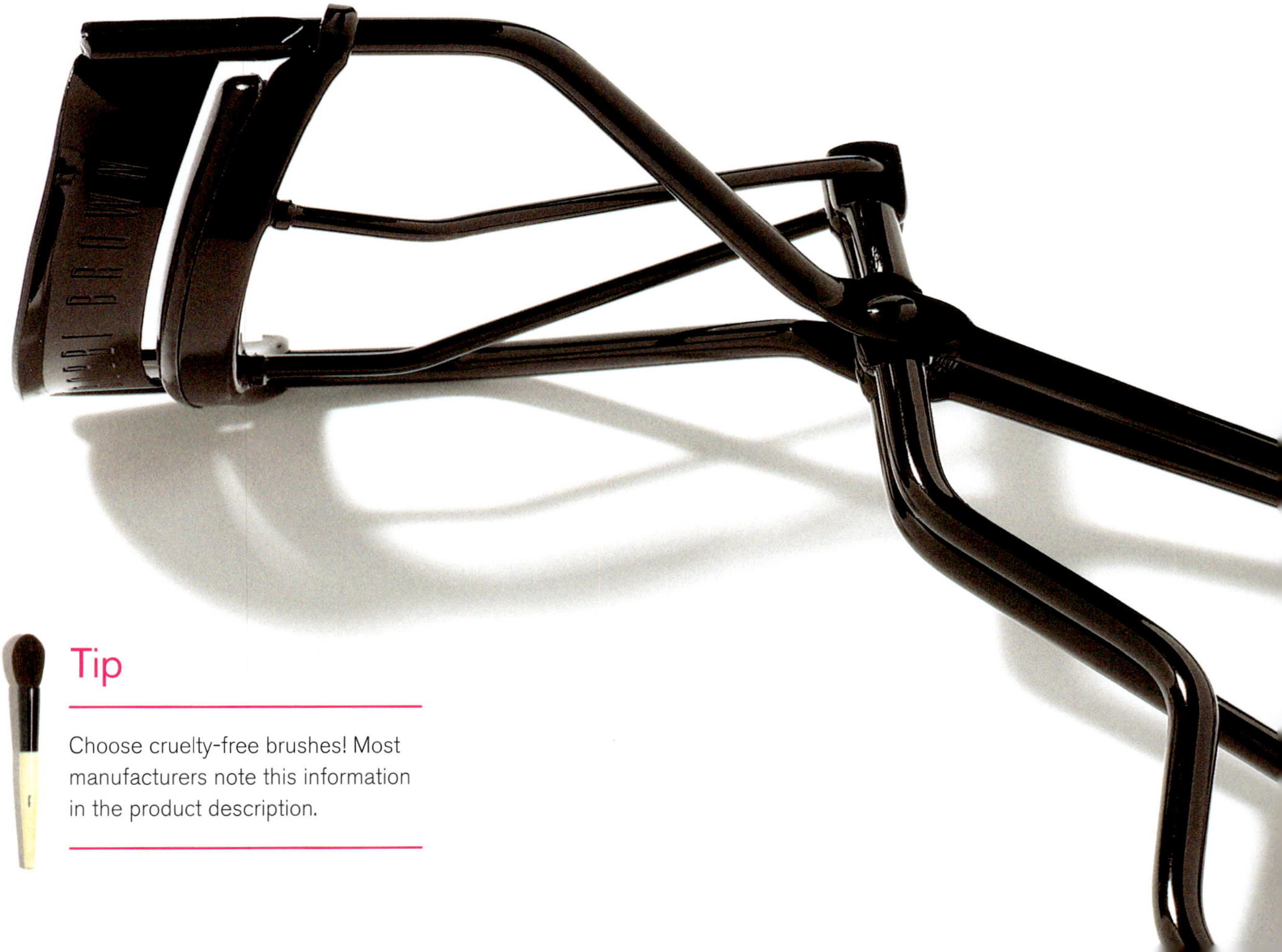

Tip

Choose cruelty-free brushes! Most manufacturers note this information in the product description.

It is a good idea to develop some shopping strategies to avoid frustration, intimidation, or impulse-buying. First, determine your budget. Makeup can be expensive. Estimate the cost of your supply needs, and add a realistic amount for trying new products. Making an inventory list of all the supplies in your makeup kit is very helpful. Use this as a shopping list, and just circle the needed items. If you want to replace something specific, you can take the container with you to the store. In a notebook, keep a page for jotting down any new products you might want to test. This is also a place to record product ingredients for comparison shopping. For the best service, shop when the stores are least crowded, generally in the mornings, early in the week. Let the makeup artist at the counter show you a new look or technique. Listen and ask questions. Be clear about your likes and dislikes. Ask for samples or trial-size containers of any products you like. Purchase a product only if you love the way the makeup looks and know that you will use it.

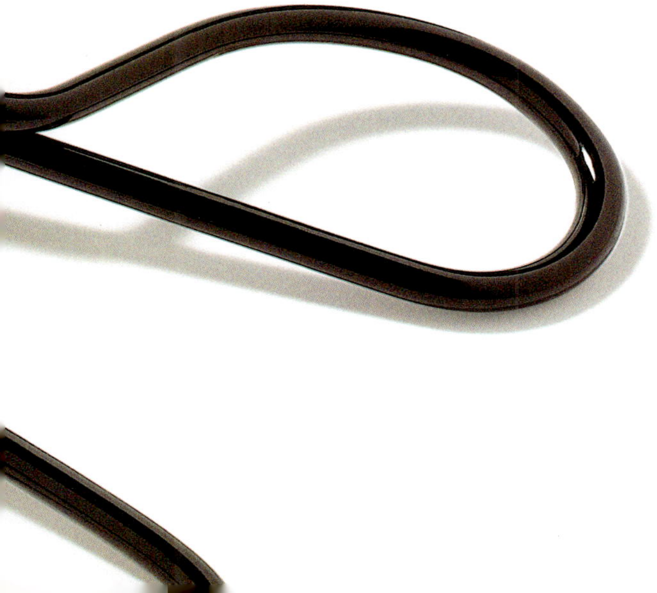

Sources

You will want to find several places to purchase makeup supplies that suit your needs and preferences. For testing and experimentation, store visits are very useful. Once you are familiar with a product line, it is faster and easier to do your shopping online. Most of the retailers and designers now have Web sites for quick and convenient shopping.

Department Stores

High-end brands are typically sold through dedicated counter areas in department stores. Most of the counter personnel are trained in makeup application and are able to provide information and advice. You can test the makeup before purchasing so you know exactly what you're getting. Some sales staff are paid on commission, so you may be pressured to make a purchase.

Drugstores and Pharmacies

These stores are convenient and carry a wide variety of mass-market products. Purchase basic supplies such as nail polish, cotton balls, makeup sponges, and cotton swabs at these retailers. Very few of the products can be tested before buying, so purchases might not meet your expectations.

Beauty Supply Shops

Makeup artists depend on these industry meccas for professional-quality products at budget-friendly prices. You will receive personalized attention and won't be rushed or pressured to make a purchase, because the sales clerks are not paid on commission. These stores will usually ship anywhere in the country.

Beauty Superstores

One-stop shops, such as Sephora and Ulta, offer a wide range of mass-market, prestige, and niche products. The staff is knowledgeable and willing to answer questions.

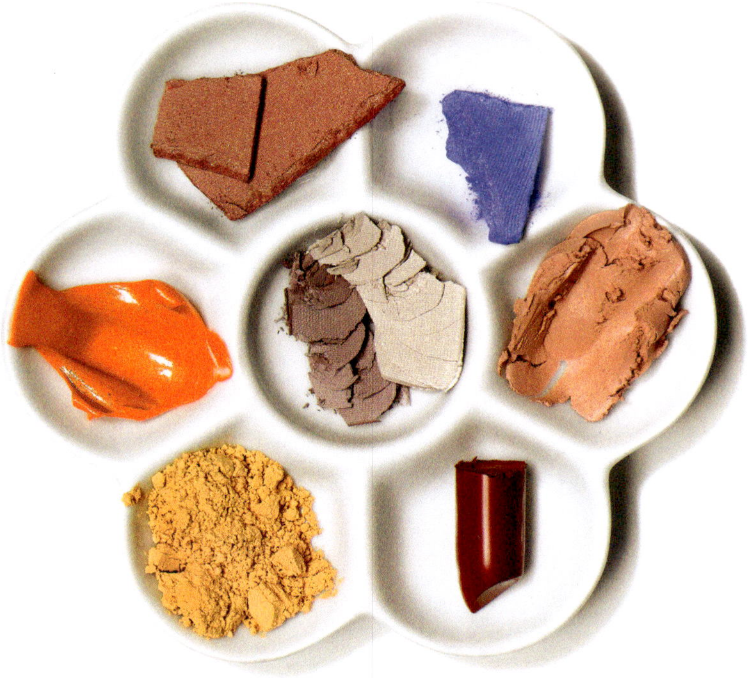

Purchasing Dos & Don'ts

Do buy multipurpose makeup, such as lip-cheek combinations.

Do shop in daylight for foundation.

Don't equate "dermatologist tested" with better quality. The claim does not guarantee that the doctor approved of the product—just that it was tested.

Do save your receipts. Many stores will refund your money within a specified period of time if you are not satisfied with a product. If any cream-based makeup smells or has an odd texture, take it back. It is probably old.

Don't toss leftovers unless the makeup is more than eighteen months old. When that lipstick or cream blush gets near the end, scoop the remainder into small, covered, compartmentalized boxes (palettes) that are available at art and beauty supply stores. Label the back of the palette with the color name for reference when you need to restock.

Specialty Stores

These freestanding stores offer a wide selection of products, often "indie" brands. This is a good place to find trend-driven shades, foundations, and concealers.

Catalogs

Shopping from catalogs specific to a brand is a convenient way to stock up on favorite shades of cosmetics. Once you are familiar with a product, this is a fast and easy way to order replacements, get a quick overview of new products, and see the latest fashion colors.

Discontinued?!?

Has your signature fragrance or favorite lipstick disappeared from the market? This happens for any number of reasons. It is possible that the product was not selling well, or it has been reformulated to meet new standards. Discontinued beauty products are available if you know where to look. Use the Internet to do your research. Visit the company's Web site first. There will generally be information available on discontinued products. Estée Lauder, for example, publishes item closings in advance on their Web site so that consumers can stock up. Specialty Web sites, outlets, and online auctions often carry these cosmetics and fragrances. Do be aware of expiration dates, however. Cosmetics have a limited shelf life and should not be used after the expiration dates posted by the manufacturer.

Finally, if you just can't locate your old favorite, make a plea. Either e-mail or write a personal letter asking the company to bring it back. Companies listen closely to their customers, and it is not unusual for specific colors or products to be resurrected thanks to consumer demand. At the very least, you will get a response from the company, usually providing reasons for the closing and often samples of similar products for you to try.

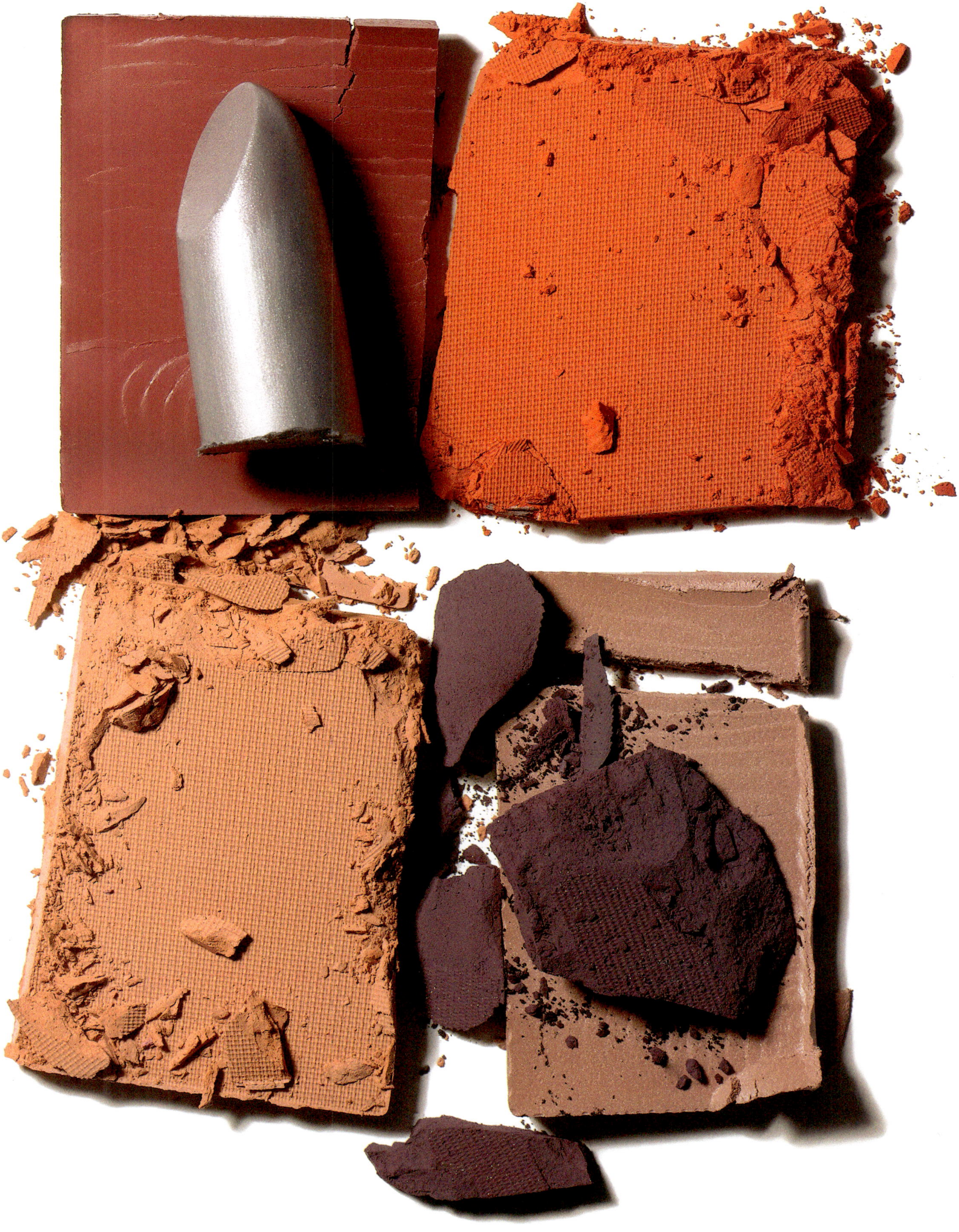

CARE & MAINTENANCE OF TOOLS & MAKEUP

Your makeup is only as good as the tools you use to apply it. Therefore, your tools must always be in their best working condition. That means clean brushes, puffs, and sponges; sharpened tweezers; makeup containers that are in perfect shape; and makeup that's not too old to use safely.

Brush Care

A good set of brushes will last several years if it is well cared for. This involves storing the brushes properly (either in a neat brush roll that has individual slots for each brush or upright in a pencil cup) and keeping them clean. To clean brushes, take a drop of brush cleaner or very gentle soap in your palm, wet the brush, and swirl the bristles around on your palm until they are covered in soap. (I love using baby shampoo.) Rinse thoroughly until all soap residue is gone. Do not immerse the brush head in water, because the hair is glued to the base, and even the most expensive brushes will come apart. Squeeze out excess moisture with a clean towel, reshape the brush head, and let it dry with the bristles hanging off the edge of a counter so the bristles dry into the perfect shape. Brushes can become mildewed if they rest on a towel while drying.

Clean all your brushes every month or two. For a quick cleaning in between washings, use a spray brush cleaner. Spritz it onto the bristles, and swipe them back and forth on a tissue until all product residues are removed from the brush.

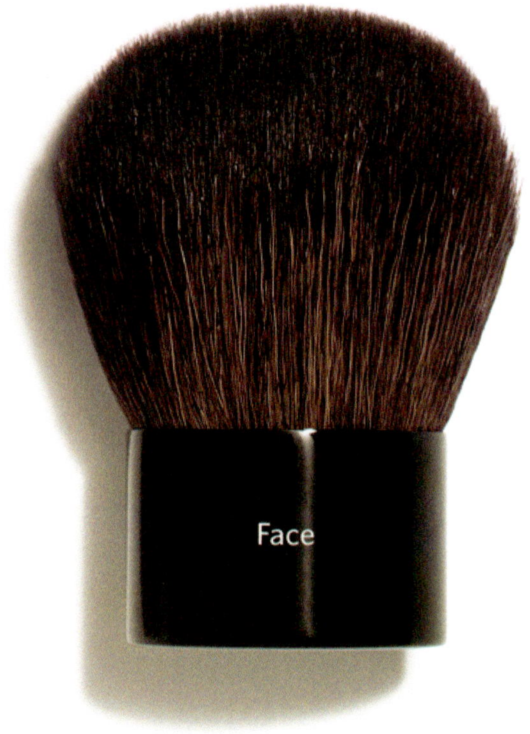

Tip

Clean the sides of messy compacts with a cotton swab to keep them looking fresh.

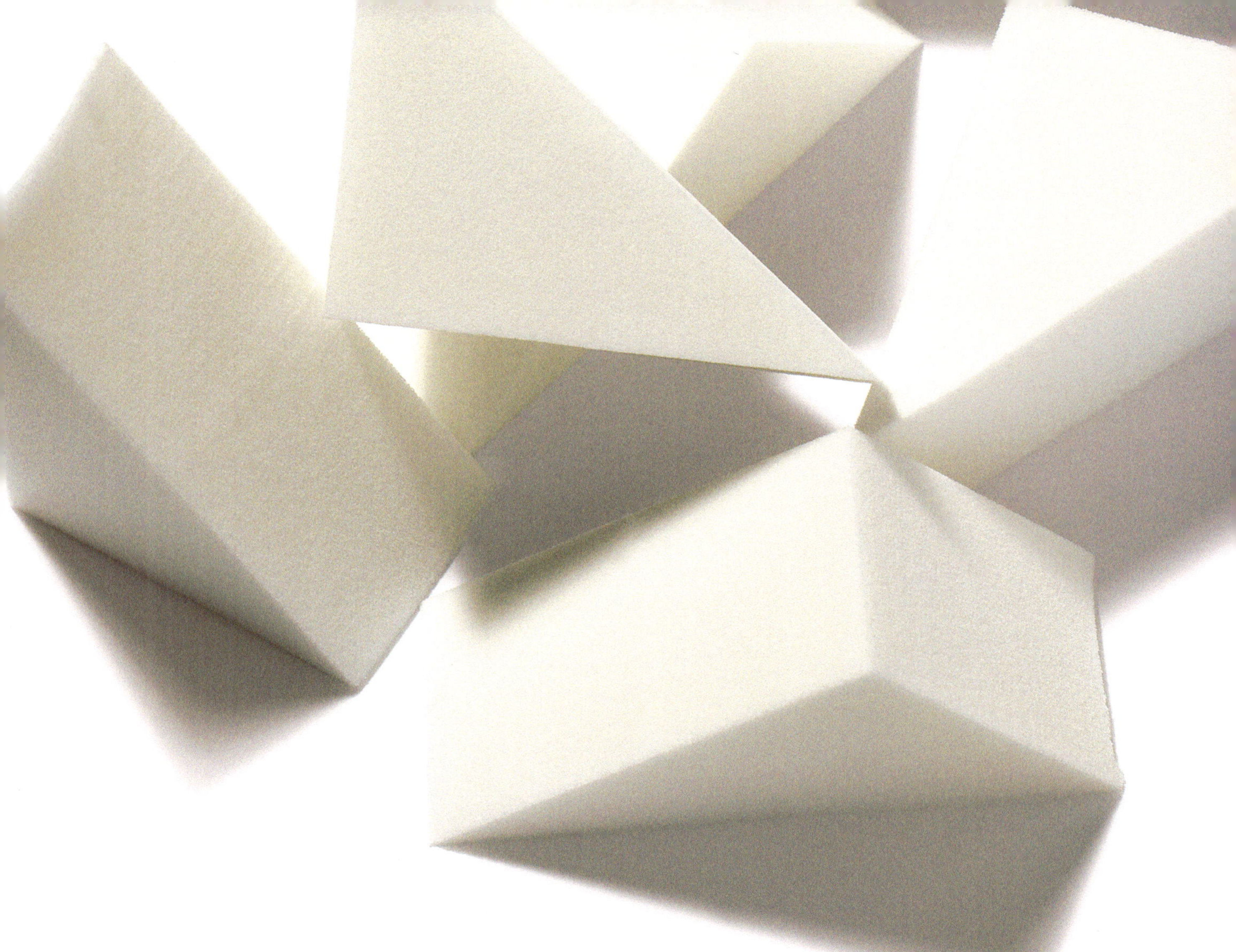

Sponge Care

High-quality sponges can be washed many times before they need to be discarded. Alternatively, you can buy disposable synthetic sponge wedges at the drugstore that work well and are inexpensive. You can wash and reuse them only a few times before you throw them out.

Powder Puff Care

While drugstores sell disposable powder puffs, it's worth investing in a better-quality one. Hand wash the puff using the same liquid soap you use for your brushes, or toss it into your next load of laundry or on the top rack of the dishwasher.

Tweezer Care

When tweezers get dull—which happens with repeated use—they are no longer as effective at grabbing on to and removing small hairs. You can take them to a knife shop for sharpening. Some of the better brands, such as Tweezerman, come with a lifetime guarantee that includes free sharpening whenever necessary.

Eyelash Curler Care

The rubber pads that line the inside of an eyelash curler are there to protect the lashes, so when the pads start to wear out or break apart, they must be replaced. Many eyelash curlers come with a set of replacement pads. Keep a set on hand.

Makeup Care

Examine the contents of your makeup bag, drawer, or cabinet. Take out anything that's in a broken container or missing a cap. You can pour liquid foundation into a fresh bottle, scoop out creams and lipsticks and transfer them to small containers or palettes, and place capless pencils in zip-top plastic bags. Broken powder blushes and pressed powder compacts are irreparable and should be tossed. Weekly maintenance is far easier than semiannual overhauls.

You also need to get rid of any makeup that's past its expiration date:

Liquid and cream foundation	2 years
Concealer	2 years
Powder	2 years
Mascara	6 months
Lipstick	12 to 18 months
Lip and eye pencils	12 to 18 months
Eye shadow	2 years
Powder blush	2 years
Cream blush	2 years
Moisturizer	2 years
Eye cream	6 months
Sunscreen	2 years
Face cream	2 years

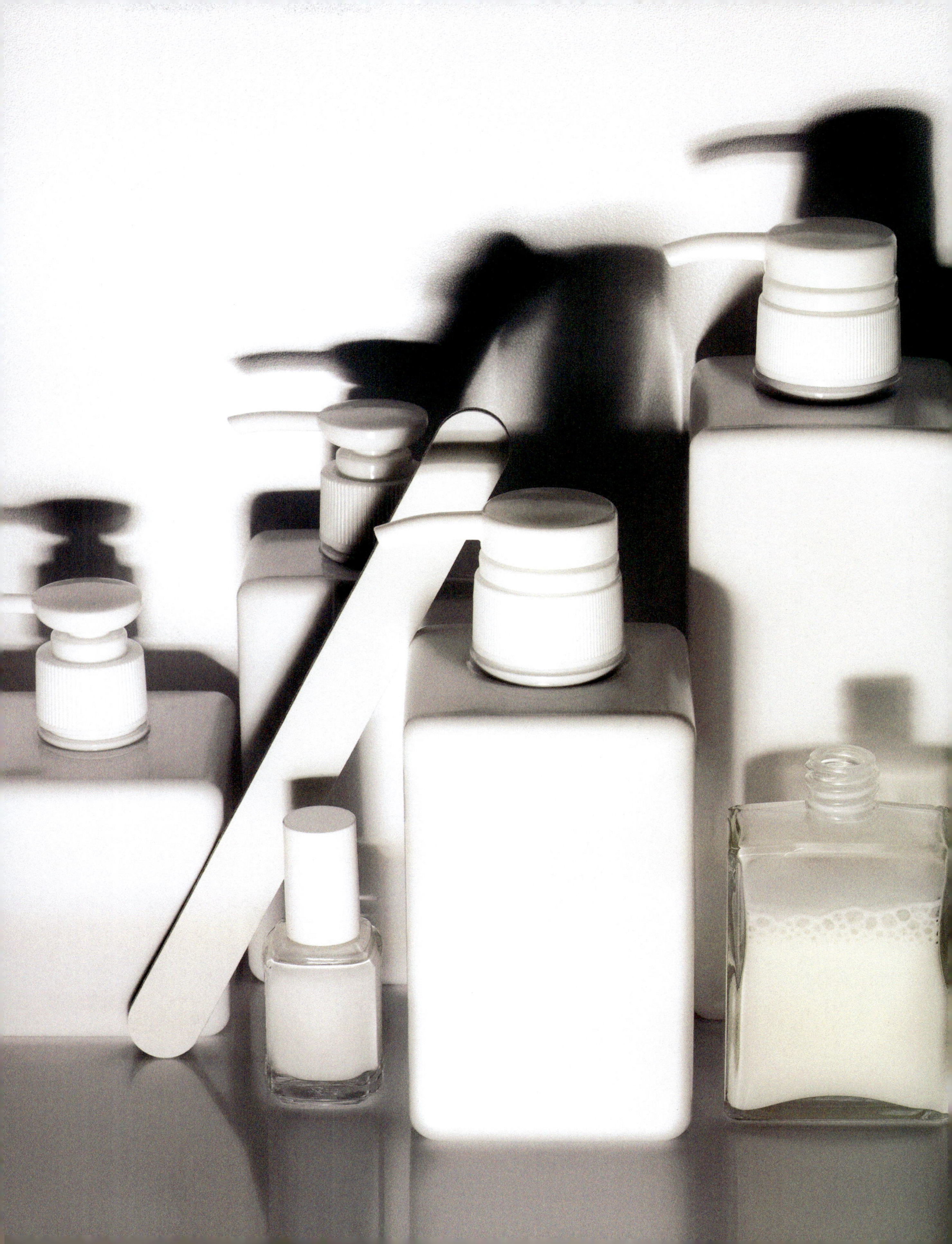

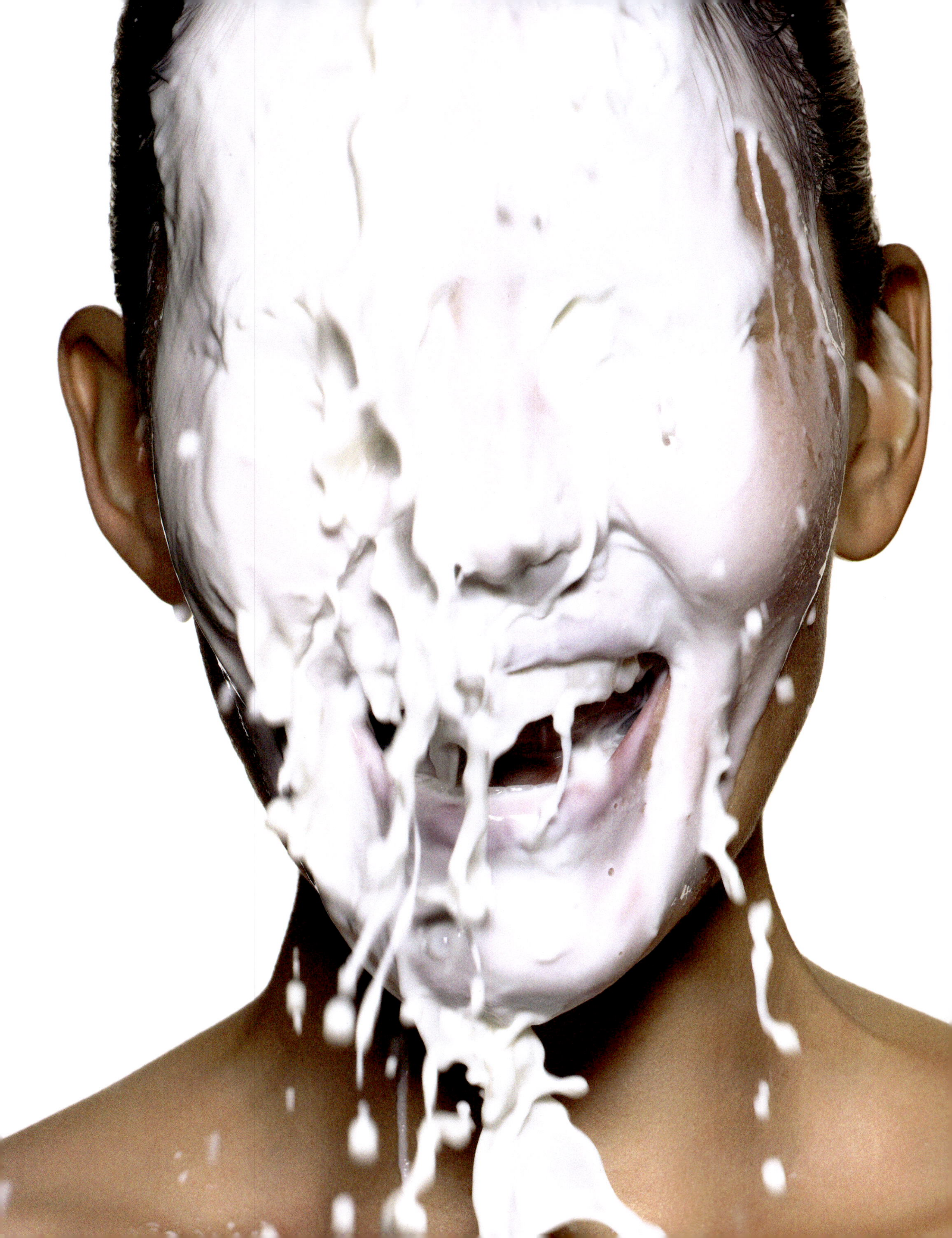

Chapter 3

SKIN

Beauty starts with smooth, healthy, glowing skin.

Anyone can learn to become a skincare expert by:

Understanding how **lifestyle** impacts the condition of the skin,

Knowing **how skin works,**

Learning the basics of skincare, including

How to **analyze** skin conditions,

How to **identify** skin types,

How to properly **care for skin,**

Knowing skincare **ingredients** and how they work in order to select and use the appropriate products.

LIFESTYLE

Beautiful skin begins with a healthy lifestyle. While heredity may determine how your skin looks, behaves, and ages, you can improve it by taking good care of yourself. Skincare basics include eating the right foods, drinking plenty of water, exercising, getting enough sleep, protecting your skin from the sun, not smoking, and limiting your intake of both caffeine and alcohol.

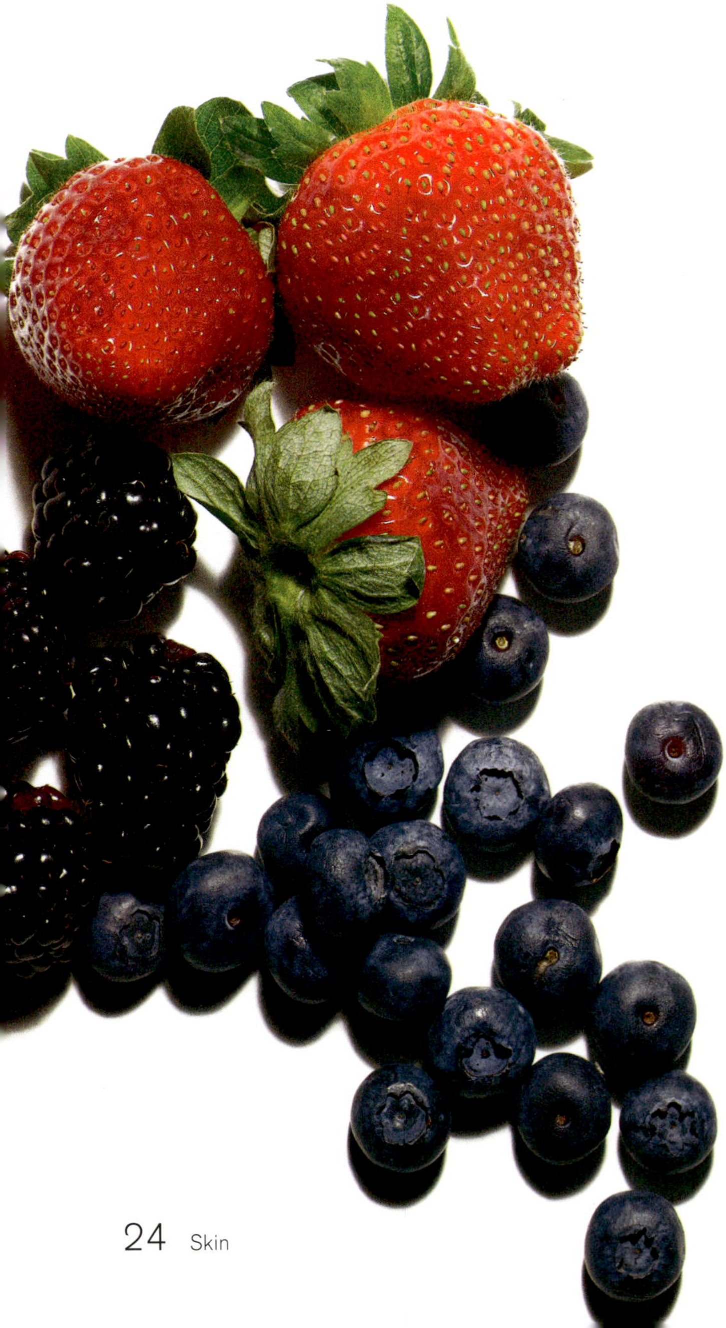

Nutrition

The health of your skin begins with good nutrition. New, living cells continually replace the dead cells on the surface of the skin. The growth of new cells is dependent on vitamins, minerals, and hydration.

Eat at least five servings of fresh fruits and vegetables each day. Remember to look for the "ACE" vitamins: A to help prevent aging, C to promote clarity, and E to protect against the environment. Vitamins A and C are most important for healthy skin and are plentiful in fruits and vegetables. Vitamin A is found in carrots, spinach, watercress, broccoli, sweet potatoes, and melons. Peppers, strawberries, oranges, grapefruit, and leafy greens all contain vitamin C. Also include whole-grain foods, nuts, dairy, fish, and beans in your diet. They are all foods rich in zinc, which promotes healing and reduces inflammation in the body.

Biotin is another nutrient needed for healthy skin, hair, and nails. It is sometimes identified as vitamin H and is part of the vitamin B complex. Foods such as peanut butter, whole grains, eggs, and liver contain biotin and can help prevent dermatitis and hair loss.

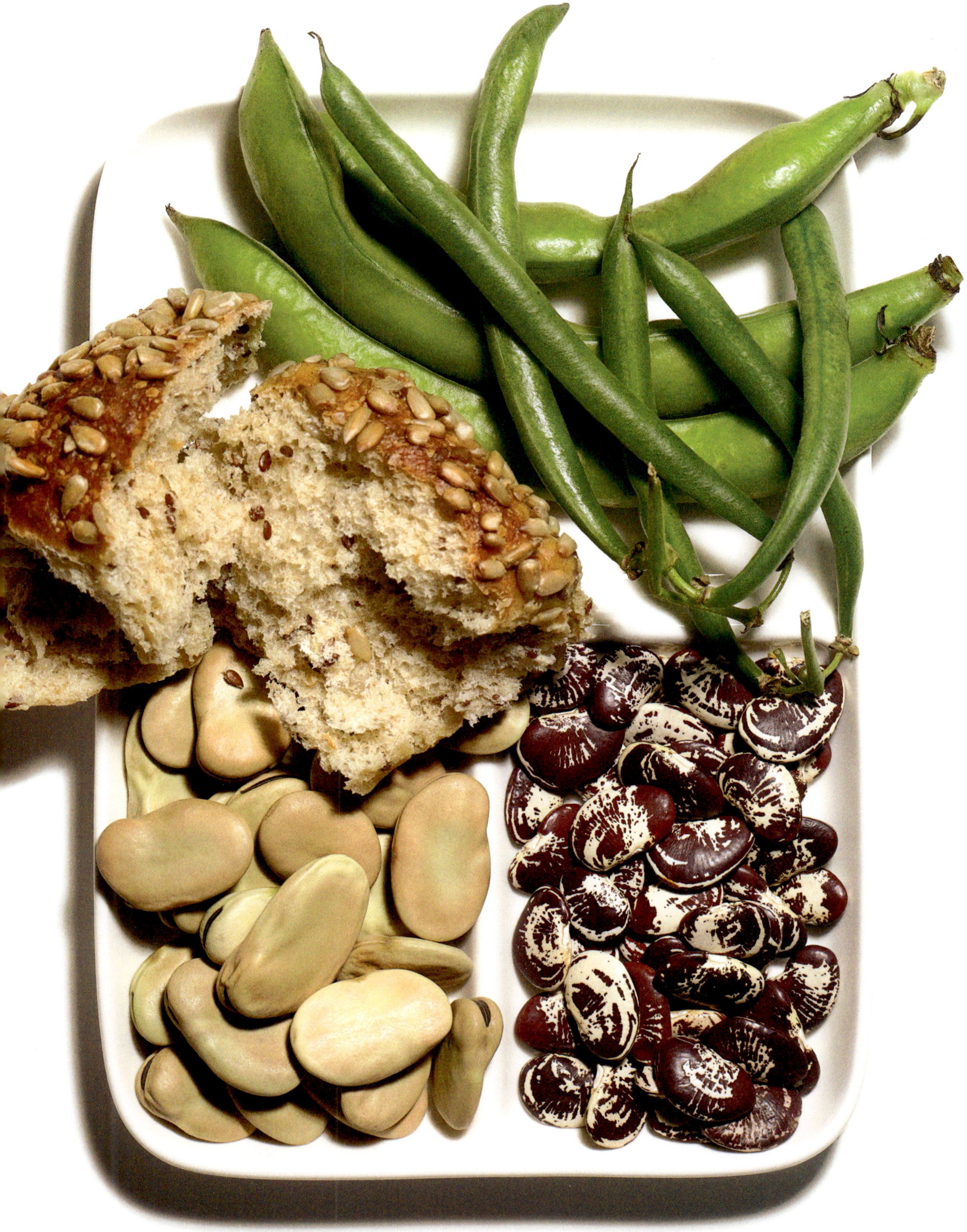

There are many advantages to taking your vitamins in food rather than in pill form. When you eat, you are never getting single, isolated nutrients. For instance, a bowl of leafy greens provides an abundance of several important vitamins, such as B, K, and E, as well as fiber and antioxidants. The fresh fruits, vegetables, and whole grains that provide fiber also naturally deliver vitamins and minerals and are low in calories. It is virtually impossible to consume dangerous levels of any vitamins or minerals through diet alone.

Your diet has a direct impact on not only your overall health and how you feel but also on how you look. Certain nutrients in particular are important for maintaining healthy skin, hair, and nails. Think of them as your beauty vitamins.

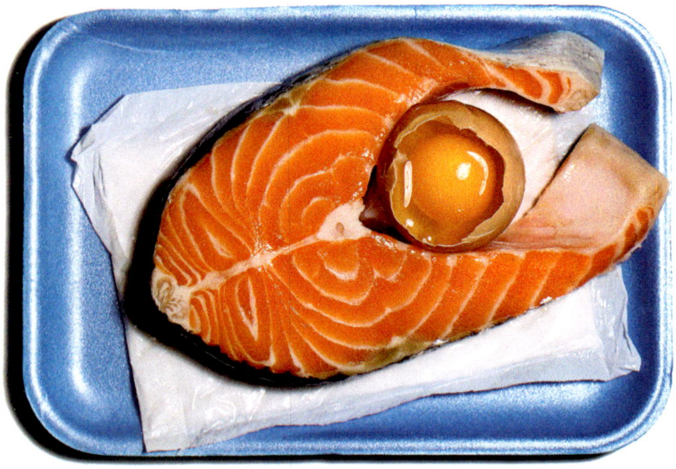

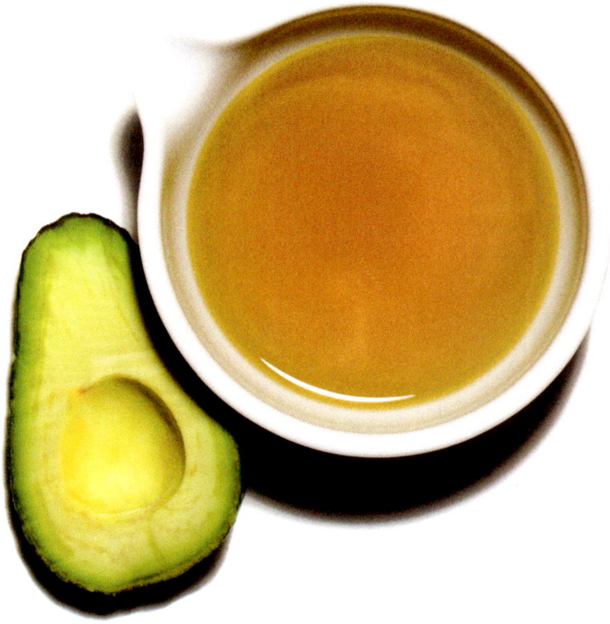

VITAMIN A

Antioxidant essential for the **growth and renewal of new skin cells. Topically applied, may boost collagen production and promote skin cell turnover.**

Egg yolks, dairy

VITAMIN B

Increases fatty acids in the skin, **promoting exfoliation and firmness.**

Yeast, eggs, liver, vegetables

VITAMIN C

Building block of collagen, the protein that gives skin its **structure, tone, and elasticity.**

Citrus fruits, broccoli, peppers, berries, tomatoes

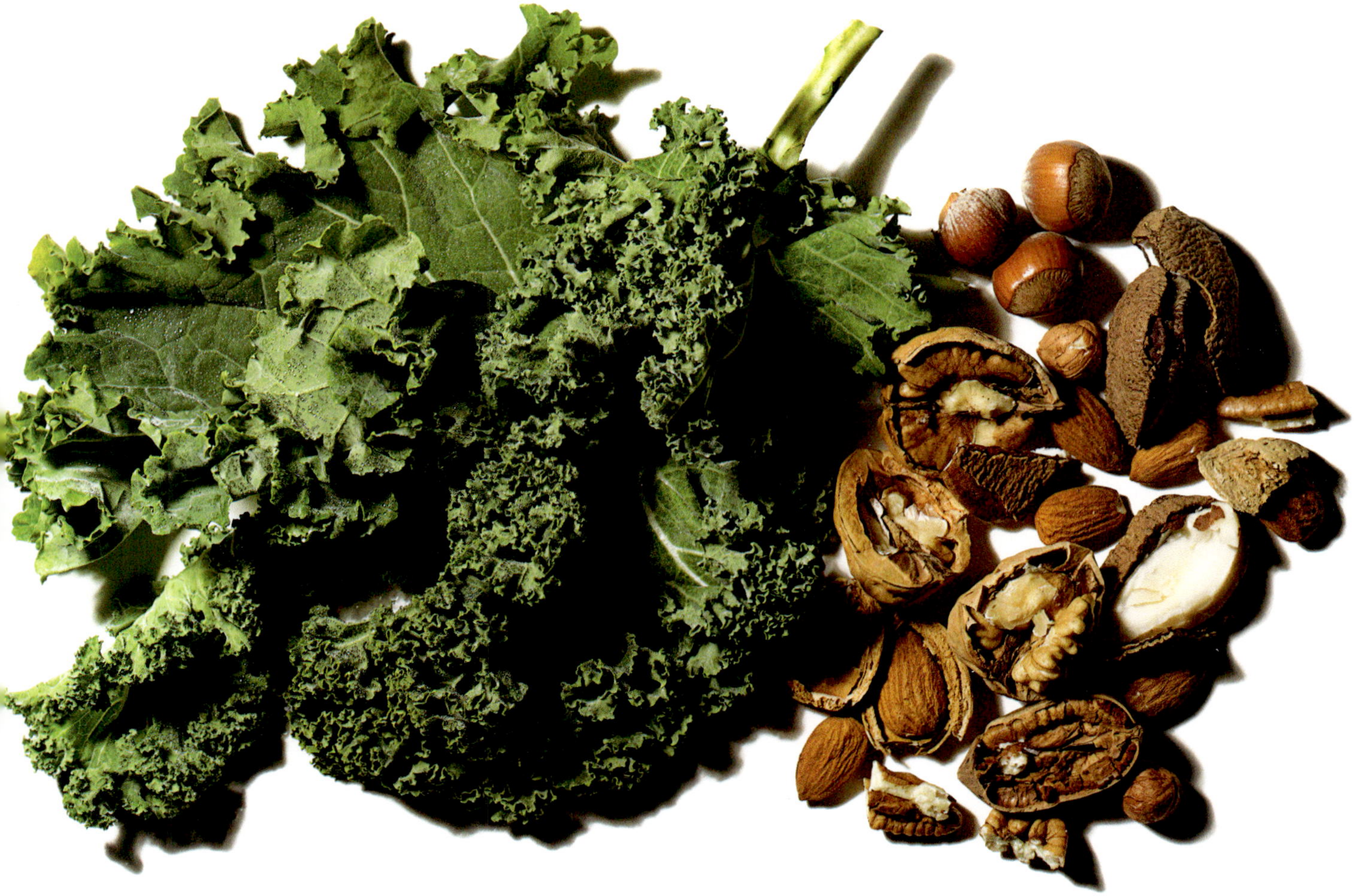

VITAMIN D

Essential for the **development of skin cells.**

Egg yolks, salmon, fortified milk, and other dairy products

VITAMIN E

Antioxidant that helps build and **maintain healthy skin tissue.**

Wheat germ, leafy greens, nuts, whole grains

FAT

Fat is also an important nutrient for the skin and the health of the whole body. **It is necessary for supple skin and soft, shiny hair.**

Incorporate unsaturated fats, such as the monounsaturated fats found in olive oil and avocado, with omega-3 fats, found in fatty fish and some seeds, into your daily diet.

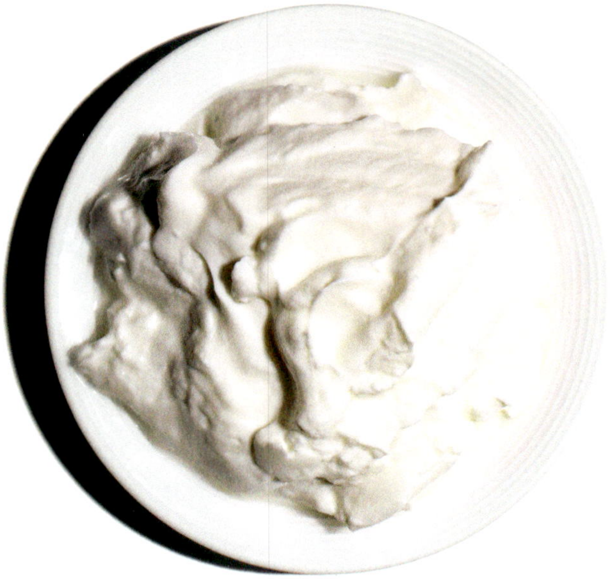

Keep these healthy foods on hand for satisfying between-meal snacking:

Almonds

Plain, low-fat yogurt

String cheese

Chocolate protein powder

Protein bars

Low-fat ricotta cheese with a dash of vanilla

Hard-boiled eggs

Water with a bit of unsweetened cranberry extract or lemon juice

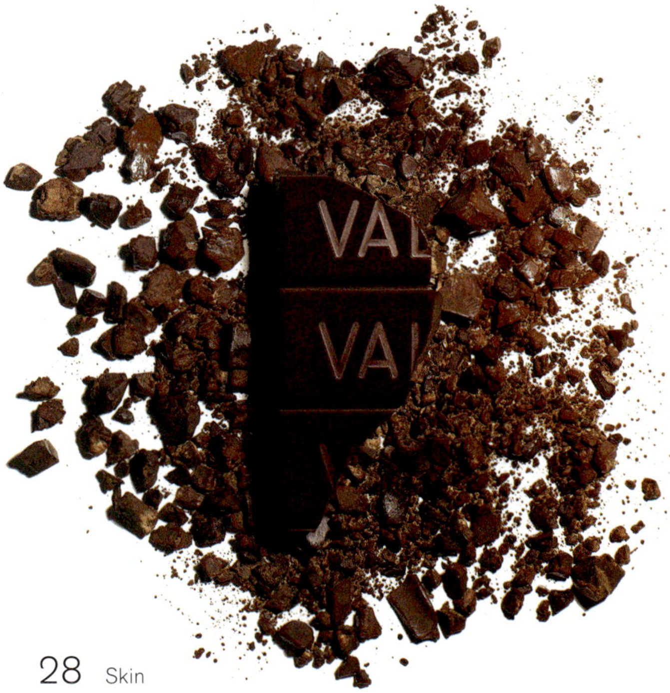

Our bodies are 80 percent water. Without sufficient hydration, the skin cells become dry and flaky. To keep the body, including the skin, hydrated, eat foods with a high water content, such as fruits, vegetables, and clear soups, and drink at least eight glasses of water a day. It is important to limit your intake of coffee and other drinks containing caffeine, as they are diuretics that remove water from the body and block the absorption of vitamins and minerals.

Exercise

Exercise is a skincare essential. Raising the heart rate through vigorous exercise increases blood flow, brings more oxygen to the skin, and cleanses impurities from the body through sweat. Just twenty to thirty minutes of exercise a day is enough to help boost your immune system, reduce stress, lower blood pressure, strengthen your heart, build stronger bones, increase your energy level, and improve your mood. Ideally, you want to do a mix of aerobic exercise and strength training. Aerobic exercise helps get the blood flowing, so take a walk, run, or swim regularly. With regular exercise, you build lean muscle mass and raise your metabolism. Since the metabolism slows with age, exercise is fundamental to weight management.

Sleep

Sleep is the time when the body's cells have a chance to repair and regenerate. Sleep deprivation stresses all of the body's systems, including the skin, and can result in headaches, irritability, lack of energy, or the inability to focus. The skin becomes less elastic and prone to outbreaks of acne or rashes.

Tip

Smile, be positive, breathe, and take a vacation once in a while.

Sun

Excess sun exposure is skin's number-one enemy. It causes premature aging, including wrinkles, loss of elasticity, and hyperpigmentation. Worse, overexposure often causes deadly forms of skin cancer. Wear a broad-spectrum sunscreen with a sun protection factor (SPF) of at least 15 in the winter and 30 in the summer.

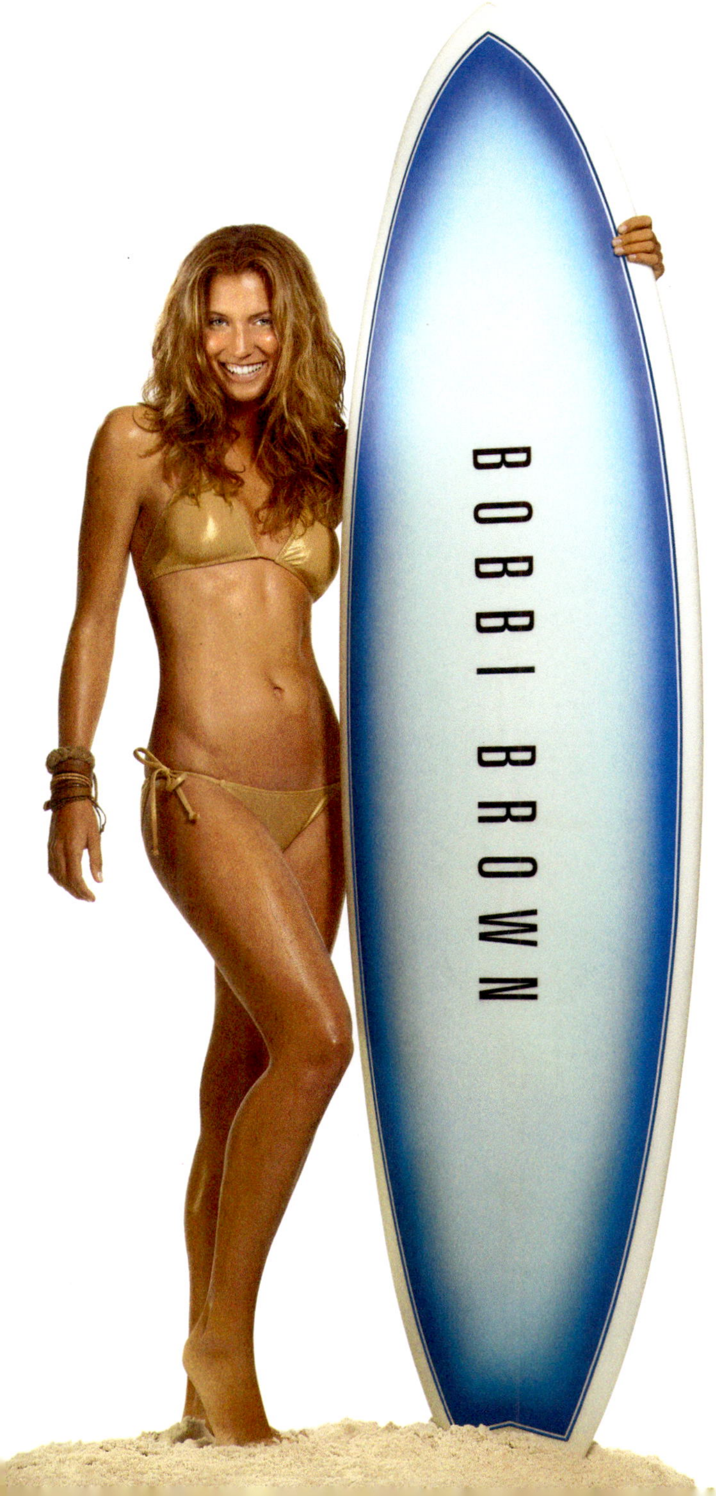

Smoking

Smoking also causes the skin to age prematurely. Nicotine impairs the blood vessels that provide skin with both oxygen and nutrients and rid the skin of impurities. It eventually robs the skin of oxygen, causing it to look dull and gray. With low levels of oxygen, the skin loses elasticity, which leads to sagging and wrinkling.

Alcohol

Skin problems can be caused by excessive alcohol intake. Alcohol can cause allergic reactions, such as hives and rashes. Some people have allergic reactions to salicylates, which occur in such foods as berries, bananas, beans, grapes, and wine. If a rash appears after you eat these foods, it is likely that beer and wine will also cause outbreaks.

Stress

Stress often shows up on the skin. Stress-related hormonal fluctuations can cause adult acne and other skin problems. While healthy eating and exercise habits help to combat the symptoms of anxiety and stress, finding mechanisms to deal with the underlying causes of stress is important.

Tips

Drinking eight to ten glasses of water a day will help flush out toxins and keep all skin types clear.

Drink one glass of water each time you have a beverage that contains alcohol or caffeine.

SKINCARE BASICS

Few people have naturally perfect skin. With some knowledge, experience, good diet, and exercise, it is possible to greatly improve the appearance of the skin. The condition of the skin changes from day to day and season to season. Hormonal fluctuations, stress, pregnancy, medication, travel, and seasonal changes are only a few of the factors that can cause skin to act up. If you learn to recognize the various skin conditions, you will be able to choose the right cleansing options and moisturizers.

How the Skin Works

The skin is composed of three layers: a deep layer called the hypodermis, a middle layer called the dermis, and a surface layer called the epidermis. The epidermis gives immediate, visual clues to the condition and health of the skin, while the dermis determines how the skin responds and changes with age. The hypodermis, the deepest layer, contains a layer of fat, blood vessels, and nerves.

Skin's middle layer, the dermis, is composed mostly of collagen and elastin, which are proteins that give skin structure, strength, and flexibility. As we age, collagen and elastin production diminishes. The results show up on the face as a loss of firmness, rougher texture, more obvious wrinkles, and sagging.

Hair follicles, nerves, blood vessels, and sebaceous glands are also part of the dermis. Sebaceous glands produce sebum. This oily substance moves through the hair shaft to the top layer of the skin, where it covers the epidermis and provides a protective barrier against moisture loss. Too much sebum results in oily skin.

The outermost layer of skin, the epidermis, is several layers deep. Basal cells are created in the lowest layer and then migrate through a hardened layer to the stratum corneum, from which they fall off the body. The skin continually sloughs off the dead cells and grows new living cells. It takes about a month for a live basal cell to move to the top layer of the epidermis. As the cell moves toward the surface of the skin, it loses moisture and oxygen content.

On the surface of the epidermis is a layer of oil transported from the dermis by the hair follicles that forms a natural barrier, helping the skin to retain water. Harsh and scented cleansing products, exposure to chemical and biological pollution in the environment, and poor diet can remove this protective oil-based layer from the skin. This layer can be replenished with moisturizer.

Moisturizers work in several ways. First, they fill in the spaces between the relatively dry, or cornified, cells of the epidermis, making the skin feel and appear smoother. They also create a barrier on the skin, helping the skin retain water. The oil content in moisturizers works with the protective lipid coating of the skin to partially protect the skin from the air. Care must be taken in the selection and use of moisturizing products, as they make a huge difference in how the skin works. Hydration is the key to smooth, even skin, and moisturization is the external way to achieve it.

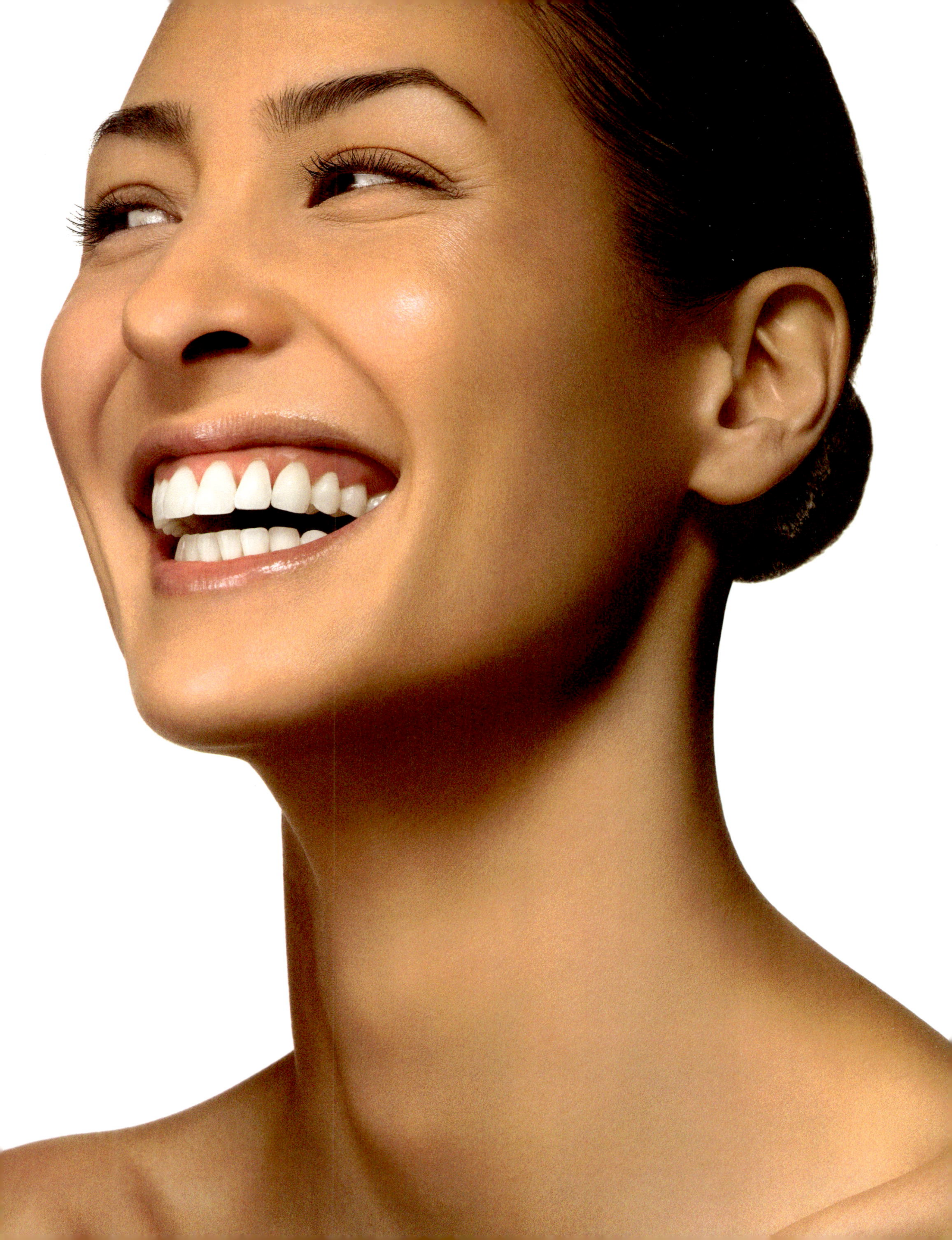

ANALYSIS OF THE SKIN

The following descriptions will help you recognize skin conditions and make decisions about skincare products.

Normal

Analysis

Comfortable-feeling

Smooth, even texture with small pores

Cheeks are the driest area, but not excessively so

May experience some shine and larger pores on the forehead, nose, or chin

Water and oil content in this skin is balanced

Care

Normal skin needs routine cleansing with a foaming cleanser, exfoliation twice a week, moisturization with lightweight lotions, and the use of a sunscreen to keep it healthy. A diet rich in vitamins A, C, and E helps keep skin smooth and soft. Sufficient fluid intake is important to maintain hydration and rid the body of toxins.

Dry/Extra Dry

Analysis

Feels tight after washing

May look dry or flaky

Feels rough and uneven; dehydrated

May be sensitive

Pores are small—almost invisible

Shows fine lines faster than other skin types

Care

Dry skin requires special care. A lifestyle that includes a healthy diet with foods high in water content, such as fruits and vegetables, and at least eight glasses of water a day keeps this skin type hydrated. Caffeine and alcohol cause dehydration, so limit intake to two cups or glasses a day. Using richer cleansers, limiting sun exposure, and using a good moisturizer can protect your skin's natural oils. Layering different textures of moisturizer can do wonders to hydrate the skin. Begin with lightweight face oil, and then layer a richer cream over that. Night creams with alpha hydroxy acids (AHA) help remove the dry, dead skin while moisturizing the new. Air-conditioning and heating create dry environments. Correct this in your home by using humidifiers.

Self-Test: Skin Analysis

Look at your own clean, unmoisturized skin in the mirror. Is the overall texture flaky (dry), shiny (oily), or smooth (normal)?

How does your skin feel after you wash it with your current cleansing regimen? Tightness through the forehead is an indication of dry skin.

How does your skin normally look by midday? Is there oil breakthrough or dryness even though you have moisturized?

What lifestyle factors are influencing your skin's current condition: stress? hormonal fluctuations? sun exposure? diet?

Does your skin have noticeable sun damage? How are you protecting yourself against the sun?

An accurate skin analysis will help you determine the most effective cleansing, hydration, and makeup products for your skin type and condition. However, when problem skin shows no improvement or worsens, see a dermatologist.

Oily Skin

Analysis

Oily skin is shiny, especially through the T-zone (the forehead, nose, and chin); it is a condition caused by overactive sebaceous, or oil-producing, glands.

May have large, visible pores

Frequent breakouts

Few signs of aging, such as fine lines

Care

Management of oily skin and the prevention of breakouts requires a healthy diet and a regular skincare routine. Cleanse the face at least twice a day to prevent dirt accumulation and to keep pores open. Use an alcohol-free astringent to remove excess oil. Use oil-free moisturizers to keep the skin from overdrying.

Combination Skin

Analysis

Oily through the T-zone

Dry cheeks or spot dehydration

Larger pores on the forehead, nose, and chin

Care

Care for this skin type requires regular cleansing, toning, and moisturizing of the oily areas and the use of a milder cleanser and denser moisturizer for the dry areas. Moisturizing products containing AHA will benefit this skin type.

Sensitive Skin

Analysis

Can range from dry to oily

Easily irritated by cosmetics, moisturizers, and cleansers

Sensitive and prone to redness

Itchy or blotchy

Care

Sensitive skin requires mild, nonperfumed cleansing products. Use an alcohol-free toner formulated for sensitive skin. Also, use cleansers and moisturizers specifically formulated for this type of skin.

Misleading Skin Conditions

Don't be fooled. The skin's condition can be quickly impacted by changes in environment, health, diet, and even current product choices for cleansing, toning, moisturizing, or makeup. There are many skin conditions that can hide your actual skin type. Redness, dryness, or flaking can be caused by a medical condition or medication. Skincare products can be overused, causing oily skin to become dry or flaky. Dry skin that is overmoisturized can appear greasy. Redness and irritation can be caused by low-grade allergies to cleansing, moisturizing, or makeup products, necessitating a change to gentler products.

CLEANSING & TONING THE FACE

Cleansers

The purpose of cleansing is to remove bacteria, makeup, and the dirt, sweat, and oil that build up on the skin each day. At *least* once a day, the skin needs to be cleaned with a formula that does not strip the skin of all its natural oils.

Makeup Remover Options

EYE MAKEUP REMOVERS remove eye makeup quickly and easily without harsh tugging or wiping. Look for oil-free, water-based formulas gentle enough for all skin types.

LONG-WEAR MAKEUP REMOVERS quickly and gently remove long-wearing and waterproof makeup. Look for products safe for contact lens wearers. These can generally be used for removal of lipstick and mascara or eyeliners.

CREAM CLEANSERS also work. See below.

Cleanser Options

Familiarity with these options will allow you to make the right choice based on your skin condition and type. Look for ingredients like wheat germ oil, which cleans without stripping, and glycerin, which attracts moisture to the skin's surface.

SOAP will deeply clean the skin and leave it feeling thoroughly cleansed and refreshed. Look for glycerin or cold cream soaps formulated specifically for the face. Glycerin creates a moisture cushion on the skin and a soft feel. Soap is best for oily skin types. Do not use body or bath soap, especially antibacterial soap. It will strip the skin and leave it feeling tight and dry.

GEL CLEANSERS typically foam or lather during use. These cleansers are formulated to dissolve oil buildup and fight blemish-causing bacteria without stripping the skin. They are best for oily or combination skin types that are prone to breakouts.

CREAM CLEANSERS are lightweight, water-based formulas that clean without leaving residue. These products contain oils and emollients along with cleansing ingredients and are recommended for normal to dry skin types.

OIL CLEANSERS work best on the driest of skins.

BALM CLEANSERS condition and moisturize the skin while cleansing. They leave a moisturizing cushion on the skin and are suitable for all skin types except oily.

EXFOLIATING CLEANSERS sometimes contain alpha hydroxy acids, such as glycolic or salicylic acid, and can be used several times a week to encourage cell turnover and dead skin removal. These products are gentle enough for all skin types. Some exfoliating cleansers contain beads or grains that loosen dead surface skin cells. These manual exfoliants should be used twice a week in place of the daily cleanser.

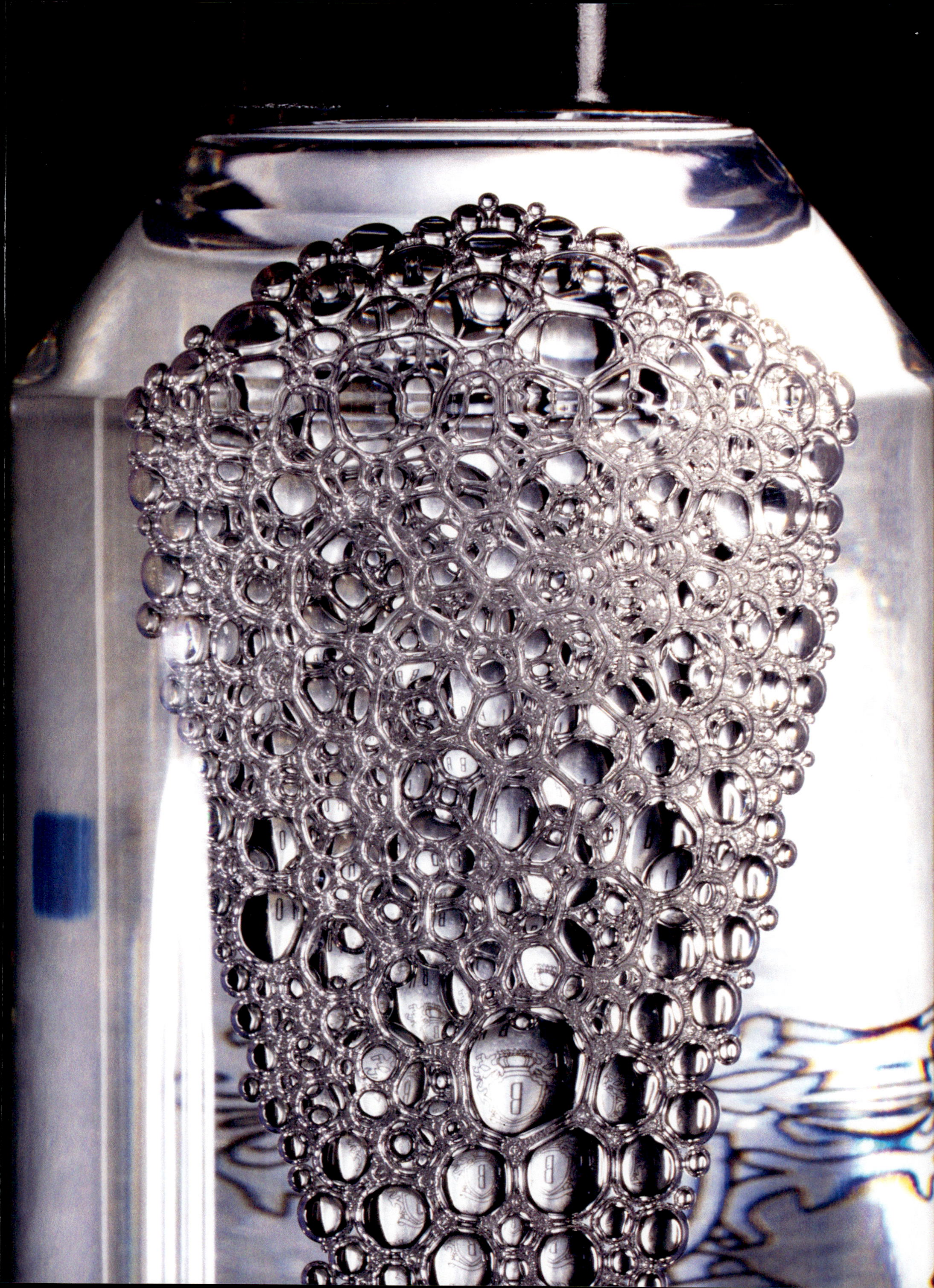

TREATMENT MASKS provide intensive supplements to the regular cleansing regimen. Oily and blemish-prone skin will benefit from the application of a clay mask, which helps to draw out impurities, reduce blackheads, and dry up excess oil. Dry skin, or any skin type that's been exposed to strong sun or wind, can be rejuvenated with a creamy hydrating mask. Masks containing cucumber, chamomile, aloe, or calendula are naturally soothing and good for irritated skin.

STEAMING THE SKIN helps remove impurities, stimulates circulation, and opens the pores. Herbs, such as lavender or thyme, added to a steam treatment stimulate the skin. Steaming can be helpful for all skin types.

MASSAGE stimulates circulation and helps to relax the facial muscles, giving the face a smooth and lifted look.

Toners

Toners stimulate circulation in the skin, remove any remaining dead skin cells or greasiness, and give the skin a smooth texture. Toners can be helpful for those who have very oily skin or who wear lots of makeup. Use a toner after cleaning the skin or as an interim cleaner to remove dirt and oil. During the summer, toners can be especially useful, as the skin is more oily and tends to attract more dirt and bacteria. Toners also help to restore the skin's natural pH balance.

While no cosmetic product can change the size of your pores, toners and astringents can make them appear smaller. These products work by very slightly irritating the skin, causing it to swell, making pores less noticeable.

To apply toner, pat the skin with a cotton ball soaked in the product of choice. You can also spray toner onto the face. Of course, cold water can just be splashed on the face instead.

Toner Options

Alcohol and water are the major ingredients in many skin fresheners, astringents, and toners. Other ingredients can include witch hazel, glycerin, rose water, vinegar, alum, boric acid, menthol, camphor, and other herbs. The major difference in the products is the amount of alcohol they contain. Alcohol strips the naturally occurring oils skin needs to be healthy, so look for a product without alcohol, especially if you have dry skin.

COLD TREATMENT with a splash of cold water is the best toner and can be used by those with any skin type. It closes the pores and improves the skin's texture.

SKIN FRESHENERS are very mild and contain water, such humectants as glycerin or rose water, and very little alcohol (less than 10 percent). Humectants help prevent the evaporation of moisture from the skin. These products are very gentle and are especially good for sensitive, dry, and normal skin.

SKIN TONICS are stronger, containing water, humectants, and up to 20 percent alcohol. Tonics are for normal, combination, or oily skin.

ASTRINGENTS contain water, humectants, up to 60 percent alcohol, and antiseptics. These are drying and only suitable for very oily skin or for application to specific problem areas. Witch hazel is an astringent.

Removing Makeup & Cleansing the Skin

Secure hair off the face with a headband or elastic.

When wearing makeup, it is often necessary to cleanse using a multistep process. Start with a makeup remover or tissue-off cream to dissolve much of the makeup, avoiding the eye area.

The skin around the eyes is especially delicate and can be easily irritated. There are makeup removers specifically formulated for this area. Take a cotton pad dampened with the product, and rest or press it gently around the closed eye. Wipe lightly. Do not tug or pull on the eye or surrounding skin.

Apply cleanser to the entire face. With a cleanser appropriate to your skin type, massage the product into your skin with an upward circular motion. Include the neck, under the ear lobes, and the chin.

Rinse the entire face, including the eye area, with warm—not hot—water.

Dry the face with the softest natural-fiber towels you can find. Pat the face dry. Rubbing or hard wiping creates small abrasions on the skin surface, causing irritation, redness, and even swelling.

MOISTURIZERS & SUN PROTECTION

Hydration

The most important skincare step is ensuring hydration. Skin's tone and flexibility depends on the presence of water in the underlying tissues—water drawn from humidity in the air and moisture added to the skin's surface. Oil is the skin's natural protectant, preventing moisture from leaving the skin. Oil in the skin functions as a defensive barrier. It smoothes the texture and helps to maintain skin-cell health. When oil glands overproduce, the skin appears greasy, and when the glands underproduce, the skin becomes dehydrated and flaky. Adding moisture to the skin helps maintain skin firmness, smoothness, softness, and luminosity.

Facial Moisturizers

Moisturizer is the true fountain of youth. Moisturizers form a barrier between the skin and the environment that holds water in the epidermis. They hydrate and plump up the skin so that it looks smooth and bright. The right moisturizer will enhance the look, feel, and health of the skin and can even help temporarily eliminate fine lines and wrinkles. Moisturizers can also protect the skin from pollution, debris, and weather. The right skincare products help makeup go on smoothly, properly adhere to the skin, and last longer.

There are two types of facial moisturizers. Oil-in-water emulsions usually contain humectants, such as glycerin, which attract water. Added water from the environment is wonderful for the skin. The second category of moisturizer is the water-in-oil emulsion. These creams and lotions work by forming a water-trapping barrier on the skin surface. Look for the ingredient sodium hyaluronate, which locks in moisture and prevents it from leaving the skin. Humectants are often added to these products as well.

The major difference between moisturizing products is the ratio of water to oil. Even products labeled oil-free sometimes have small amounts of oil in them. You can sometimes find the ratio of water to oil on the label of a moisturizer.

PETROLEUM-BASED MOISTURIZERS are very effective at locking in moisture. They can, however, block pores and feel sticky.

VEGETABLE OILS are sometimes used as the base for moisturizers but in general are not as effective as mineral oils or animal fats.

INGREDIENTS SUCH AS VITAMIN E, COLLAGEN, PROTEINS, HORMONES, PLACENTAL EXTRACTS, AND AMINO ACIDS are sometimes added to moisturizing products.

VITAMIN A DERIVATIVES are added to anti-aging products.

CHEMICALLY ENHANCED products contain agents such as urea, glycolic acid, or lactic acid. They are formulated to improve the moisture-retaining ability of the moisturizer and are often recommended for dry skin.

FRAGRANCES are added to products to provide a pleasant aroma and to mask the odor of other ingredients.

All skin types benefit from the use of some type of moisturizer.

DRY SKIN needs a heavier, oil-based moisturizer that will absorb completely into the skin, leaving it feeling soft and supple. Oils are more effective than creams at preventing water evaporation. Look for the ingredients urea or propylene glycol, chemicals that keep skin moist.

NORMAL SKIN has a healthy moisture balance. Water-based moisturizers containing lightweight oils, such as acetyl alcohol, or silicone-derived ingredients, will help maintain healthy, normal skin.

OILY AND COMBINATION SKIN types benefit most from an oil-free, water-based moisturizer. Oil-free products are made from synthetic chemicals and contain little to no oils or animal fat. If you have oily skin, use all moisturizers sparingly. Look for products labeled "noncomedogenic," which means they are formulated to prevent clogged pores. Test moisturizers to find one that leaves a matte finish on the skin. This will minimize shine and the appearance of large pores.

SENSITIVE SKIN needs a moisturizer that does not contain fragrances or dyes and is designed for this skin type.

EXTRA DRY AND MATURE SKIN requires more moisture. Nourishing oils, dense creams, and balms are formulated specifically for both these skin types. These products help to temporarily plump up the skin, making it appear smoother and reducing the appearance of fine lines. Look for petrolatum-based moisturizers that also contain ingredients such as lactic acid or alpha hydroxy acids, which help to prevent dry skin.

Specially formulated moisturizers are needed for the area under and around the eye. The skin surrounding the eyes has smaller pores, is thinner than the rest of the facial skin, and is more sensi-

Tips for Moisturizing

Use a fast-absorbing eye cream under concealer to help skin look smooth, not crepey. The skin around the eyes is more delicate than the rest of the face. For puffiness and wrinkles under the eye, try using a richer formula containing shea butter or beeswax at night.

If your skin is very dry and dehydrated, use a super-rich moisturizing balm with ingredients like petrolatum, glycerin, or shea butter for better texture and for smoother application of foundation. Warm the balm in your palms before applying it to your face.

Layer different textures of moisturizers to achieve maximum results. For instance, use an absorbing cream with balms or oils.

If you have oily skin, try using an oil-control lotion on the forehead and nose to tone down shine. Oil-free formulas hydrate while helping to control overactive oil glands. Foundation applied over the lotion will hold better, too.

For dry, chapped, or cracked lips, apply a balm formulated specifically for lips.

Try patting a moisturizing balm onto your cheeks after completing your makeup. It will give a glow to your face and help the foundation look natural.

To create your own sheer, tinted moisturizer, mix face lotion with foundation.

These tests will help you to determine the ratio of oil to water in a moisturizing product.

Apply moisturizer to your skin. If the skin under the moisturizer is warm, there is a greater percentage of oil in the product. If the area is cool, there is a greater percentage of water. The science behind this is that evaporation cools, and water evaporates. Oil does not evaporate and therefore traps heat in the body.

Put a small amount of moisturizer on a tissue, and hold it over a lightbulb. Products with higher oil content will melt. The wider the area of melted oil, the greater the percentage of oil in the moisturizer.

tive. It is important to keep this area as hydrated as possible. Products on the market target specific problems. Before you go shopping for an eye cream, decide whether you want an eye cream that hydrates and prepares for concealer, or an overnight cream that is rich and emollient. Anti-wrinkle or anti-aging creams contain caffeine, retinol, alpha hydroxy acids, or vitamin C. Anti-darkening creams contain vitamin K or hydroquinone. Also decide if you want two different creams, one for night and the other for day. To avoid possible irritation of the eye, look for an eye cream that does not contain fragrance and has a pH close to that of tears (about 7.5).

Lips are often the first area of the face to wrinkle. Dry and chapped lips are a clear sign that you need to drink more water. While hydrating the body is the first step toward beautiful lips, there are many products that help keep them plump and smooth.

For personal use, have on hand two facial moisturizers, one lighter than the other. On those days when the skin needs more moisture, apply the lighter product first, and then layer the heavier moisturizer over that. Also find a moisturizing product formulated specifically for the under-eye area, lip balm, body moisturizer, and sunscreen. As your skin changes in response to lifestyle, season, or climate, you can treat it with the right hydrating product. Makeup artists carry a full range of moisturizers in their kits.

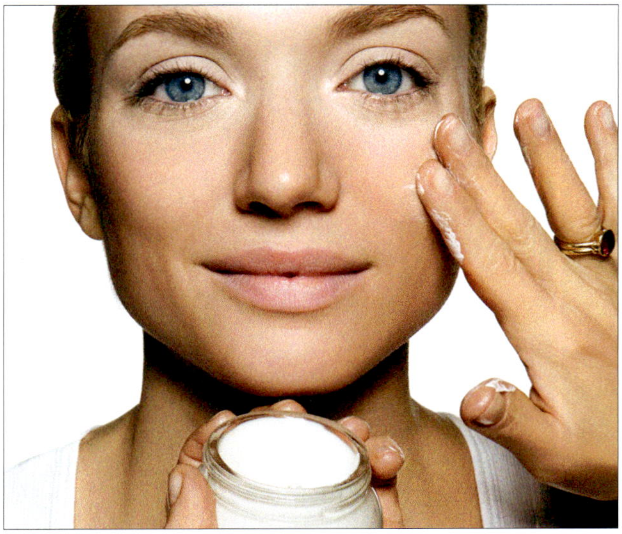

Moisturizer Application

Once the face is thoroughly cleansed and toned, and while it is still slightly damp, apply moisturizer using a clean sponge or your fingers. (Note: dense balms will work only on dry skin.) If you are using your hands to apply any makeup products, always wash them thoroughly so you don't transfer oils and bacteria to your face. Bacteria on the hands or makeup tools often cause breakouts.

Use about a nickel-size amount of moisturizer.

Warm the balm or moisturizer between your palms.

With firm, upward strokes, gently press the product into the skin until it is completely absorbed.

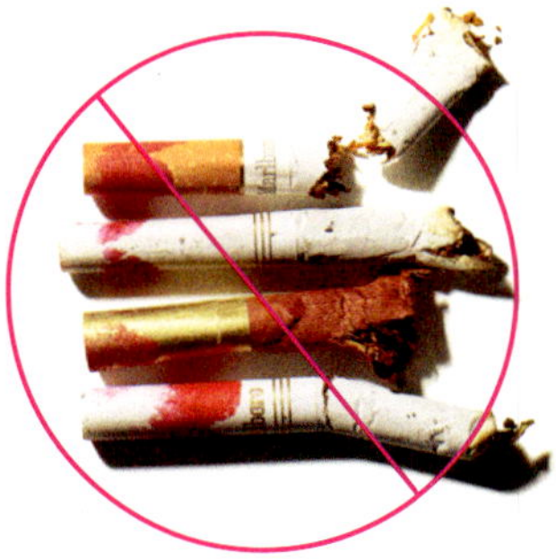

Smoking is always a horrible idea.

It severely damages your skin and lungs and is a common cause of cancer. It makes you smell and robs color from your skin and lips. Smoke breaks down the skin's defenses, depriving it of the oxygen it needs for healthy cell renewal. Repeated exposure to cigarette smoke causes the skin to lose its luster and tone and to wrinkle. Smokers often develop permanent wrinkles around the lips. Smoking is the one lifestyle choice for which balance and moderation are not options.

Sun Protection

Lines, dark spots, and uneven skin texture are *not* the inevitable effects of aging but are often the result of too much sun exposure. Overexposure to sunlight can also cause cancer. Too much sun is the skin's worst enemy. The only way to prevent premature aging and skin damage due to overexposure is to stay out of the midday sun when possible, wear protective clothing and hats, and always use the proper sunscreen.

Three types of radiation reach us from the sun. Visible and infrared light rays provide light and warmth. Ultraviolet rays are harmful. The sun's ultraviolet (UV) light falls into three wavelength bands: UVA, UVB, and UVC.

UVA RAYS have the longest wavelength and remain high in intensity all day. They penetrate through the epidermis and deep into the dermis, damaging newer cells. UVA rays are very dangerous and can cause cancers and sensitivity reactions.

UVB RAYS have a midrange wavelength, and like UVA rays penetrate the epidermis and continue into the dermis. These rays break down the organization of skin cells, causing wrinkles and broken blood vessels. They are highest in intensity from 10 a.m. to 2 p.m. and near the equator. Glass protects skin from UVB rays.

UVC RAYS have the shortest wavelength and are usually absorbed by the ozone layer. They are absorbed by the epidermis and can be very dangerous in

Tips for Protecting Your Skin from the Damaging Effects of the Sun

Whenever possible, stay out of the sun for long periods of time, especially between 10 a.m. and 2 p.m., when rays are strongest.

Protect exposed skin all year round. Wear sunscreen with an SPF (sun protection factor) of 15 to 30, depending on the season and length of exposure. Long-sleeved shirts and wide-brimmed hats provide some protection. Remember, the sun penetrates through loosely woven and wet clothing very easily, so wear sunscreen even when covered.

Avoid tanning beds. There is no such thing as safe tanning.

Wear sunglasses that wrap around the eyes and have 100 percent UV-blocking lenses. Most sunscreens are too harsh to use on the sensitive area around the eyes.

Select a sunscreen that protects against both UVA and UVB rays, sometimes labeled as broad-spectrum sunscreen. Many popular sunscreens will not adequately protect your skin from these harmful rays.

Apply liberally—about one teaspoon of sunscreen to your face and at least one ounce (about a shot glass) to your body each day. The face and hands are high-risk areas for cancer, so apply liberally to those areas.

If you have sensitive skin, use a cream-based product, and avoid sunscreens with tretinoin (Retin-A, Stieva-A, Retisol-A, Rejuva-A, Renova, Vitamin A acid), which dries the skin. Look for a fragrance-free, hypoallergenic sunscreen if you have any allergies to skin products.

Waterproof and water-resistant sunscreens are good if you are involved in swimming or sports. Waterproof products work for ninety minutes; protection with water-resistant sunscreens lasts thirty minutes. They need to be applied/reapplied twenty minutes before entering the water so that the product can bond with the skin.

Those who work out of doors might need frequent application of a sunscreen with a high SPF.

UVA rays are reflected from all light surfaces, including water, sand, snow, ice, and even concrete.

Children younger than six months old should not wear sunscreen but instead be covered and kept out of the sun.

large amounts. As the ozone layer thins, attention will need to be paid to these UVC rays.

Exposure to the sun produces the formation of molecules in the skin called free radicals. These molecules attack healthy skin cells, damaging and interfering with the production of new collagen. With the destruction of collagen fibers and hyaluronic acid molecules—both of which are responsible for preserving the volume and resiliency of the skin—skin loses its firmness, resulting in wrinkles. The sun can also damage the eyes and affect the immune system. UV rays can damage white blood cells and Langerhans cells, both essential to the skin's ability to fight viruses and other diseases.

For more information and to learn of new developments in sunscreen protection, these Web sites, listed recently in a *New York Times* article, might prove helpful.

Environmental Working Group
(lists products with UVA protection)
www.cosmeticsdatabase.com

The Skin Cancer Foundation
www.skincancer.org

American Cancer Society
www.cancer.org

American Academy of Dermatology
www.aad.org

British Columbia Centre for Disease Control
www.bccdc.org

Sunscreen Application

Apply sunscreen at least once a day, and use an adequate amount of the product.

Clean the skin before application.

Apply to cool, dry skin twenty to thirty minutes before exposure. Cool, dry skin allows sunscreen to bind effectively. When sunscreen is applied to warm skin, the open pores can become irritated, and rashes can develop.

Two applications help cover any missed spots.

Apply moisturizer and makeup over sunscreen.

Reapply during the day, depending on your rate of perspiration and the amount of sun exposure you get.

Tip

Use the equivalent of a shot glass of sunscreen—that's two tablespoons—to cover skin from head to toe.

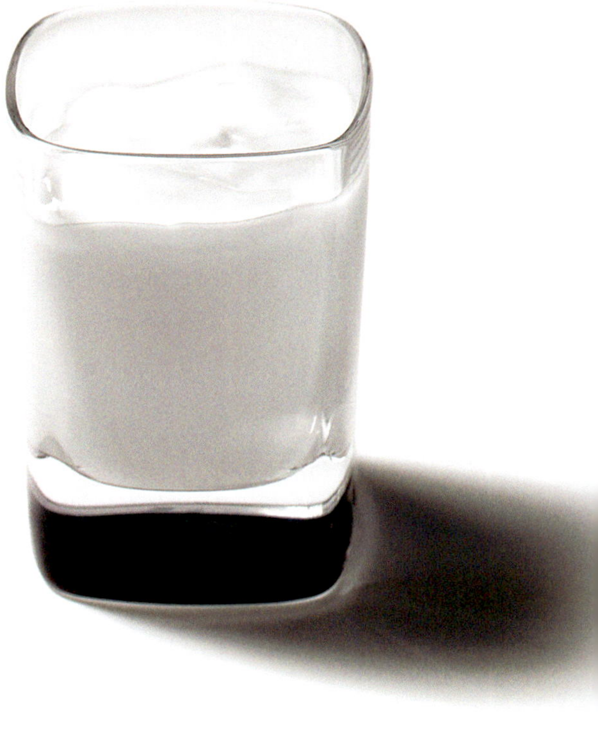

Skincare Glossary

There are many terms and ingredients associated with skincare products. What follows is only a basic list. While there are no miracles when it comes to the skin, a clear understanding of how ingredients function will help you select the right skincare products.

ALPHA HYDROXY ACIDS (AHAS) are naturally occurring acids found in fruits and milk, used topically to reduce the appearance of fine lines. AHAs help speed up the skin's natural exfoliation process, helping it shed dead skin cells. They can improve the texture of skin, unclog pores, and help prevent breakouts. Glycolic acid is one of the commonly used AHAs. Do not use products containing salicylic acid (a beta hydroxy acid), which is too harsh for general exfoliation, as they are intended for use only on problem skin areas.

ANTI-AGING: The best anti-aging formula is a healthy lifestyle. Nothing will stop the clock. Poor diet, excessive drinking, smoking, lack of exercise, and sunburn all accelerate the effects of aging on the skin.

ANTIOXIDANTS help protect the skin from damage caused by free radicals, molecules with an unpaired electron. They cause oxidation that can damage cellular material. Vitamins A, C, and E, beta-carotene, green tea, and grape seed extract are all highly effective antioxidants.

BALMS are super-rich moisturizers that target dry patches of skin on face, hands, feet, and body. Look for ingredients such as avocado extract or shea butter. For a subtle glow, I warm some in my hands and pat on the cheeks after applying makeup.

BASE is a term that generally refers to a product applied under foundation to smooth and protect the skin. Bases often contain a mix of vitamins, antioxidants, and anti-aging ingredients. Previous generations referred to foundation color as base.

BRIGHTENER: Makeup products sometimes contain light-diffusing particles and/or ingredients that inhibit oxidation. Both of these are referred to as brighteners.

COLLAGEN is a fibrous protein found in skin. When collagen levels in the skin are high, the skin appears firm. Levels of collagen decline as we age. As the support provided by the collagen is reduced, wrinkles begin to form. Injections temporarily replace lost collagen. The topical application of peptides may have a similar effect.

EMOLLIENTS (squalane, avocado oil, wheat germ oil, glycerin, lanolin, petroleum, shea butter, and others) hold moisture in the skin and make the skin soft and supple.

EXFOLIATORS are designed to help slough off dead skin cells. Look for scrubs designed for the face.

FIXERS are sprays that set makeup. Makeup is also typically set with powders.

GREEN TEA EXTRACT (*Camellia sinensis*) is a powerful antioxidant found in many anti-aging products that may slow down photo aging.

HUMECTANTS (glycerin, algae extract, sodium hyaluronate, urea, lactic acid, panthenol and others) absorb water from the air and help the skin retain moisture.

HYALURONIC ACID (sodium hyaluronate) is a fluid that surrounds the joints and is found in skin tissue. Aging slows the production of this acid, so it is often supplemented as an anti-aging treatment. It is used as filler for wrinkles (injection) and can be applied topically or taken in pill form. It is often added to moisturizer and works to hydrate skin.

OXIDANTS are unstable molecules caused by pollution, smoke, ultraviolet light, toxins, and other environmental factors. Also known as free radicals, they attack and damage the skin, leading to premature aging.

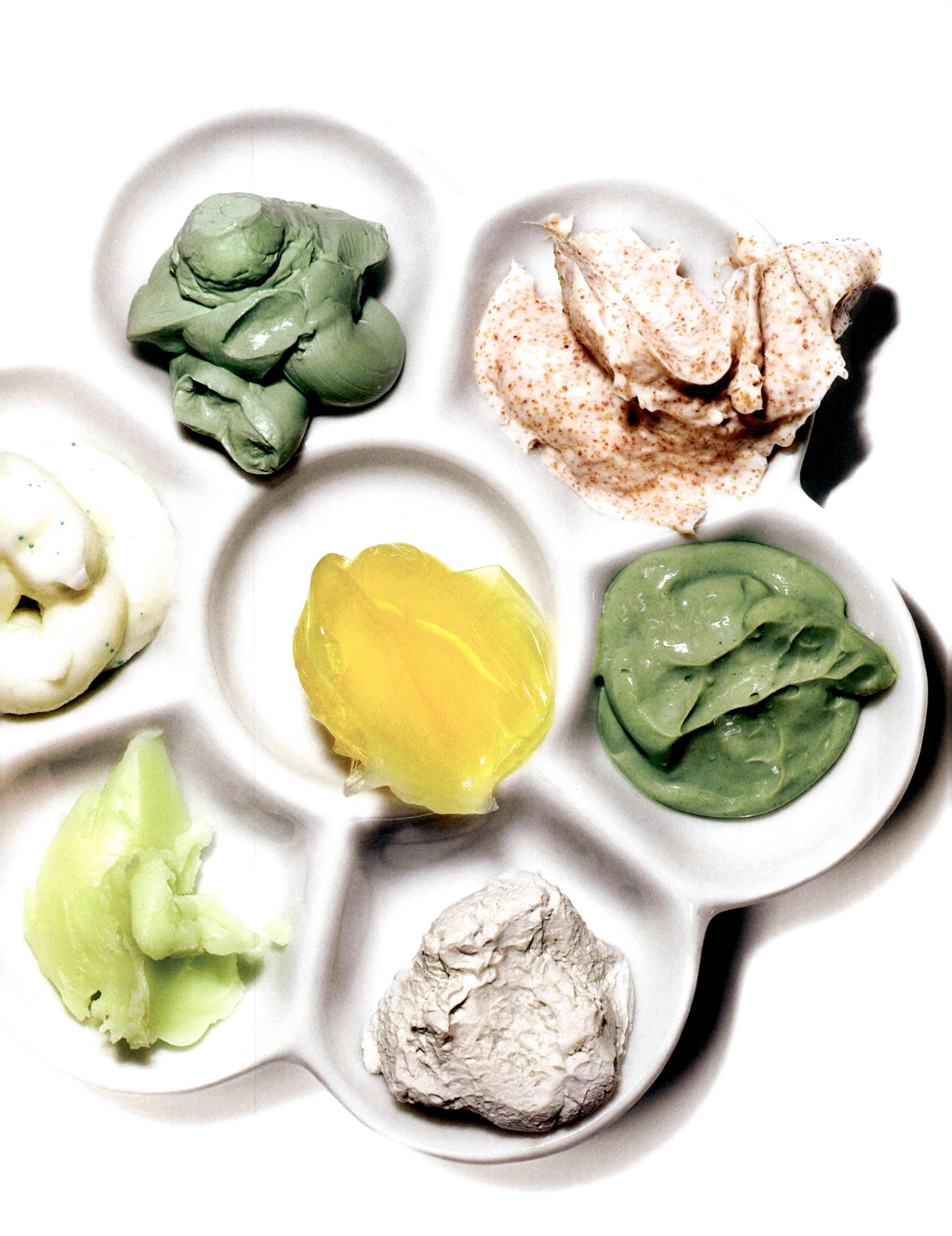

PEPTIDES are two or more amino acids bonded together, forming a linear molecule. The molecules can transfer biologically active agents (green tea, vitamin E, copper) to cells, renewing them. Algae peptides are used in some firming formulations. Copper peptides have been used for years to aid in wound healing. Labels might indicate that a product contains pentapeptides (five peptides) or polypeptides (many peptides).

PHOTO AGING is sun damage.

RETINOIDS (Retin-A, retinal, Renova) are powerful vitamin A derivatives used to fight acne and help build collagen to reverse visible signs of aging. The drug is effective in reducing fine lines around the eyes and mouth, not deep wrinkles. Inflammation and peeling are common side effects from use, which can last from two weeks to months. Because the drug makes skin more sensitive to the sun, use of a sunscreen is essential. Pregnant women and those planning a pregnancy should avoid this drug, since it is not known how much Retin-A is absorbed through the skin, and high doses of vitamin A can cause birth defects. Natural sources of retinoids include yams, tomatoes, fish-liver oils, melon, squash, and leafy green vegetables.

SERUMS are concentrated, corrective skin treatments that are packed with highly effective active ingredients that address specific skin concerns like dullness and uneven skin tone. Ingredients commonly found in serums include vitamin C, green tea extract, and white birch extract. For best results, serums should be applied after cleansing, before moisturizer.

SPF (sun protection factor) measures the degree of protection a product provides against the sun's UVB rays. The formula used divides the minutes it takes to burn wearing a thick application of the product by the minutes the same person takes to burn without any sunscreen. There is no current rating system for UVA protection.

SQUALENE (natural, unsaturated) is derived from shark-liver oil. It is very emollient and has some germicidal benefits.

TYROSINASE INHIBITORS (kojic acid, hydroquinone) all prevent browning or age spots on the skin. Licorice (*glycyrrhiza glabrd*) has been used for centuries to lighten and brighten skin.

VITAMIN B3 (niacinamide) is a water soluble vitamin found in yeast, eggs, liver, and vegetables that helps increase the amount of fatty acids in the skin, promoting exfoliation and firmness.

VITAMIN C (ascorbic acid) is an antioxidant that can reduce the appearance of hyperpigmentation and create a more even skin tone. It protects the skin from atmospheric pollution and from ultraviolet light. Vitamin C also helps convert inactivated vitamin E back to the active, antioxidant form of vitamin E. Vitamin C is involved in the formation of elastin and plays a role in converting proline, an amino acid, into collagen. Vitamin C increases collagen manufacture, reducing the appearance of wrinkles. The production of melanin is an oxidative process that causes pigmentation. As an antioxidant, vitamin C counteracts the oxidative process. High doses of vitamin C reduce the pigmentation of scars and make them less noticeable. Vitamin C is found in fresh fruits and vegetables.

VITAMIN E (tocopherol) provides antioxidant protection. All the cells in the body contain fatty acids that need protection against oxidation, which causes disease and symptoms of aging. Vitamin E protects the fatty acids (oils) against oxidation and rancidity. Vitamin E has been shown to act as a mild sunscreen, with a sun protection factor (SPF) of 3.

VITAMIN K helps to reduce ruddiness and promotes faster healing of bruising, swelling, and skin irritation.

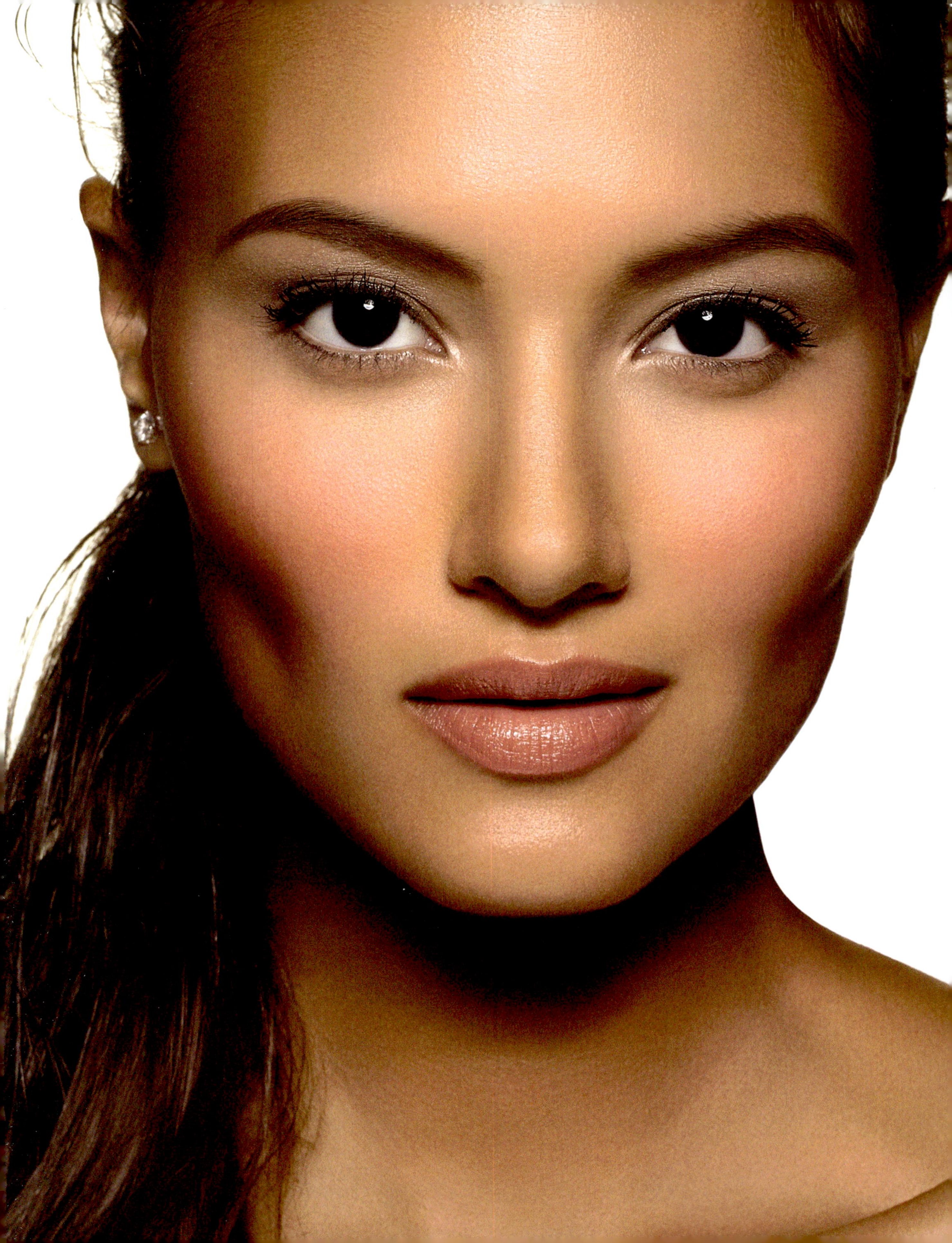

Chapter 4

FACE

The basics—**under-eye concealer, foundation, and powder**—are the secret to a great look. If the basics aren't right, the makeup won't be either.

PREPARING THE FACE FOR MAKEUP

Begin with these steps before applying any makeup.

Analyze the type and condition of the skin. This will determine the combination of skincare and makeup formulas to use. The condition of your skin changes each day, so make an assessment each morning.

Decide which products will improve the skin's current condition. That includes determining what weight moisturizer(s) are appropriate and whether an oil-controlling gel, a skin-soothing lotion, or a combination of skincare products is needed. Understanding how various ingredients work and the range of options available to you is important.

Choose the right foundation formula for the skin type and condition. Options include stick foundation, lightweight tinted moisturizer, denser tinted balm, fuller-coverage liquid foundation, powder, and oil-free formulas.

Select the correct foundation shade for the skin tone. It is important to select the foundation shade first.

Select an under-eye concealer one to two tones lighter than the foundation, and determine if a corrector is needed.

Select the perfect shades of powder to ensure that makeup stays fresh looking and lasts for hours. Choose a lighter powder to set concealer and that will double as an eye primer, and a deeper shade that works with the foundation tone. Test the color of the powder on the skin after applying foundation.

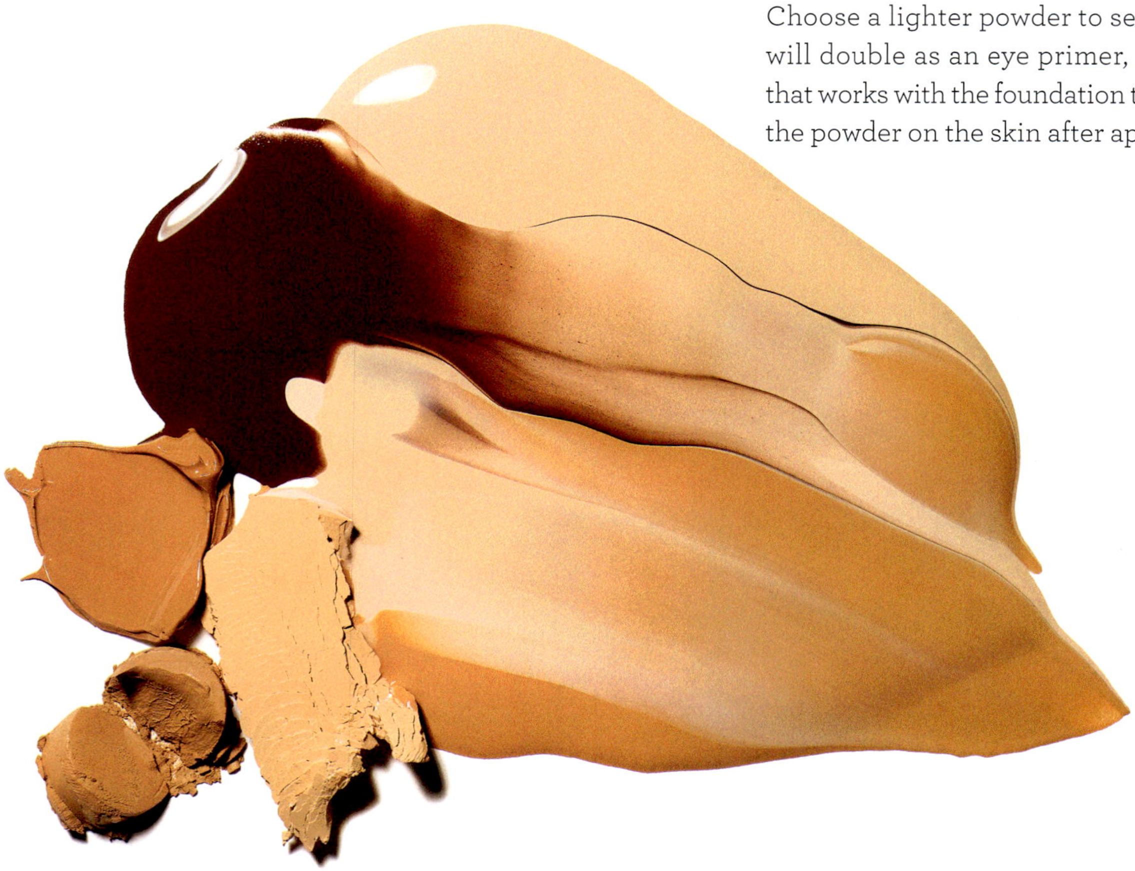

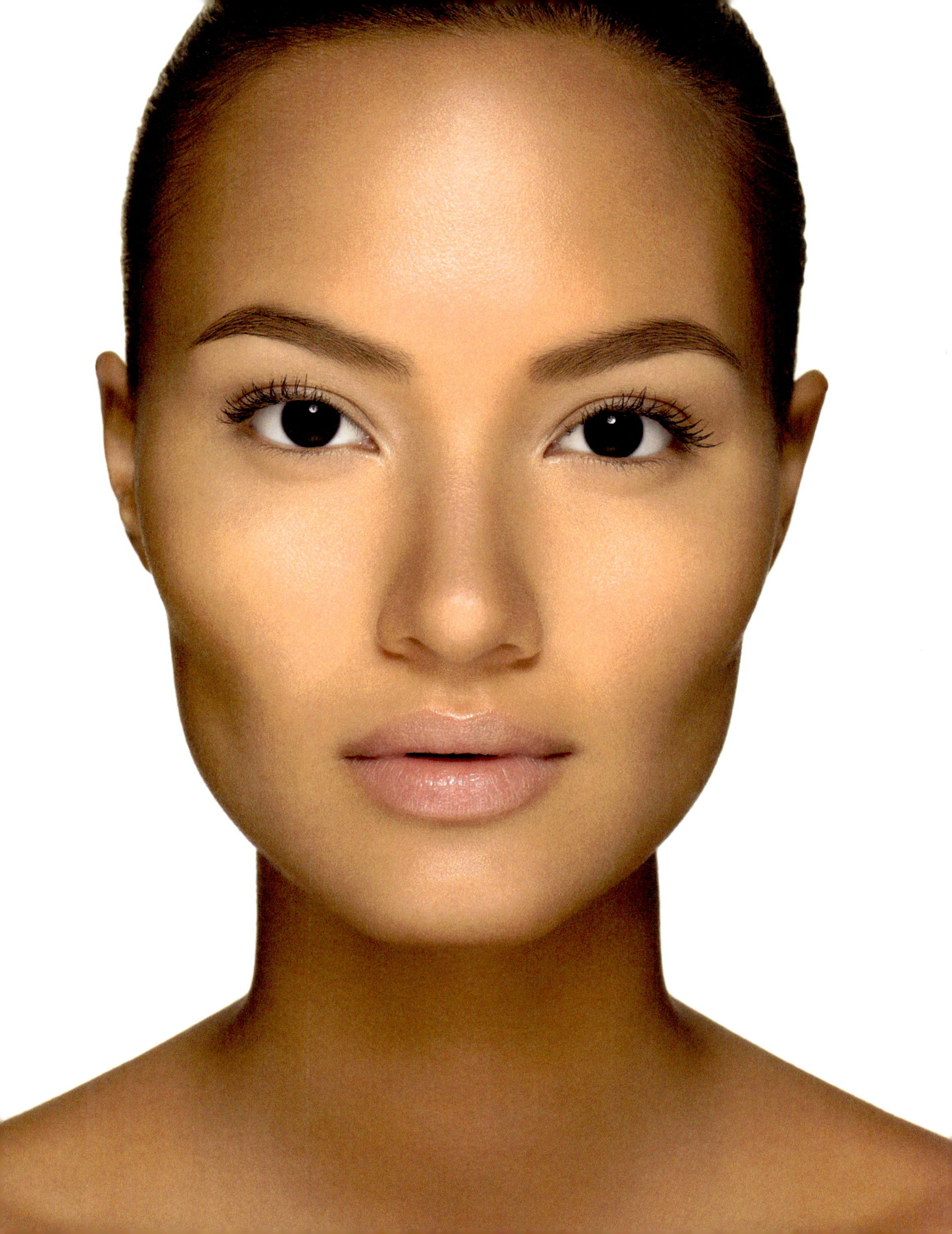

CONCEALERS & CORRECTORS

Correctors brighten the darkest areas under your eyes, allowing concealers to both lighten and blend. Concealers should blend into your skin, lightening dark circles and instantly making you look better.

Concealers are the secret of the universe.

While concealers are available that cover tattoos, spots, blemishes, scars, redness, and bruises, most people use a concealer to lighten dark circles under the eyes. Different concealers and correctors are formulated for each specific use. Pick a concealer and, when needed, a corrector designed for each of your problem areas. Under-eye concealers are not formulated for use on blemishes or areas of redness. They are creamier in consistency and lighter than the skin tone. Using under-eye concealer on areas of redness will only highlight the imperfections. Yellow-toned foundation that matches the skin tone is the best way to adequately cover blemishes, scars, and tattoos.

The application of under-eye concealer is the most important step in any makeup routine. Concealer is the one product that, when chosen and applied correctly, can instantly lift and brighten the face. Choose a color one to two shades lighter than the foundation. The skin under the eye is very thin, so the blue of the fine veins just under the surface tend to show through. A light yellow-toned concealer masks this blue discoloration and brightens the skin. For those with alabaster skin, a porcelain-toned concealer will work. Sometimes a stick foundation one or two shades lighter than the face can serve as an under-eye concealer for those who need very little coverage.

Correctors are available for extreme under-eye darkness. When a regular concealer cannot fully lighten the under-eye area, a peach or pink corrector is used to counter the purple or green tone. A regular yellow-toned concealer is usually lightly layered over the corrector to lighten the under-eye area. Occasionally, those with extremely deep purple or green coloration under the eye will not need the layer of regular concealer.

Tips

Some women need between two and four colors that can be mixed and blended to accommodate changes in skin tone under the eye, which can vary with the time of day, amount of rest, and hormones.

Sometimes a corrector is enough to solve the under-eye problem. Rules should be followed, but there should be flexibility for what works where. Sometimes something as bold as a bright pink or peach cream blush will work for very intense darkness.

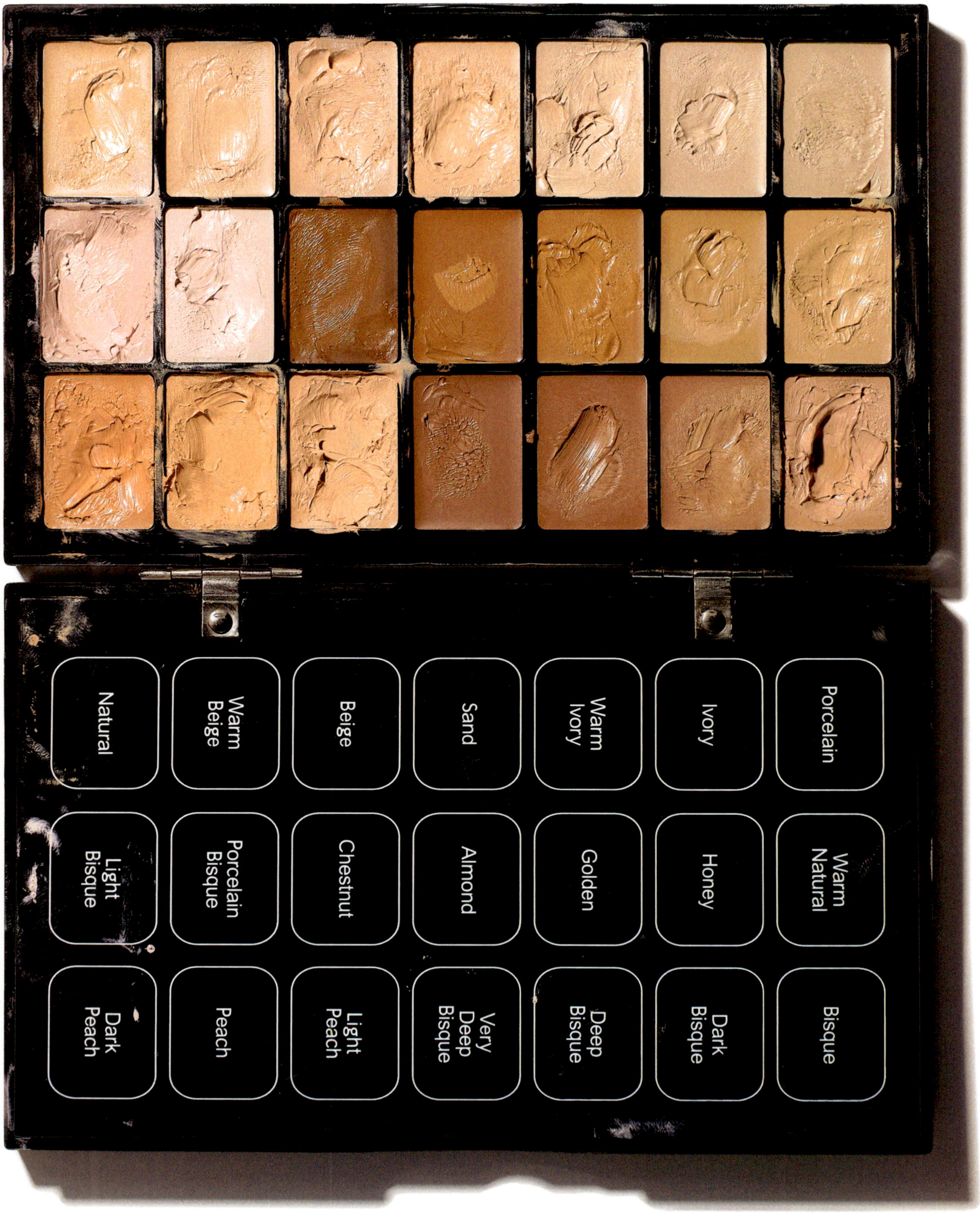

Natural
Warm Beige
Beige
Sand
Warm Ivory
Ivory
Porcelain
Light Bisque
Porcelain Bisque
Chestnut
Almond
Golden
Honey
Warm Natural
Dark Peach
Peach
Light Peach
Very Deep Bisque
Deep Bisque
Dark Bisque
Bisque

CHOOSING CORRECTOR COLOR

Correctors are for extreme under-eye darkness. If your skin is pale, choose the lightest colors, beginning with bisque or light pink. For deeper skin tones, choose peach or darker peach.

Pink

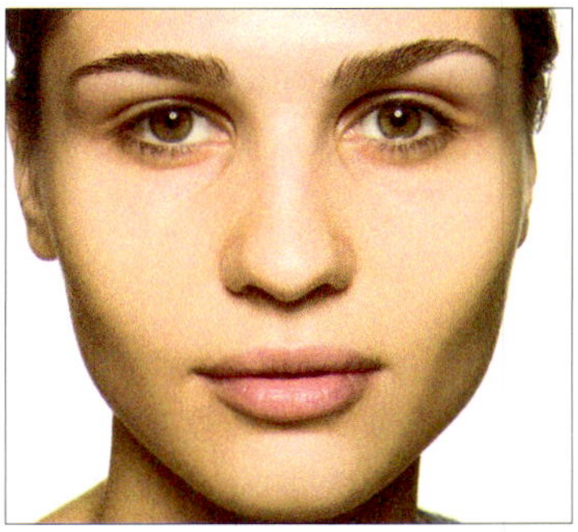

1

Begin with a clean face.

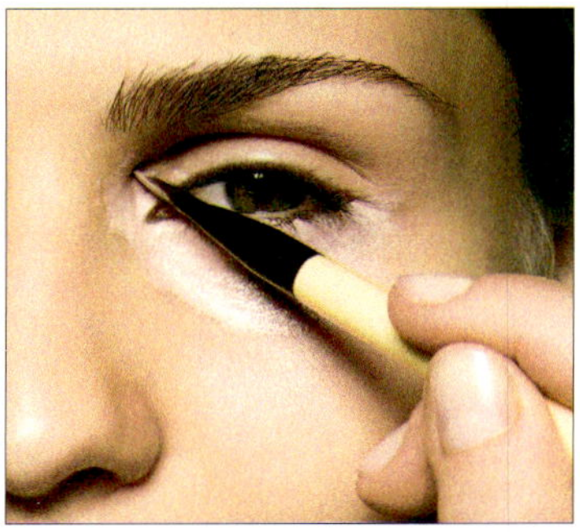

2

Apply corrector beginning at the inner corner of the eye and continue underneath close to the lashes, where there is darkness.

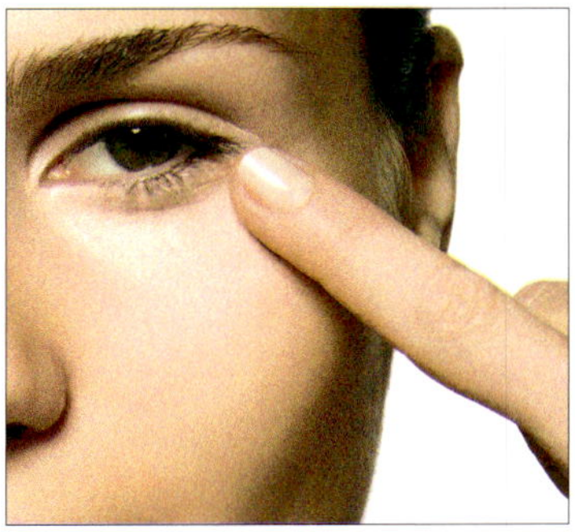

3

Gently blend by pressing with your fingers.

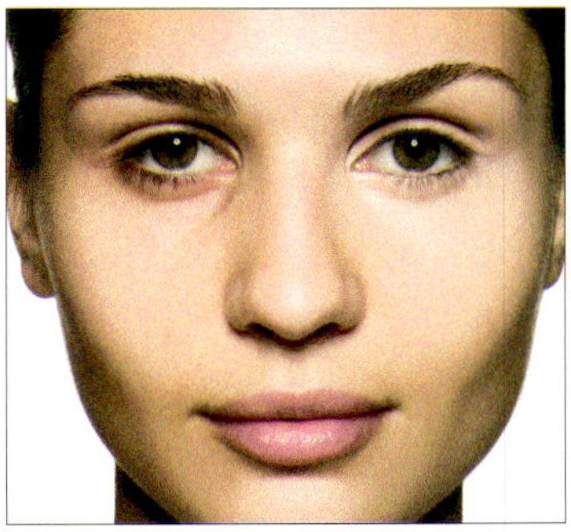

4

The corrector is complete on the right.

Peach

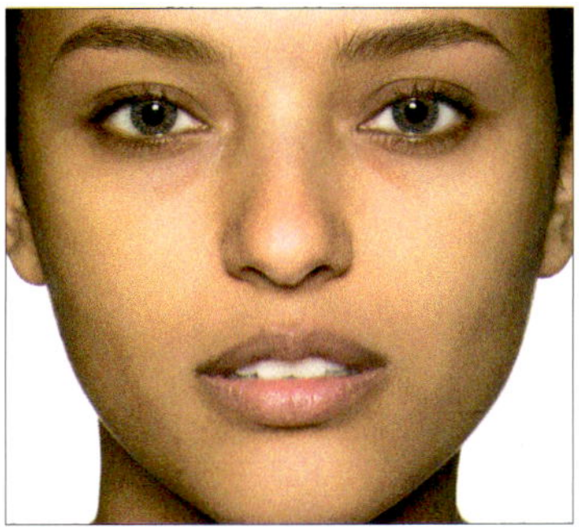

1

Begin with a clean face.

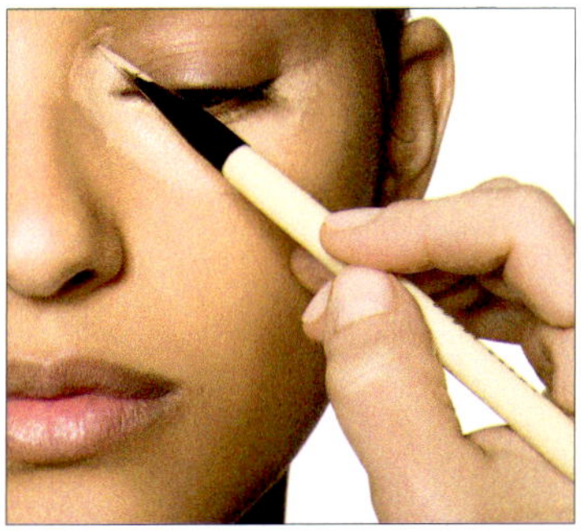

2

Apply corrector at the innermost corner of the eye and underneath to cover the darkest areas. Apply corrector generously, making sure there is enough to block the darkness.

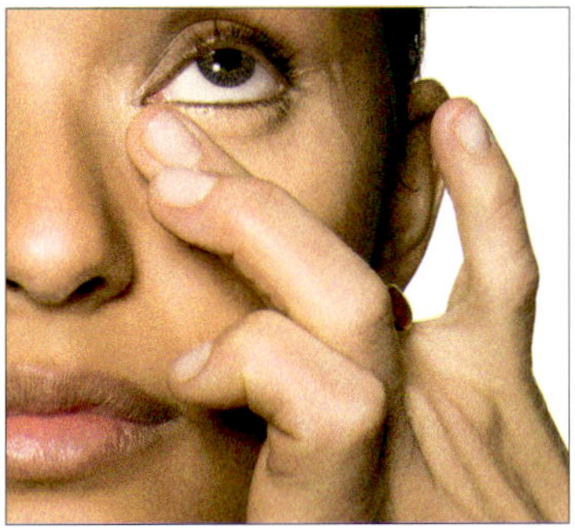

3

Gently blend and tap with your fingers.

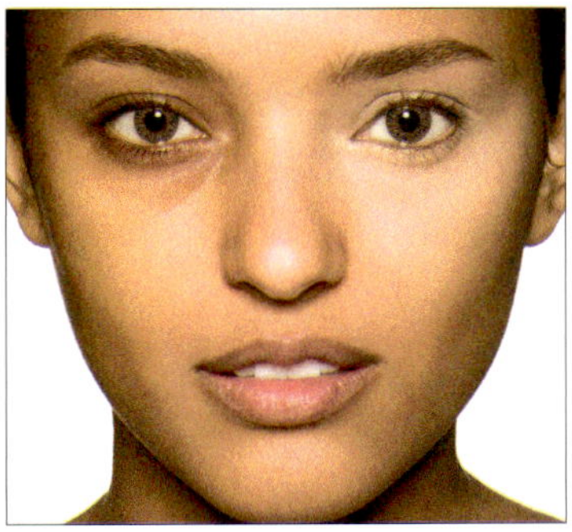

4

The corrector is complete on the right.

Darker Peach

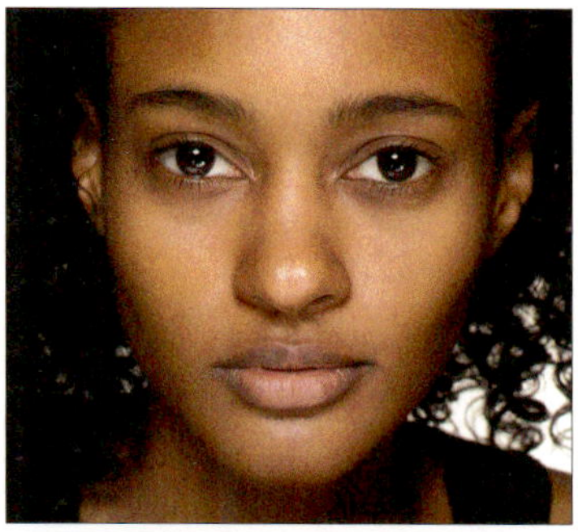

1

Begin with a clean face.

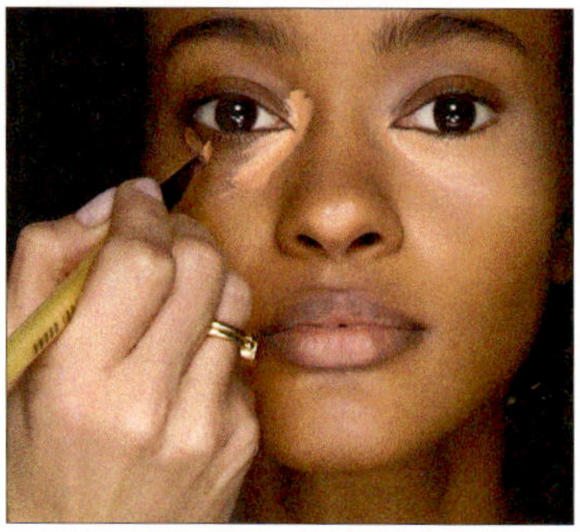

2

Begin at the innermost corner of each eye. This is the deepest, darkest area of the face, so apply the corrector densely.

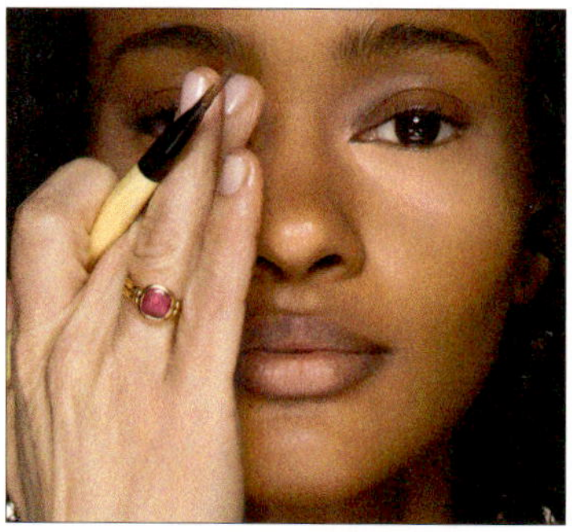

3

Blend with your finger and press the corrector into the skin. Never rub or drag your finger across the skin.

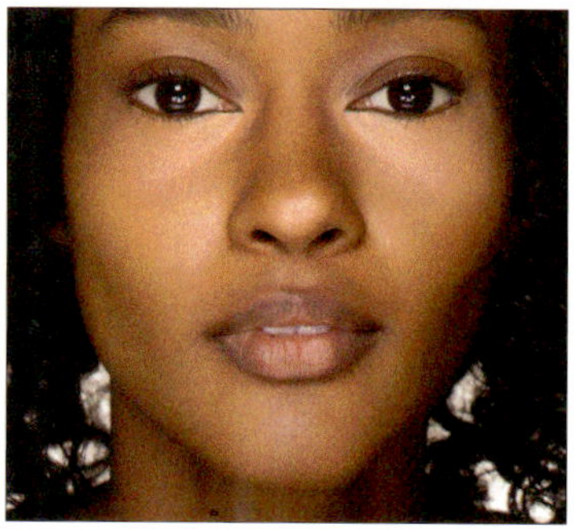

4

The corrector is complete.

CORRECTOR APPLICATION FOR ASIAN EYES

Even if you don't have a lot of darkness corrector still brightens the eyes.

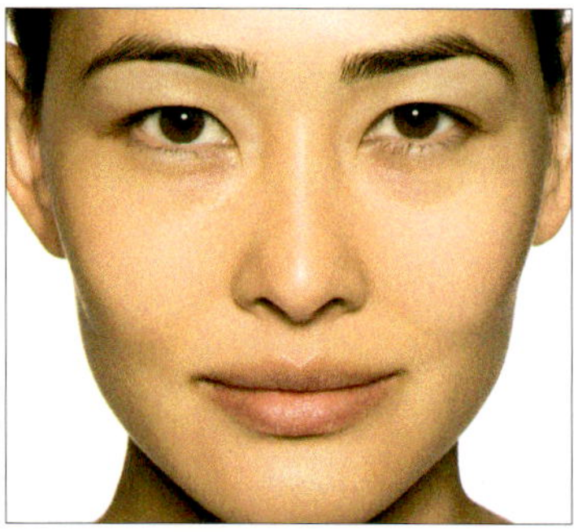

1

Begin with a clean face. Note the darkness is not severe.

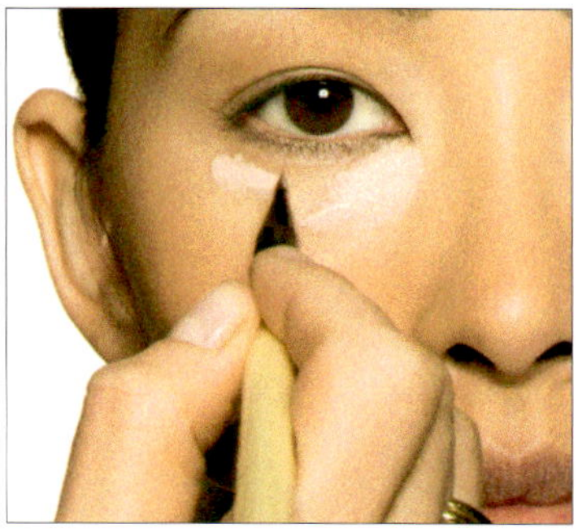

2

Cover the entire area with corrector.

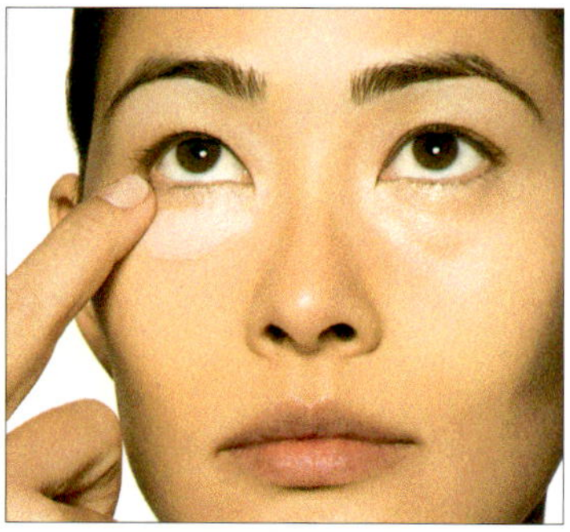

3

Gently blend with your fingers.

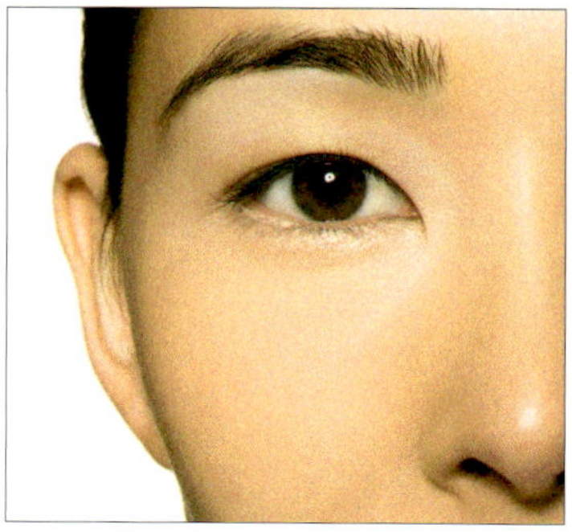

4

Note the difference even when the darkness is subtle.

CORRECTOR BRIGHTENS

Corrector can be pink or peach toned. Make sure it is applied up to the lashes and in the inner corner space between the eye and the bridge of the nose.

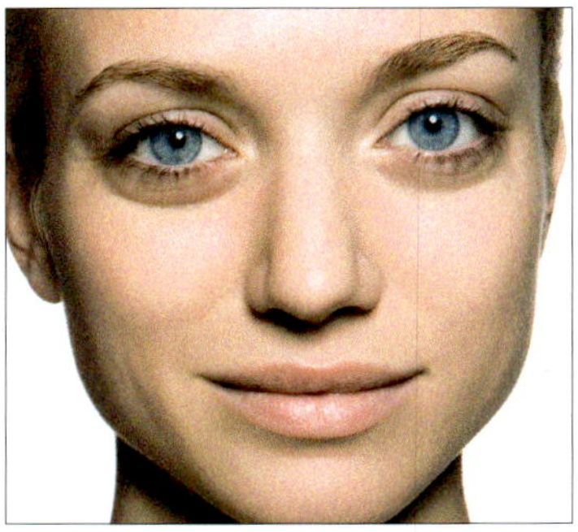

1

Determine whether corrector is needed to counteract deep purple or green coloration under the eye.

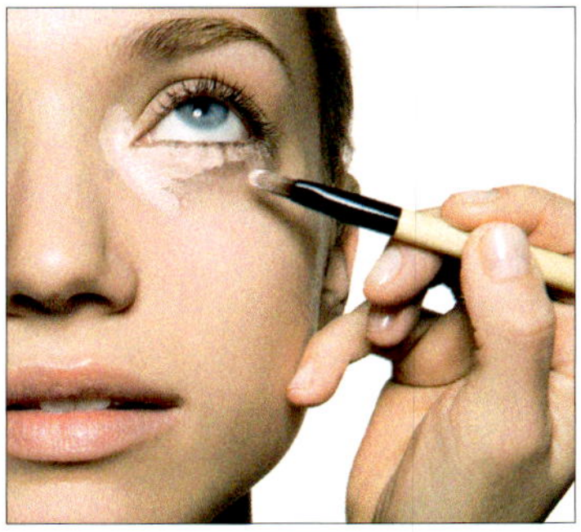

2

If corrector is needed, choose the color according to the directions on page 52.

Apply corrector using a small concealer brush and starting at the inner eye.

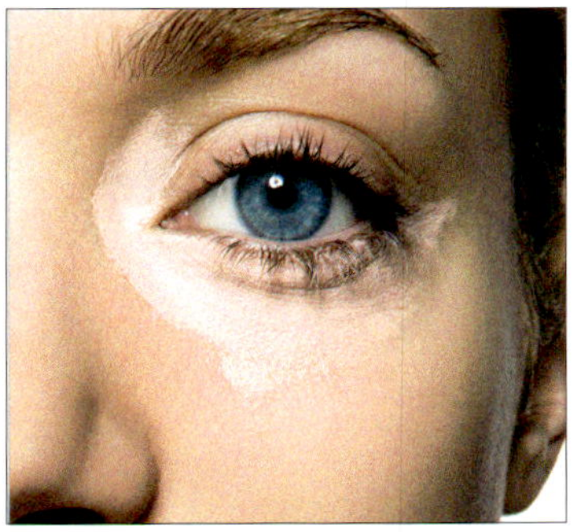

3

Apply corrector to all areas of darkness.

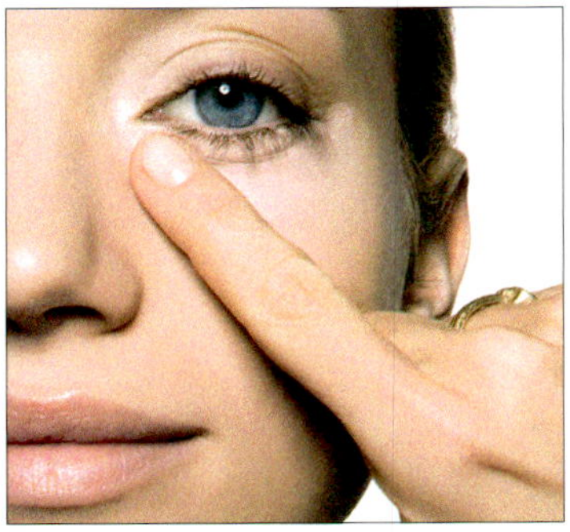

4

Gently press the corrector into the skin with your fingers.

Troubleshooting: Corrector or Concealer

If it creases
Using enough powder applied correctly is key. If you skimp, it will end up creasing.

If it's cakey
The ratio of eye cream to concealer is off.

If it's too light
Use an extremely light dusting of light bronzing powder to warm up the area.

If it's not bright enough or if it's too dark
Try to add a bit of fast-absorbing eye cream, then repeat corrector and concealer.

If the eye makeup transfers to the concealer
Use eye makeup remover, a cotton swab, or a sponge and remove all under-eye product. Start over with eye cream, and let it absorb before applying other eye makeup.

Clean brush between corrector and concealer steps.

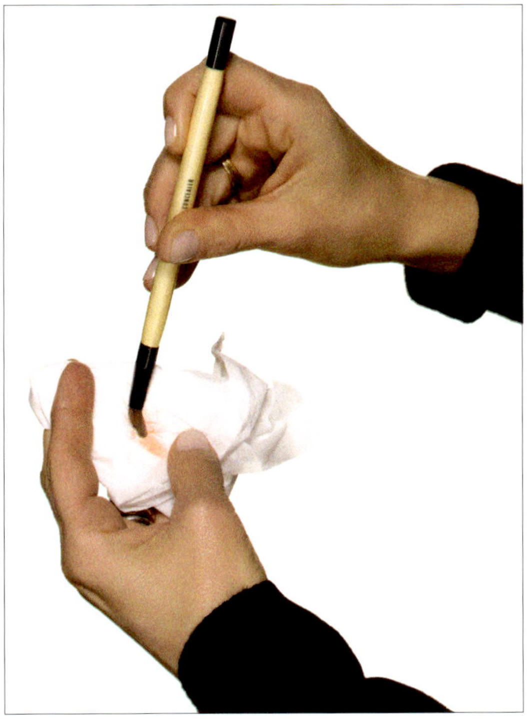

CONCEALER LIGHTENS

Concealer should be one or two shades lighter than your foundation and yellow in tone to blend as it lightens. Apply after corrector in most cases.

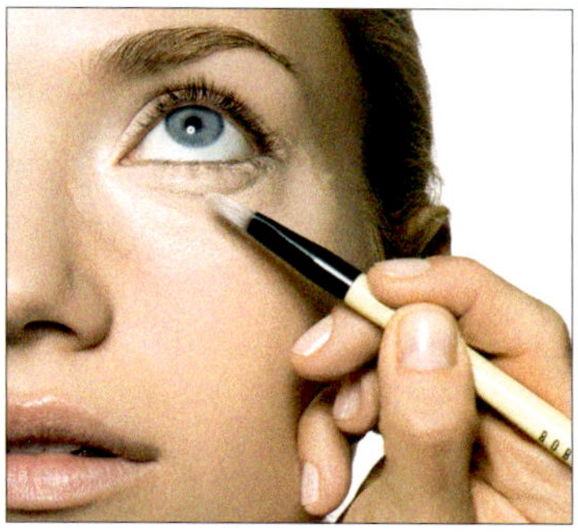

1

Apply concealer generously under the eyes starting at the recessed area at the innermost corner of each eye.

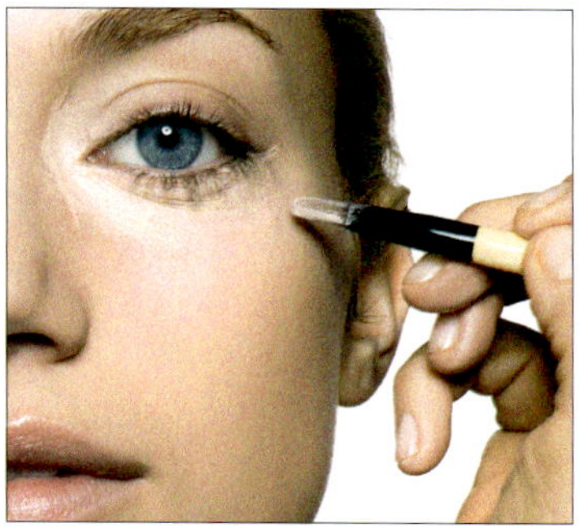

2

Cover the entire area below the lower lash line to cover any darkness or redness.

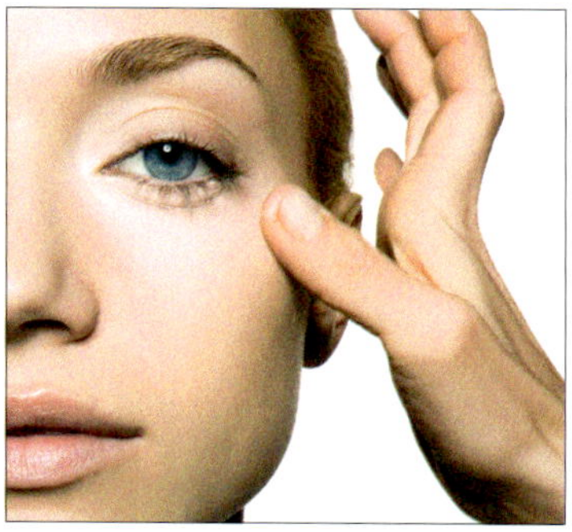

3

To blend the concealer, gently warm it between your fingers and then press it into the skin.

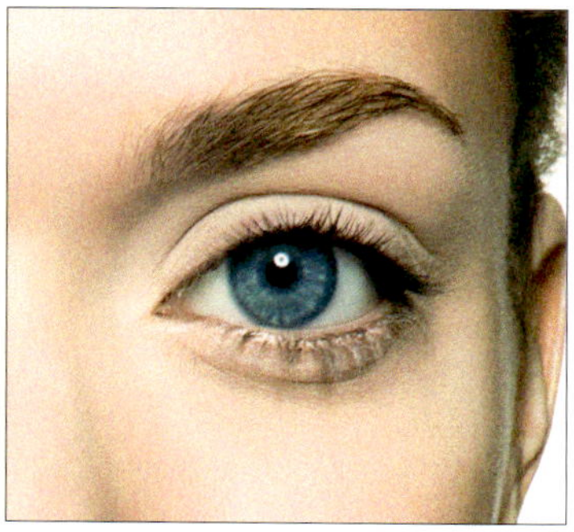

4

Set the concealer in place with a sheer loose powder.

POWDER SETS CONCEALER

Most women can use a yellow-toned, loose powder, but those with extremely fair skin may need a white-toned powder.

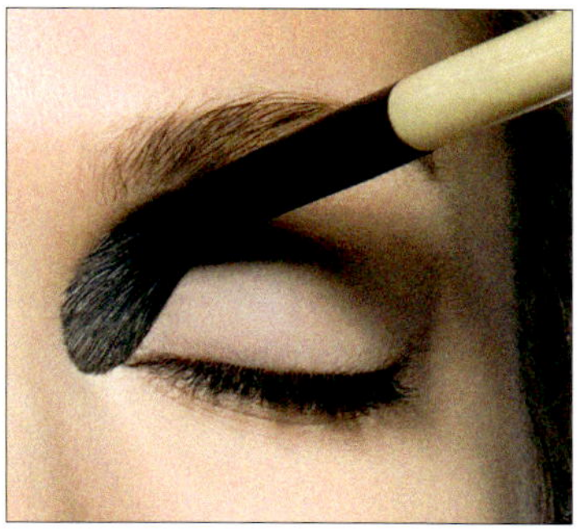

1

Using a brush that fits in the corner of the eye, dust the powder onto the skin.

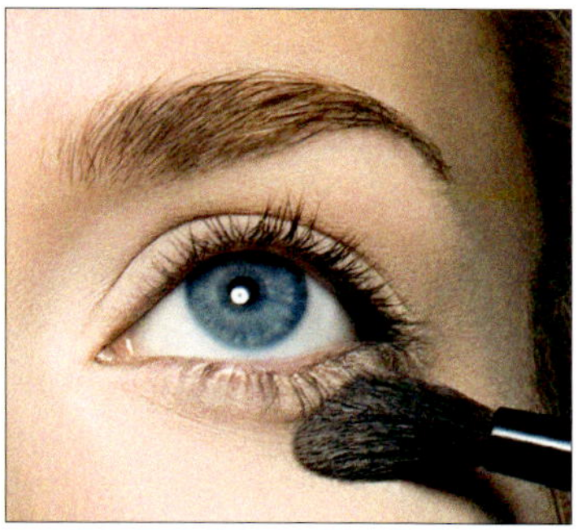

2

Brush the powder across the under-eye and sweep off any excess with the brush.

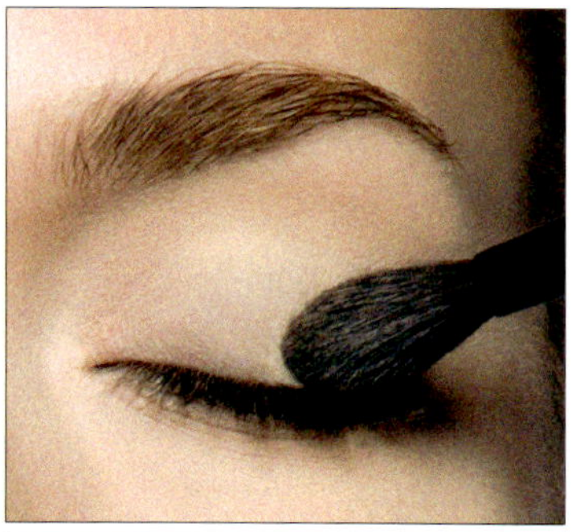

3

Sweep the powder across the eyelid.

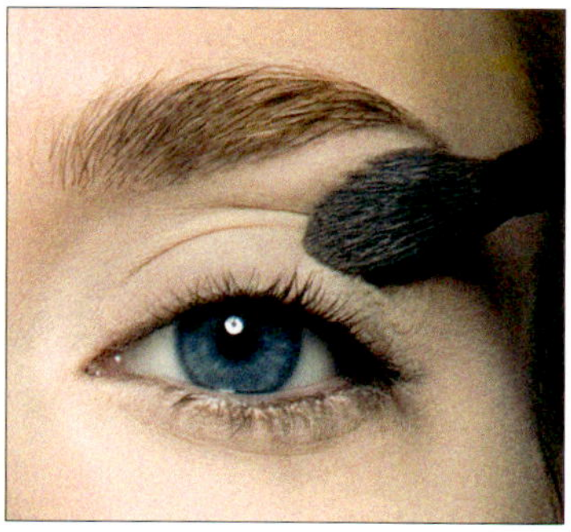

4

Apply the powder under the brow bone. Repeat two times if necessary.

FOUNDATION

Beauty starts with great skin. The right foundation will make you look like you're not wearing any foundation at all. You'll just have even-toned, great-looking skin.

The reason we wear foundation is to even out our skin tone and texture. When applied correctly, the result is skin that looks clear and smooth. But, what is most important is that the skin look better than it did without foundation.

Some women shy away from foundation because they associate it with thick pancake makeup that sometimes looks like a mask. But even the strongest makeup should have a natural-looking base.

Formula

Foundations are available in many different formulas. Choose one that is right for your skin and style and has a consistency you like to use. Use the following guidelines to choose your formula.

TINTED MOISTURIZER
For normal/normal-to-dry skin. Gives a sheer, lightweight coverage and is an alternative to foundation. Provides a totally natural look. Great for weekends.

TINTED FACE BALM
For extra-dry skin. Provides sheer coverage. Intensively hydrates and gives skin a dewy finish. Balm actually plumps the skin and reduces the appearance of fine lines.

STICK FOUNDATION
For all skin types except oily. Provides easy spot coverage and is also buildable for medium to full coverage. Best foundation for photography.

LIQUID FOUNDATION
For dry to extra-dry skin. Hydrates and smoothes, providing medium to full coverage.

MOISTURIZING COMPACT
For dry to extra-dry skin. Hydrating formulas provide medium to full coverage.

WHIPPED FOUNDATION
For combination skin and great for skin with texture. Balances the skin by hydrating dry areas and absorbing oil in the T-zone. Provides medium to full coverage.

OIL-FREE LIQUID FOUNDATION
For oily skin. For combination skin in the summer. Absorbs oil and smoothes while providing light to medium coverage.

OIL-FREE CREAM FOUNDATION
For normal-to-oily skin. Absorbs oil, providing medium to full coverage. A good choice to cover acne and large pores.

OIL-FREE POWDER COMPACT
For oily skin. Provides medium to full coverage. Because of the portable packaging, compact foundations are great for touch-ups.

MINERAL POWDERS
Suggested for very oily skin. (Be careful when choosing color. Oily skin can change color of powders, and they may appear dry and pasty.)

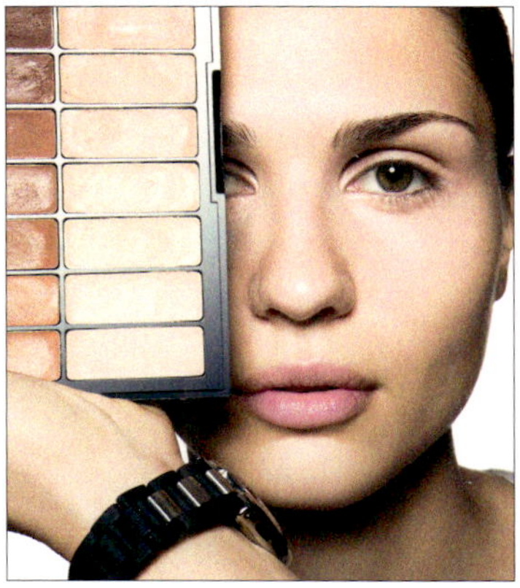
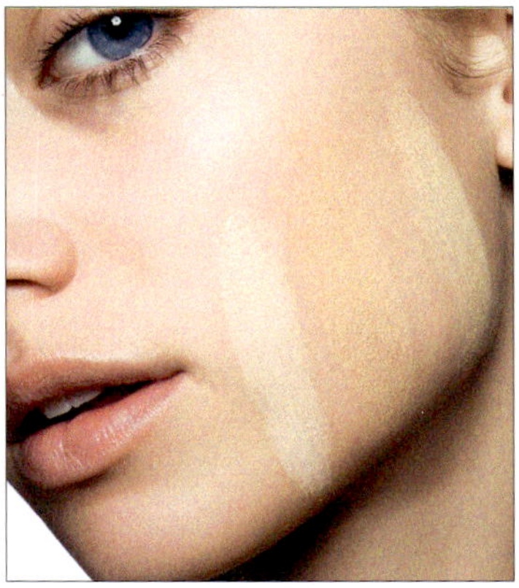
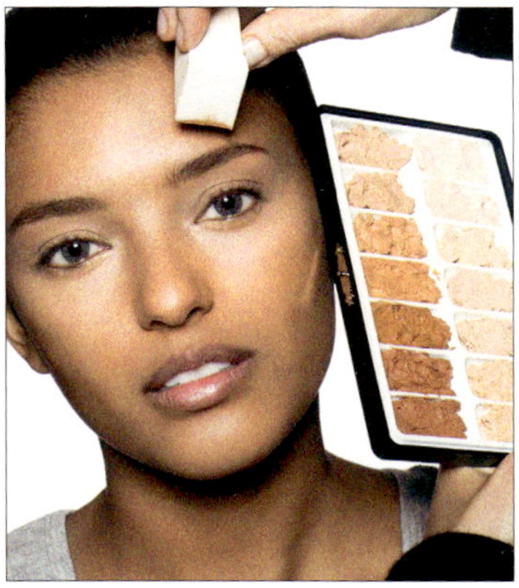

Finding the Perfect Shade

Once you have decided on the right formula of foundation, you need to find the right shade. The correct shade will disappear on the skin.

Make sure the foundation is yellow-based. Everyone has yellow undertones in their skin. Pink-based foundations look like a mask on most people. Only 1 percent need a pink tone: those who sunburn even in the shade. Foundation should not change the color of the face but simply even out the tone.

Test several shades of foundation on the side of your face, between the nose and the side of the cheek. Make a stripe of foundation in the preferred formula from cheek to jawline, gently blending into the skin. Also test a shade lighter and a shade darker for comparison. The correct shade will disappear.

Double-check the selected color on forehead. Sometimes women have darker skin on the forehead, and the foundation shade that matches here will work better for the whole face.

Always test foundation in natural light. Walk to a window or doorway to check the match. The swatch that disappears into the skin is the right shade. Do not test foundation on the hand or arm, as the face is rarely the same color as the rest of the body.

If your skin tone gets darker in the summer or on a vacation, you may need to adjust the foundation tone. Keep a deeper shade of foundation on hand to accommodate changes in skin tone. It can be blended with your regular foundation if you are between shades or used alone when skin is darkest.

Oily skin sometimes turns foundation darker. Check and adjust accordingly.

Stick foundation that is a shade or two lighter than the skin tone can be used for light under-eye coverage instead of concealer.

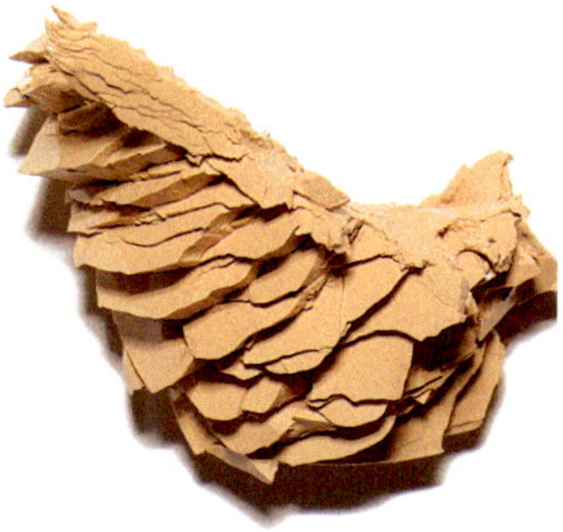

Tip

For those with combination skin, foundations are now available with both silica beads, which soak up oil, and lecithin, which hydrates skin. Moisturizers and oil-control lotions can be applied to parts of the face that need it to counterbalance the foundation choice.

Tools

The right tools help you apply foundation quickly and easily, with great-looking results. Sponges, also called makeup wedges, are used with foundation. Makeup can be applied directly to the sponge or face and gently blended into the skin. Some prefer to use a foundation brush. The synthetic bristles of this brush type can be used with all foundation formulas for a smooth and even application. Fingers are the best tool for warming and blending makeup into the skin.

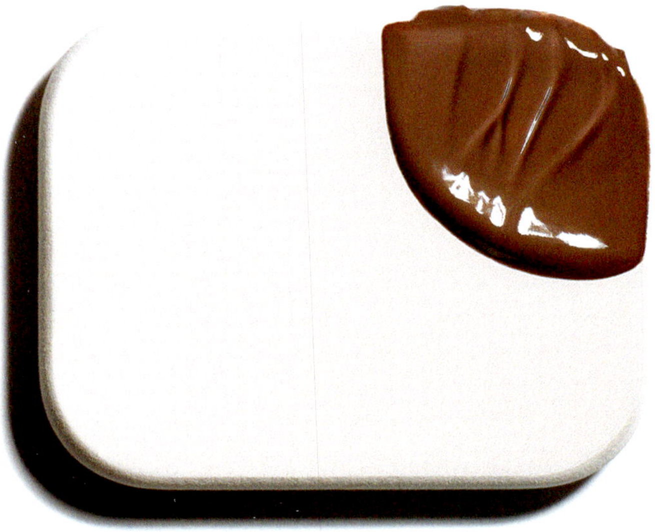

Tips

While sponges are a convenient and sanitary way to apply makeup, they can't replicate the direct control and warmth of using the fingers and hands. You can use the hands to warm a product before application. Foundation, concealer, lip color, and even pencils spread more easily on the skin if they are at body temperature. Use the fingers to apply makeup for complete control over placement of the product. Always thoroughly clean the hands and nails before applying makeup.

To see the true effect of the foundation, let it settle for a few minutes. Then blend or layer in more foundation in spots where it is needed.

FOUNDATION APPLICATION

To get the even-toned, great-looking skin you want, you need to choose the right color, texture, tools, and formulas. Always begin with a test to choose the color that's the closest match to your natural skin tone, and then follow the simple steps for proper application.

Troubleshooting: Foundation

Wrong color
Add a layer of darker foundation or darker powder bronzer or face powder to balance the face color. Select the tone properly. Sometimes the skin needs yellow, red, orange, or blue. The face color should match that of the body.

Color doesn't match neck
Instead of lightening the face, darken the neck with warm bronzer.

Face has a lot of redness
Use a sheer coat of foundation, making sure the skin tone can be seen through it. Use bronzer lightly on the face, neck, and chest to blend.

Orange-peel texture coming through
First try a light moisturizer on your palms to warm it up. Then press it into the skin. Layer with more foundation. If this doesn't work, take the foundation off. Greatly hydrate the skin. Wait two minutes and change the foundation formula to work with the skin.

Pasty-looking skin
The color is too light. Check the color following the tips below.

Yellow-looking skin
The color is too dark. Recheck the color on the forehead and cheek. Switch to another color and correct with bronzer. Some women need to use two shades on different parts of the face during different times of the year.

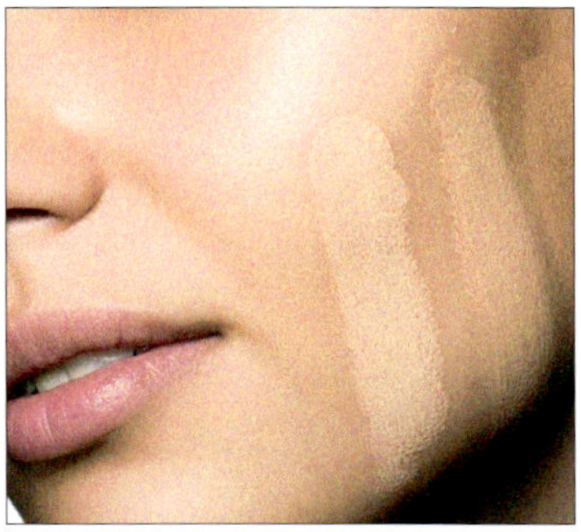

1
Swipe each shade to choose a color. Gently blend into skin. The correct color will look like your natural skin tone.

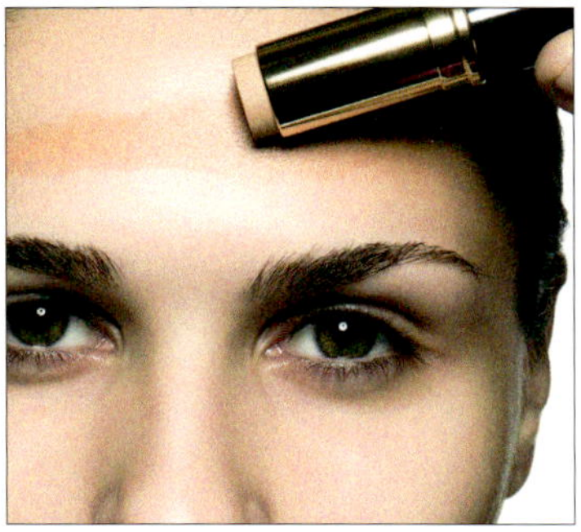

2
Check the color to be sure it matches the forehead.

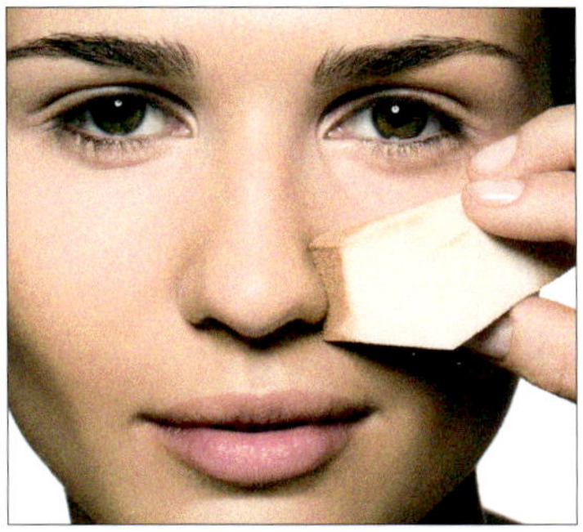

3
Begin applying a small amount of foundation around the nose.

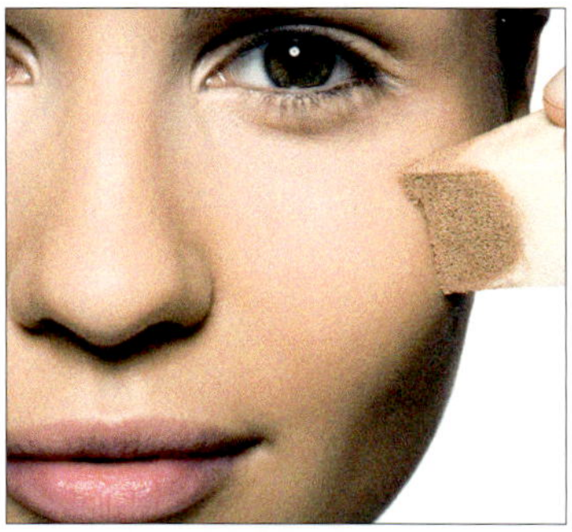

4
Blend the foundation upward into the hairline. Apply foundation all over or only to the parts that need it. Use your fingers to press the foundation into the skin to fully blend.

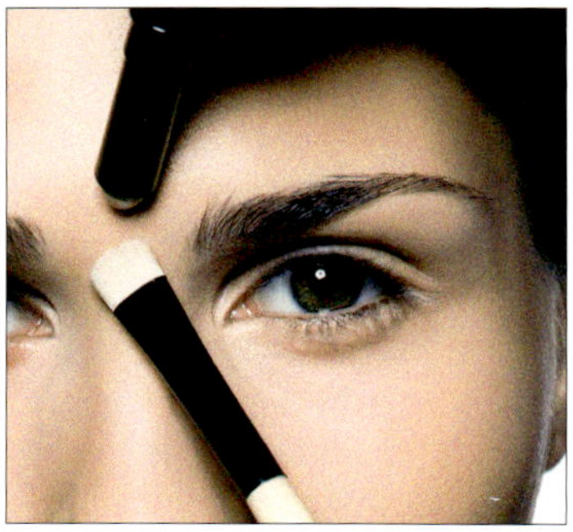

5
Use a blemish stick after the foundation to cover red spots or blemishes.

THE BEAUTY OF DIVERSITY

Through my work as a makeup artist I've had the good fortune to travel around the world and meet women of diverse backgrounds. Through these travels I've learned that women of all ethnicities—from Asian to Middle Eastern and Latina—want the same thing when it comes to their skin. They want their skin to look smooth, even, and flawless. Each ethnicity has its own unique (and beautiful) traits and I believe in using makeup that enhances, rather than masks, these traits.

Asian Skin

"Isn't yellow foundation going to make my skin look more yellow?" is a question that I often hear from my Asian customers when I recommend foundations with yellow undertones. I've experimented with countless foundations over the years and I've found that yellow-toned foundations always look the most natural—especially on Asian skins.

Many Asian women are prone to and concerned about sunspots, which are the result of sun damage. Aside from wearing sun protection every day, the best way to deal with sunspots is with corrective peach- and pink-toned concealers. Some women have skin with yellow undertones and yellow surface tones. For them, I suggest covering the sunspots with a medium-toned peach corrector. If the concealer is too light in tone it will look gray on the sunspot, so you may have to try a few different tones to find the right one. Other women have skin with yellow undertones and pink surface tones (often the result of skin irritation due to using bleaching agents). The best way to cover their sunspots is with a medium-toned pink bisque corrector. As I mentioned earlier, you'll know the concealer is too light if it turns ashy when it's applied on the sunspot. After applying the corrector, gently smooth on a yellow-toned foundation in a shade that matches your skin perfectly.

Black Skin

There are many variations in skin tone among black women, so consider the following advice as general guidelines rather than hard and fast rules. Black skin tends to be darker across the forehead and perimeter of the face, and lighter on the middle parts of the face, including the cheeks. The trick when applying foundation is to create a seamless look between the light/golden and dark/warmer parts of the face. Some women like enhancing the golden tones in their skin, and other women like playing up the warmer tones in their skin. It's a matter of personal preference and it's important—whether you are doing your own makeup or you

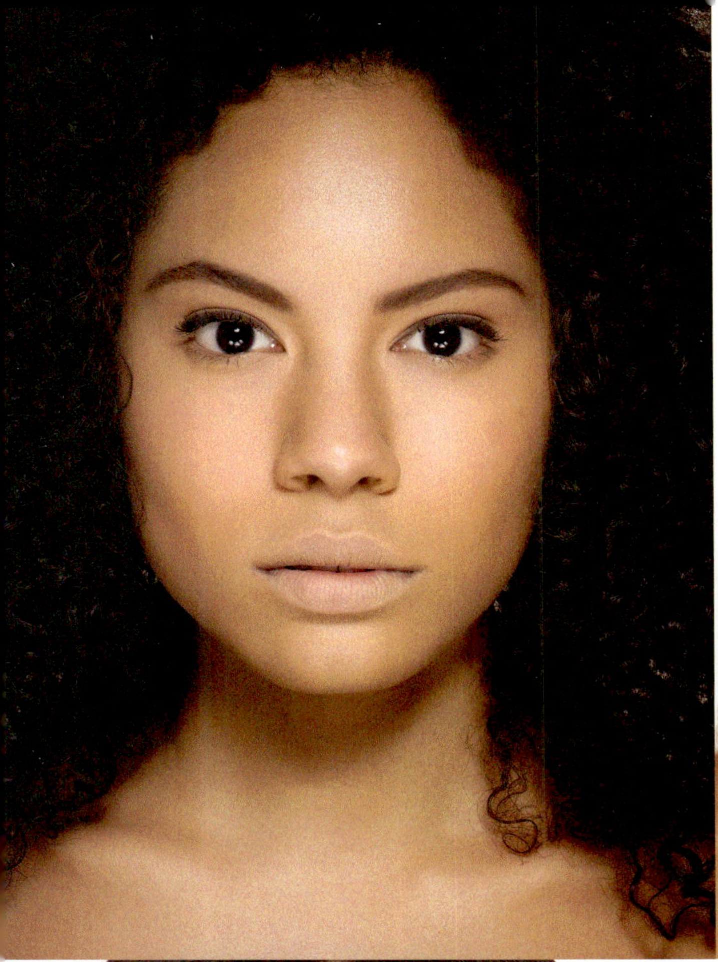
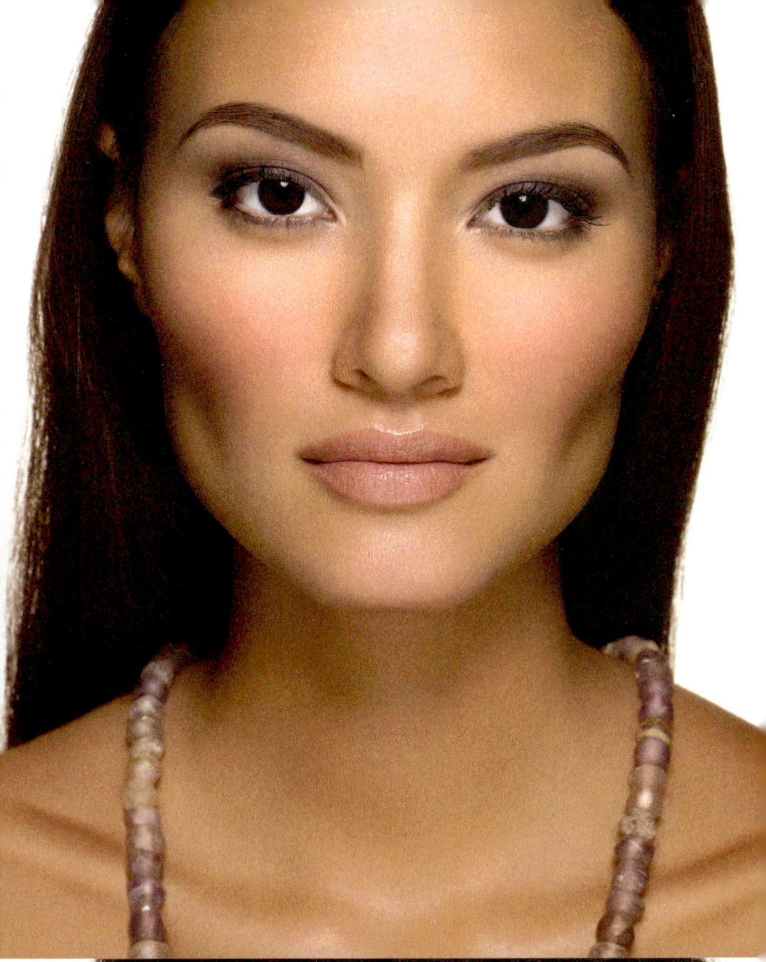
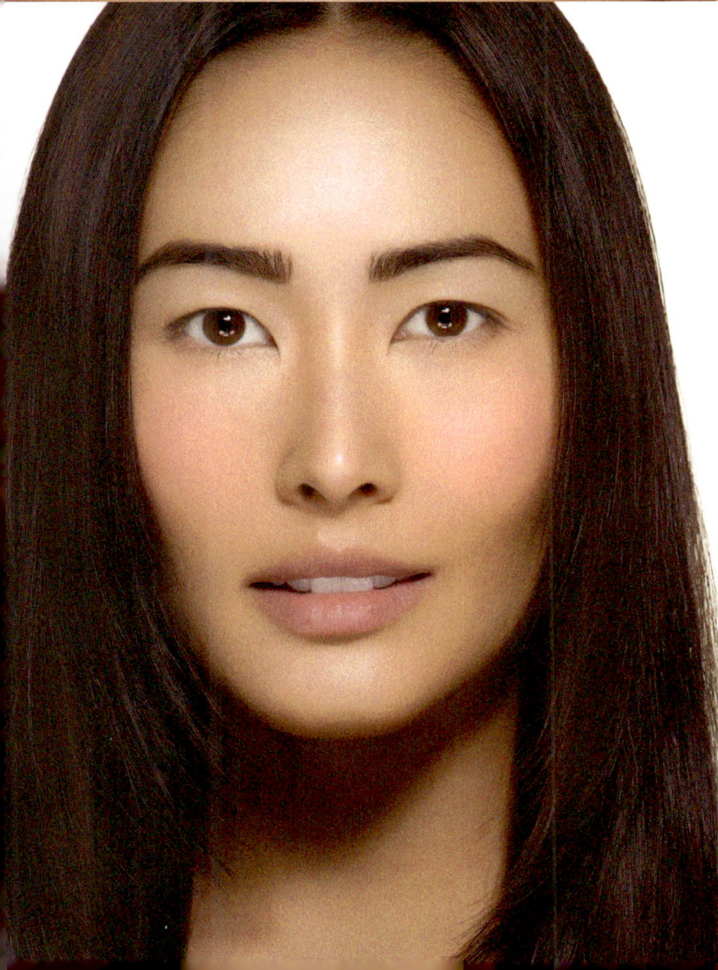
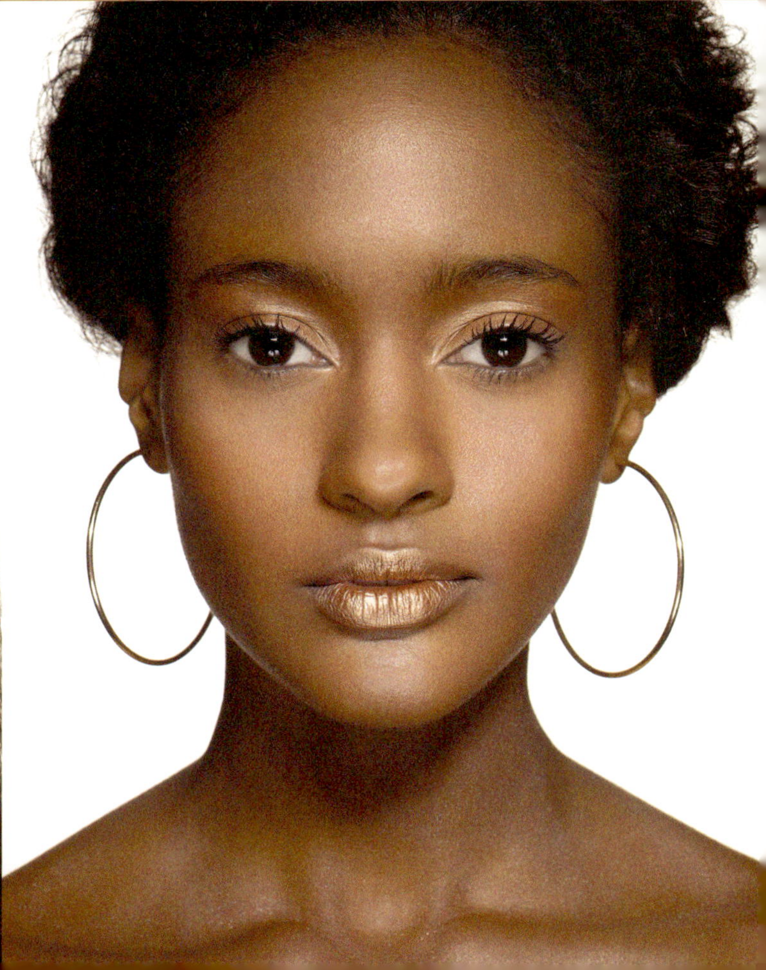

are a makeup artist working with a customer—to know which tones you're going to focus on.

If you want to go golden, choose a tinted moisturizer or sheer foundation that matches the skin on the center of your face. Apply the tinted moisturizer/sheer foundation just on this area, then use a coppery bronzer on the other parts of the face to diffuse the transition between the lighter and darker areas.

If you want to go warm, choose a tinted moisturizer or sheer foundation in a shade that falls between the lighter and darker parts of the face. Applying a dark shade of foundation all over the face will look unnatural so the idea here is to tone down the difference between the light and dark areas. Look for a yellow-based foundation that has a bit of orange, red, or blue to it, depending on how deep the color of the skin is. Lighter black skin looks most natural with yellow-based foundation that has a touch of golden orange. Very dark skin looks best with yellow-based foundation that has warm cinnamon tones. In all instances, if the foundation looks ashy or gray on the skin, it's not the right shade.

Latin Skin

Latin women generally have golden skin with olive undertones. Some women have pink surface tones (around the nose and mouth, and on the cheeks) due to skin irritation and sensitivity. Latin skin tans very easily, turning a golden cinnamon during summer months. Alternately, in the winter months, skin tends to take on a yellow-green cast.

Bronzer is a great year-round beauty staple for Latin skin because it can be used in the summer to add warmth to your foundation, and in the winter to counteract sallow coloring. Latinas range in coloring from fair to dark so one shade of bronzer does not fit all. If you are fair, choose a bronzer that has pinky-red tones to it. If you are darker, choose a brownish-red bronzer. When shopping for foundation, look for a yellow-based golden shade to complement the natural tones in your skin. Be careful not to go too golden with your foundation, however, because skin will start to look orange.

Middle Eastern Skin

Middle Eastern skin is very similar to Latin skin in that it is golden with olive undertones. Many women complain of extreme darkness under the eyes. The best way to cover their purplish-green and brownish-green under-eye circles is with corrective peach- and pink-toned concealers. If you have golden surface tones, use a peach-toned concealer one shade lighter than your foundation to cover your dark circles. If you have pink surface tones (due to sensitivity), start with a peach-toned concealer to cancel out the darkness, then layer on a pink-toned concealer to brighten the under-eye area and make it similar in tone to the rest of the face. In most instances this combination of concealers will offer enough coverage. If you still see under-eye darkness, you may have to layer on a third concealer—a yellow-toned one in a skin-tone-correct shade

Multiethnic Skin

Many beautiful mixed-race women need to be open and observant about what makeup looks natural. Basic rules apply, but sometimes these women need multiple products or bronzers as mix-ins to make foundation look great.

MULTICOLOR FOUNDATION & POWDER APPLICATION

Some dark skins need two colors of foundation and two powders to create the perfect foundation to even out skin tone.

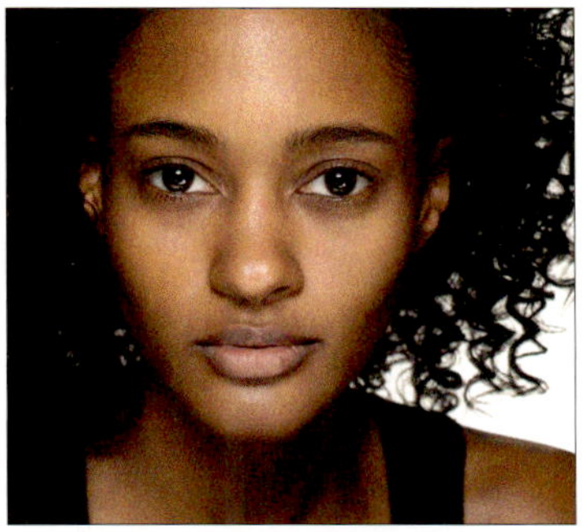

1

Check if forehead is darker than the rest of the face.

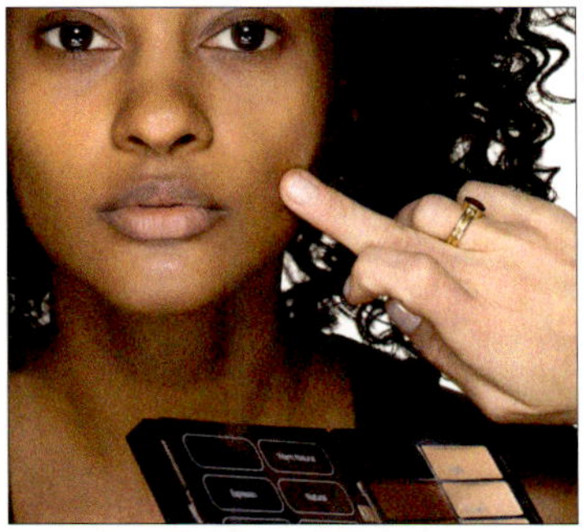

2

Check the side of the face as well as the forehead.

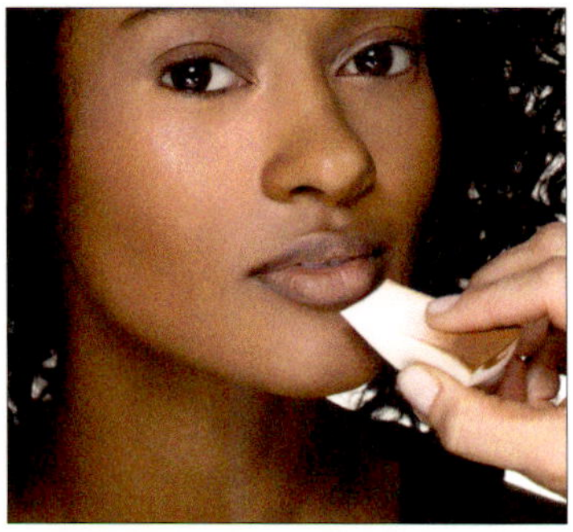

3

Apply lightest foundation color around the mouth.

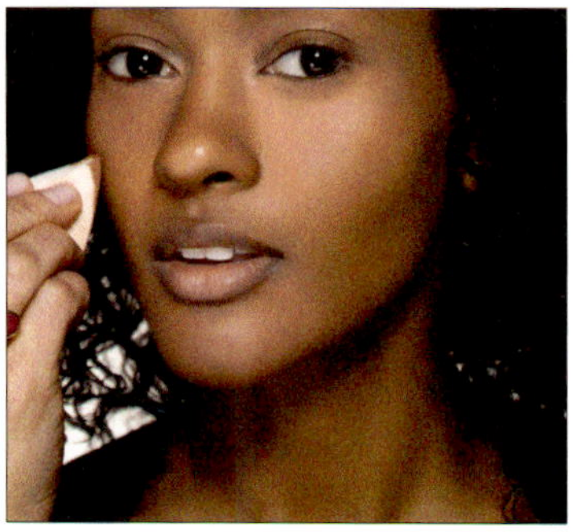

4

Use lighter color or mix light and dark foundation for cheeks.

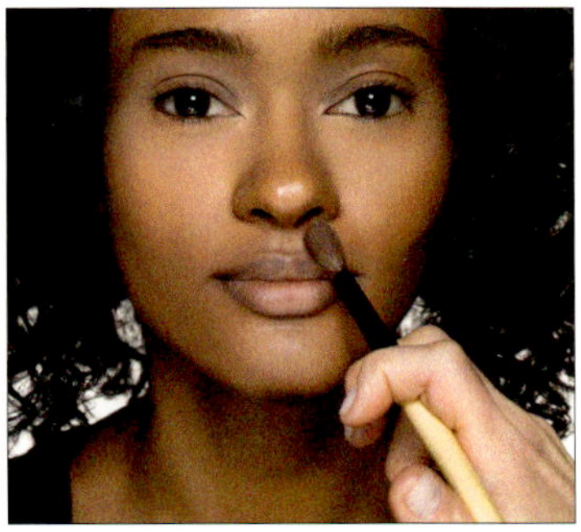

5

Apply warm-color face powder all over the face to set the foundation.

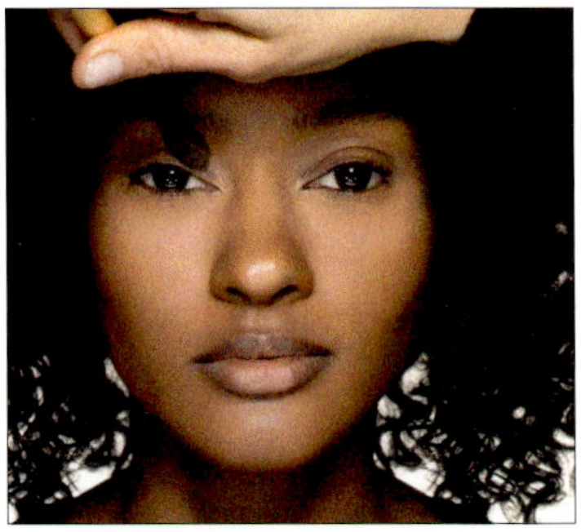

6

Apply yellow powder on lids.

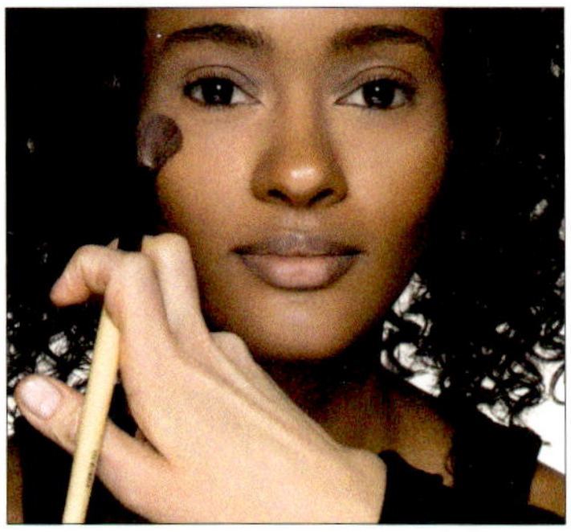

7

Apply yellow powder over concealer.

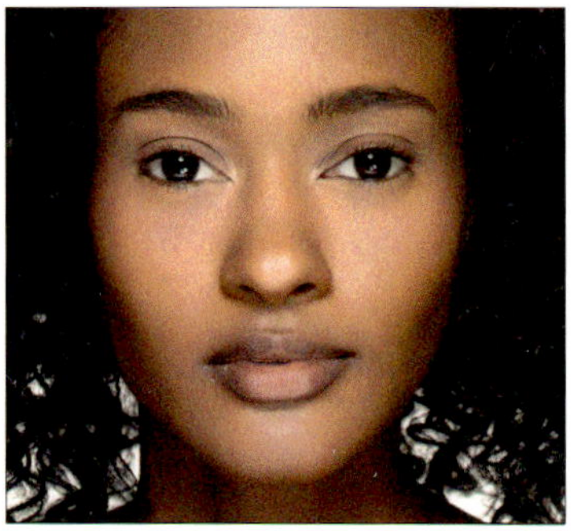

8

The end result is skin that is even and one tone.

SPECIAL SKIN CONDITIONS

Some faces need more than the basic application of foundation to look fresh and flawless. Others do best with the thinnest layer of expertly blended foundation. In special cases, you will need a skillful hand and specific application techniques. The best makeup artists recognize skin conditions, treat them appropriately, and use the perfect combination of product and technique to make the skin look its best. These product suggestions and techniques for various special skin conditions are basic guidelines. The trick is knowing when the makeup is working and when it needs to be changed. Experimentation is usually needed to achieve the desired results.

ROSACEA

A sheer, tinted moisturizer will diffuse redness. Too dense a product can make the face look masklike. Correct with a bronzer.

COMBINATION SKIN

Use moisturizer on areas of dry skin and an oil-absorbing lotion on the T-zone. Use an oil-free foundation all over the face during the summer, consider a more moisturizing formula for the winter. Either formulation can be used on specific areas of the face as needed.

EXTREMELY DRY SKIN

Use rich moisturizer followed by a creamy, moisturizing foundation. Don't use powder. Balm or oil can be applied lightly on top of foundation.

BLEMISHES

Using a concealer brush, apply oil-free cover stick or foundation to the blemish. Try to match the skin tone exactly. Concealers, which are a shade or two lighter than the face, should not be used on blemishes. Pat the area lightly. Do not rub. Blend into a small area directly around the blemish. Powder to lock the product(s) in place. Continue with foundation.

HYPERPIGMENTATION (IN GENERAL)

Apply a foundation tone or spot concealer a shade lighter than the skin to the affected area with a small brush. A bronzing gel can be blended into the skin starting at the cheek area, working around the face. This will help blend the more pigmented skin. Layer foundation that matches your skin tone over the concealer and/or gel for a flawless finish. Experiment, as concealer alone is often too light and will highlight the spot rather than cover it effectively. Set foundation with powder.

BIRTHMARKS AND PORT-WINE STAINS

Several layers of concealer are needed to cover areas with very dark pigmentation. First, apply a pale yellow-toned foundation or concealer that is three to five shades lighter than the skin tone. Then, apply one that is only slightly lighter than the overall skin tone. Finally, apply a full-coverage foundation that matches the skin tone. Set with powder. Again, experiment to find the right tone and formulations to effectively cover very dark spots.

SCARS AND TATTOOS

It may not be possible to cover scars and tattoos completely. If stick foundation or cover stick does not cover them, try using Covermark, a heavy-duty concealer designed for tattoos and scars. Apply foundation that matches skin tone to the whole face, and set with a powder that matches the skin tone.

UNEVEN SKIN

Skin is sometimes darker through the forehead or through the area of the lower mouth. Two different tones of foundation can be used to match each of the skin tones. Blend well to create an even transition between tones. Bronzer can be used over foundation to even out skin tone. A gel bronzer applied to moisturized skin prior to foundation evens the skin as well. Foundation can then be applied where needed.

FRECKLES

Rather than using a heavy foundation to conceal freckles, let them show through. Use a tinted moisturizer that evens out skin tone, and consider using a bronzer to finish.

ACNE

Start with the right skincare regimen, and use oil-free moisturizers. Apply blemish cover stick with a small, clean brush, or spot conceal with an opaque foundation only in those areas where needed. Use a tinted moisturizer or lightweight liquid foundation to even out the skin tone. The trick is to blend away the discoloration without applying heavy coverage.

WRINKLES

Hydration is the key to creating smooth-looking skin. Exfoliate regularly with a gentle scrub or an alpha hydroxy acid cream. Use water-infused hydrating ultrarich moisturizers and creamy makeup formulas. For lines around the lips, use a lip balm. Choose a creamy lipstick and matching pencil to prevent feathering.

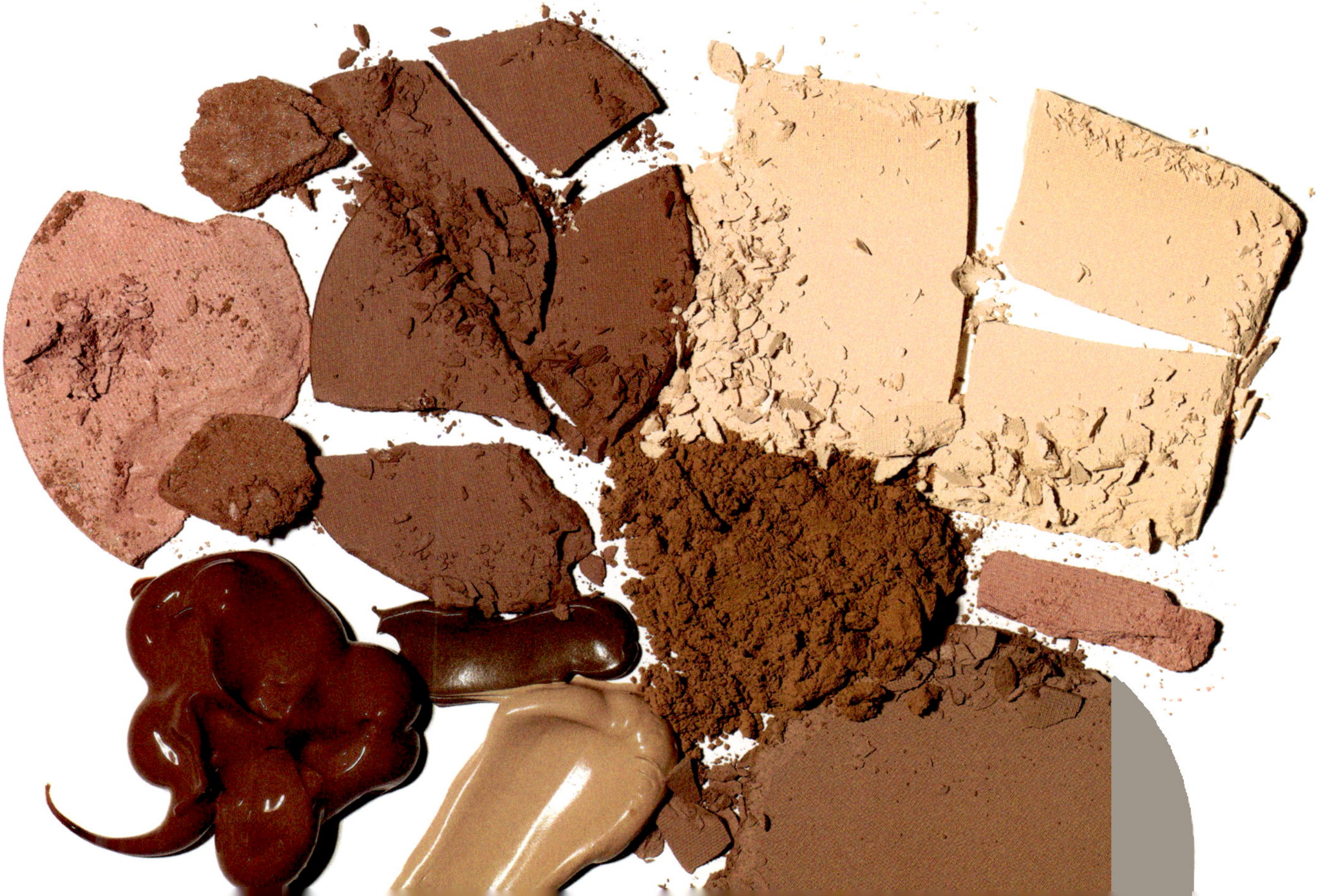

POWDER

A light dusting of powder sets concealer and foundation for hours, keeping the skin looking fresh.

Choosing the Right Powder

Color

Like foundation, powder works only when it is the right shade. For most people, the right powder has a yellow undertone. While the color of the powder will vary to match the foundation, it is the yellow-toned base that will give warmth to the skin. White powder is right only for those with alabaster skin. Translucent powder is not invisible or transparent and only makes skin look ashy.

Texture

Pressed powder is best for touch-ups. It dispenses a small amount and comes in a convenient compact. It is great for those who like a very natural look. Loose powder is denser and provides more coverage. Depending on the application technique, loose powder can be matte or sheer. Not everyone needs powder. Those with very dry skin might use powder only to set under-eye concealer.

Tools

The right tools will supply the perfect amount of powder. Using a powder puff will give powder a smooth, opaque finish. A powder brush will allow a sheer finish. A clean powder brush is also used to remove excess powder after an application with a powder puff. A small concealer brush can be used to apply powder to the corners of the face—under and around the eyes and around the mouth and nose.

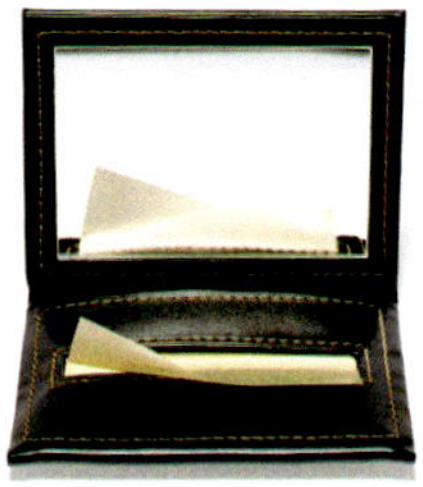

Tip

Oily skin can turn powder yellow or orange with time. Sometimes you have to choose a lighter color.

To avoid powder buildup on oily skin, use an oil-blotting paper before touching up.

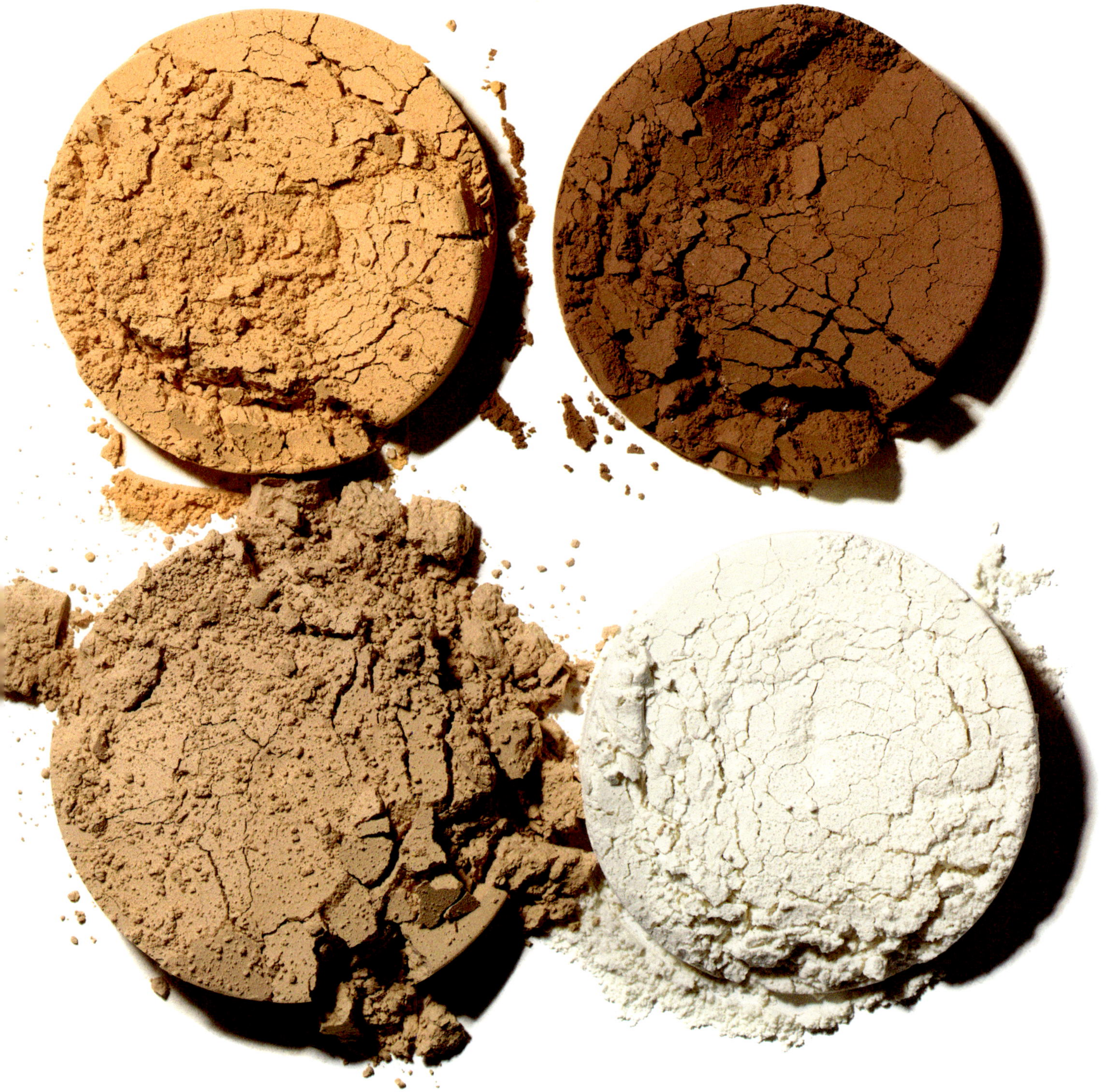

FACE POWDER APPLICATION

Some people with very dry skin can skip putting powder on the face. But everyone needs powder over concealer.

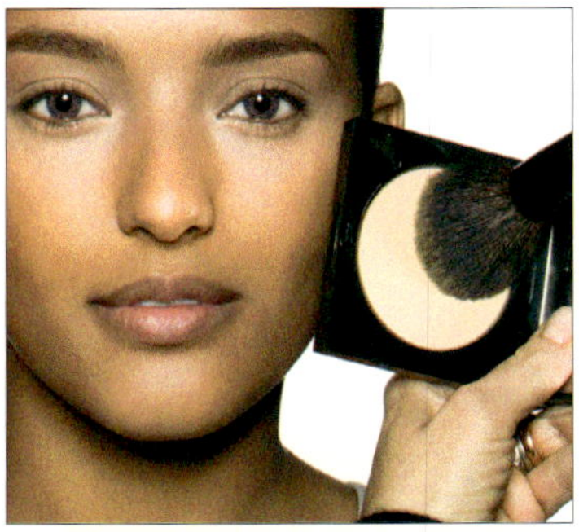

1

Choose the color according to the directions on page 66.

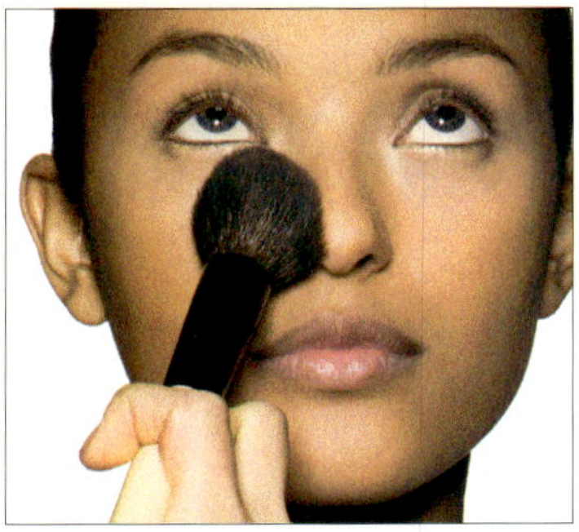

2

Apply powder with either a brush or a fluffy powder puff.

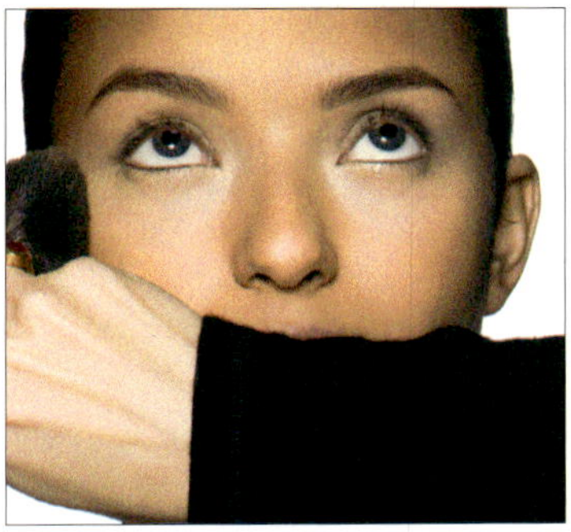

3

Dust the powder across the cheek and forehead.

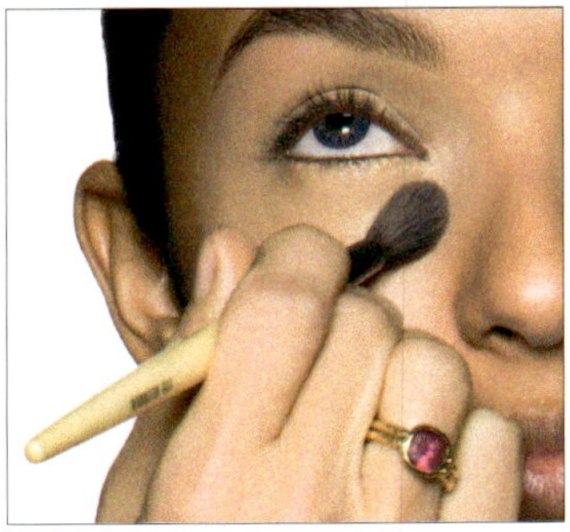

4

Switch brushes to apply powder on top of the concealer. This powder is often lighter in color than the face powder.

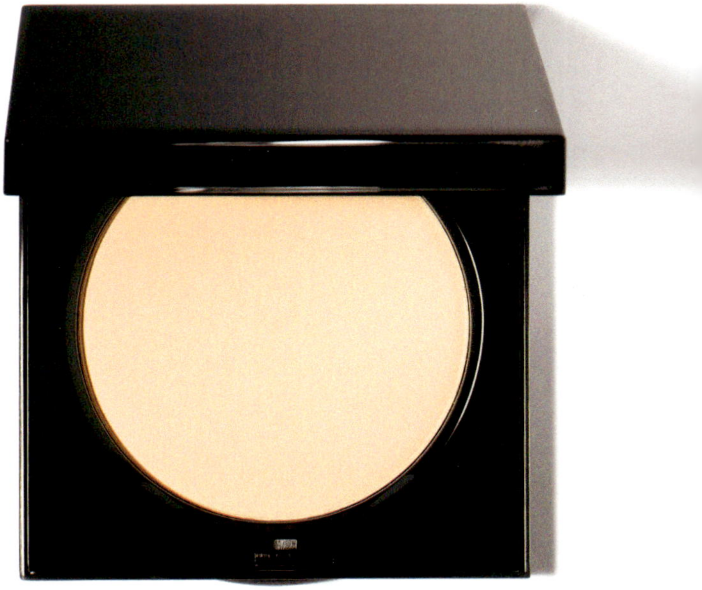

Troubleshooting: Powder

After an application of concealer, foundation, and powder step back and observe what you have done. Do the products blend seamlessly and invisibly into the skin? Do you see any darkness or redness? Do *not* continue with any other makeup until the skin looks the best it can. If you need to improve how the skin looks, stop and look. Can it be corrected with a bronzing product? Or should you begin again using a different product?

Ashy
Warm up the powder color and/or add bronzer.

Orange
Is the skin oily? Did it change? Switch to paler powder and wait to check the results.

Flaky
The skin is too dry.

Cakey
Make sure you have enough moisturizer on the skin. It's also possible to have too much. The foundation-to-moisturizer ratio may be giving the powder too much grab.

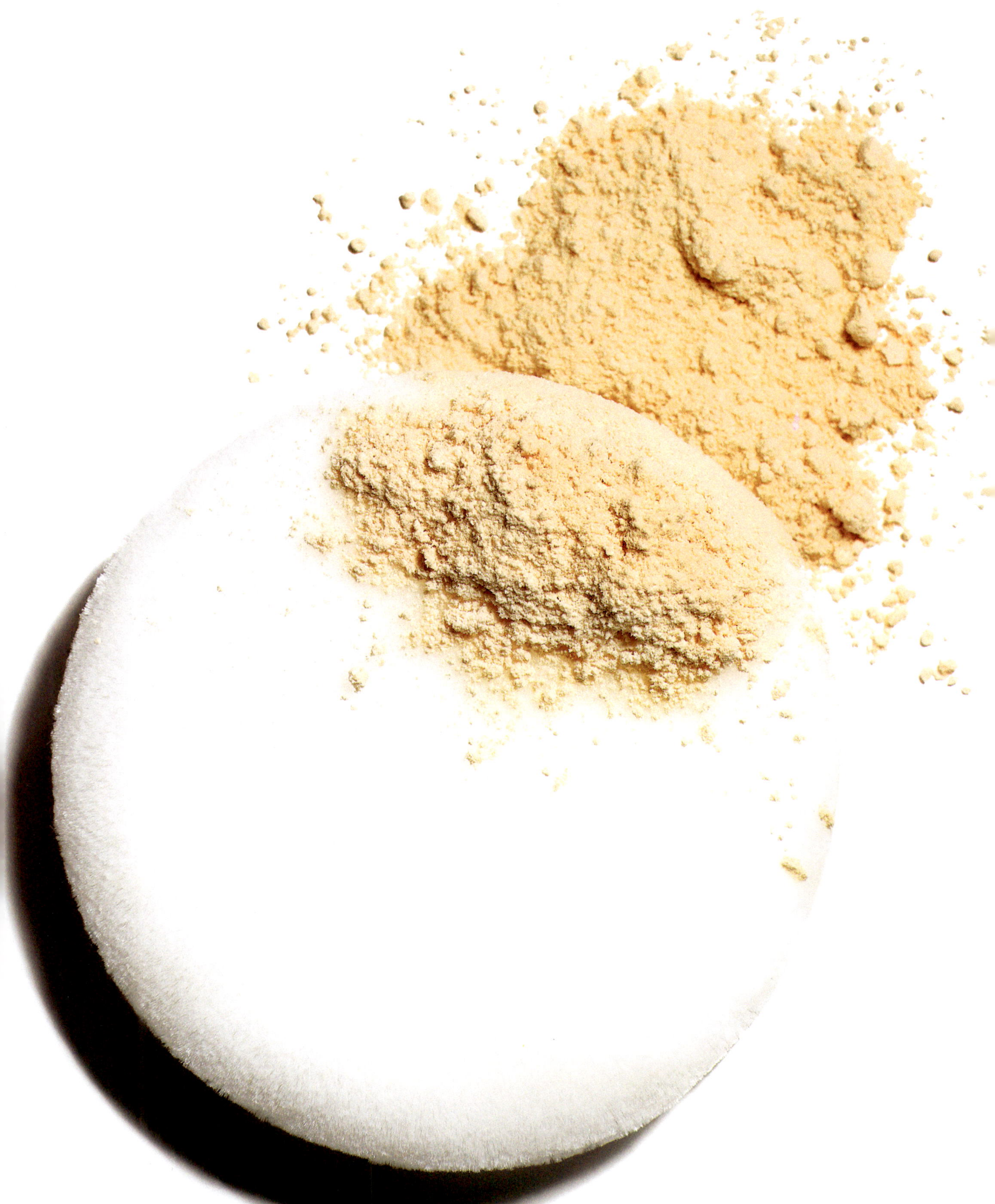

BRONZER & SELF-TANNER

Bronzers and self-tanners imitate the healthy look of the sun. They are also used as correctors to warm up the complexion. Applying bronzer is a great way to add a healthy glow all over the face and to even out color differences, especially through the neck. Bronzers work on all skin tones except porcelain because bronzer can make porcelain skin look dirty. Self-tanners can be used on the face and body to add color and hide flaws. When used on the face, apply self-tanner several hours before applying makeup, and don't forget your neck and ears (and remember to wash your palms with soap and water). Bronzer works as a blush for very dark skin. On all other skin tones, blush should be used over bronzer to add a pop of bright color.

Color: How to Choose

Bronzers work best when the skin looks natural. They can be brown-, red-, blue-, orange-, and sometimes yellow-based.

ALABASTER SKIN (Gwyneth Paltrow skin color)
Pinky shimmer or peach

LIGHT (Drew Barrymore)
Beigy brown with a bit of pink

MEDIUM (Sienna Miller)
Browny pink with only a bit of orange for warmth

MEDIUM-DARK (Jennifer Lopez)
Brownish orange

DARK (Vanessa Williams)
Brownish red

DEEPEST (Venus Williams)
Brownish blue

Formulas

Bronzers are available in flat or shimmering powder, gel stick, and cream formulas. Self-tanners are available in cream, gel, and spray, and are often mixed with moisturizer to get the best results.

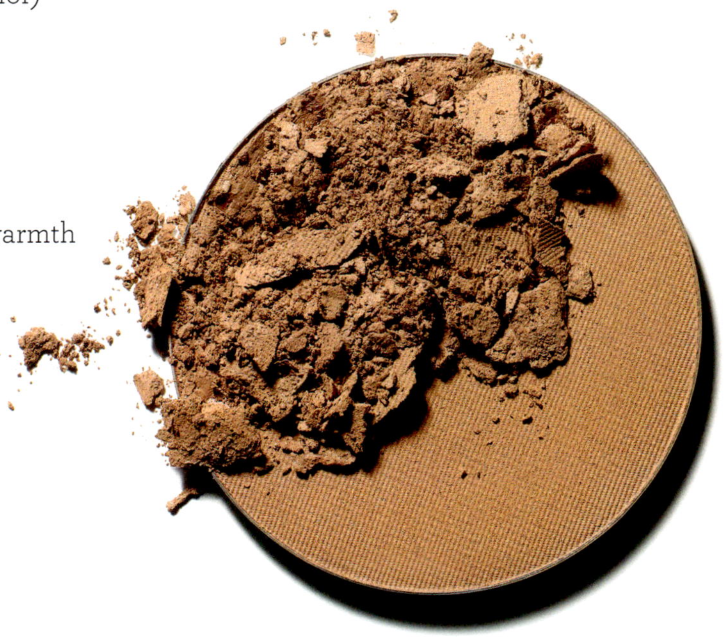

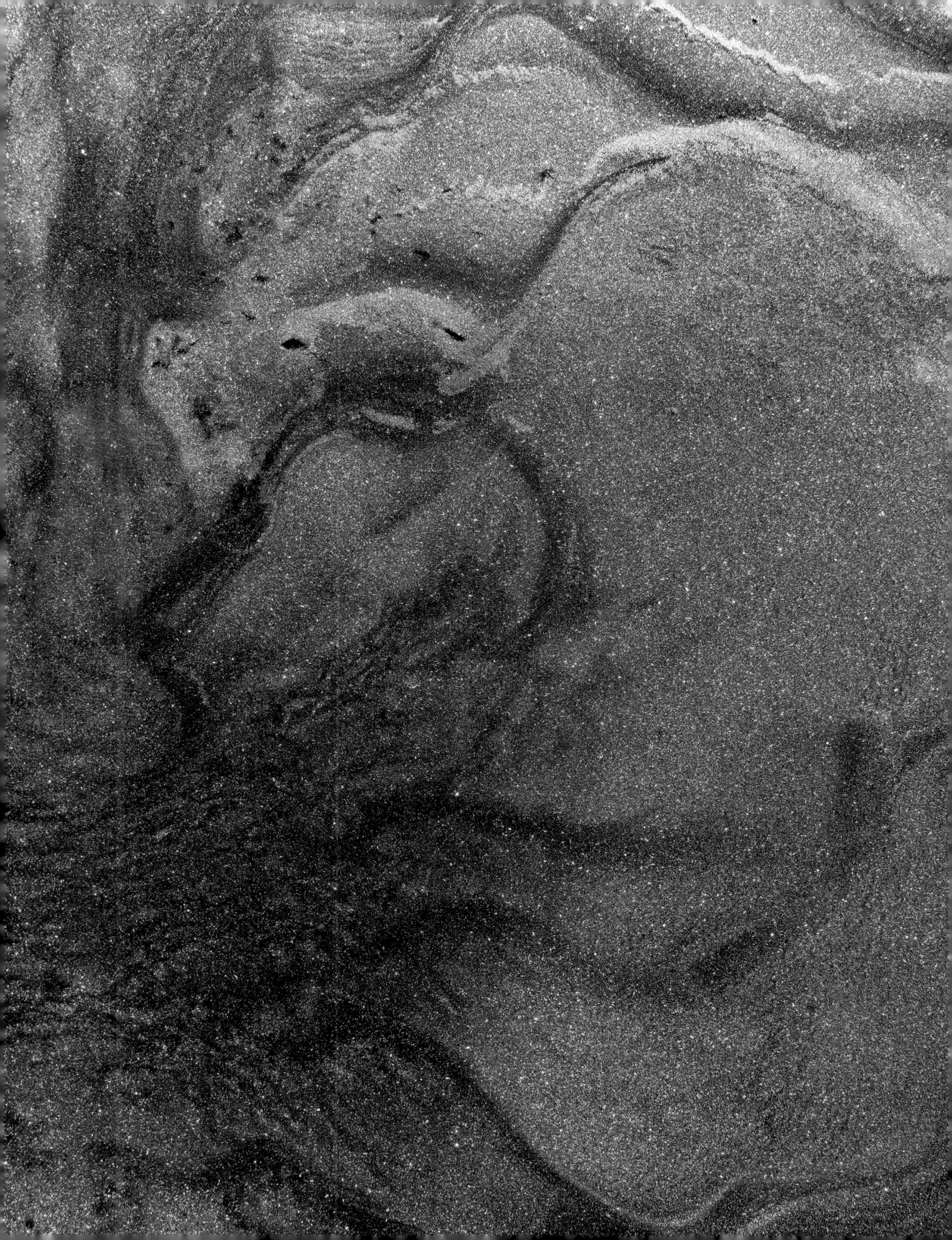

POWDER BRONZER APPLICATION

Powder bronzer is the easiest to apply. I use it to add a tint of color to the skin and to correct light foundation or red skin.

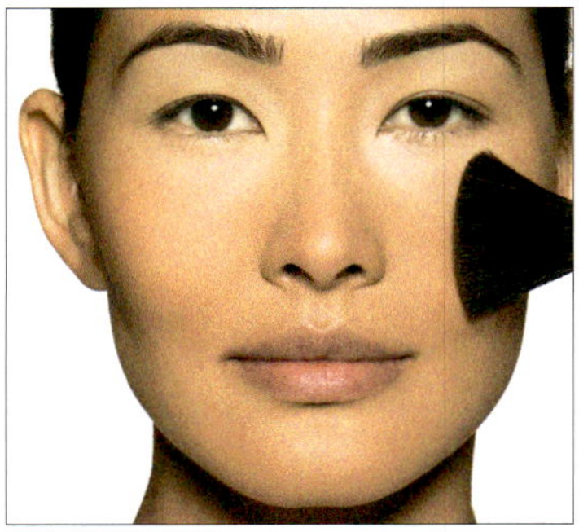

1

Using a large, flat brush, apply a small amount of bronzer for even distribution. Start on the apples of the cheeks.

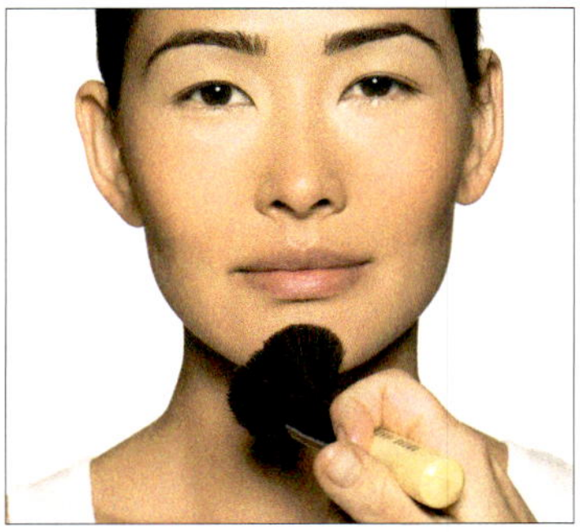

2

Next, dust over the nose and chin.

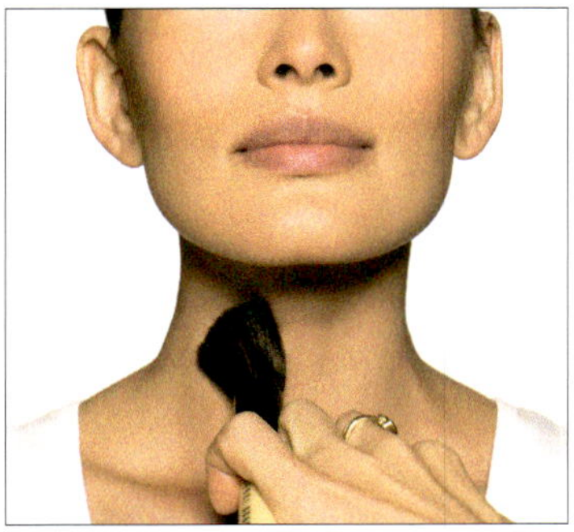

3

Brush bronzer onto the neck area.

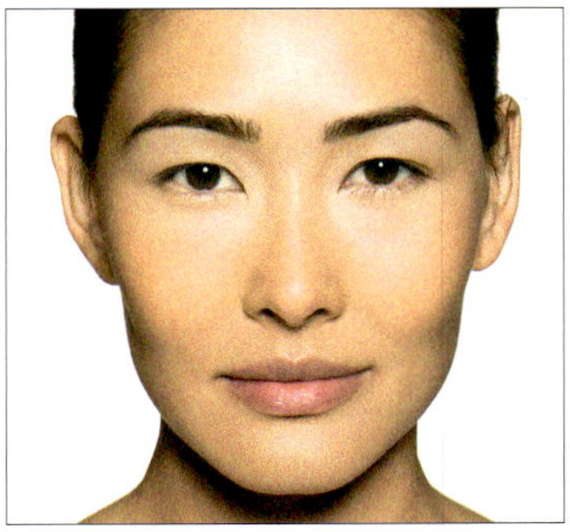

4

Turn the face to either side to make sure the color is well blended.

GEL BRONZER APPLICATION

This formula is sheer and can correct foundation if necessary, but it is a bit harder to blend than others. It works well on men.

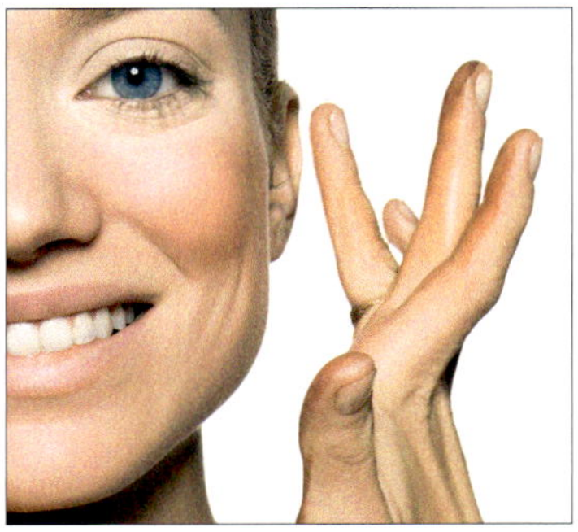

1

Choose the color to enhance your natural shade.

Begin at the apple of your cheeks.

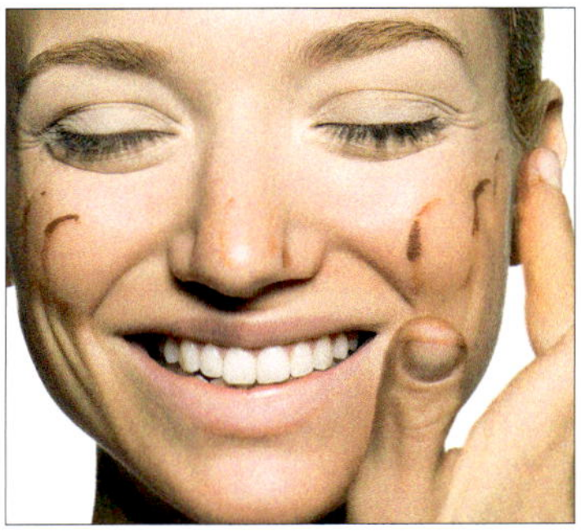

2

Gently apply bronzer to the cheeks, forehead, nose, and chin. Apply lightly. You can always add more.

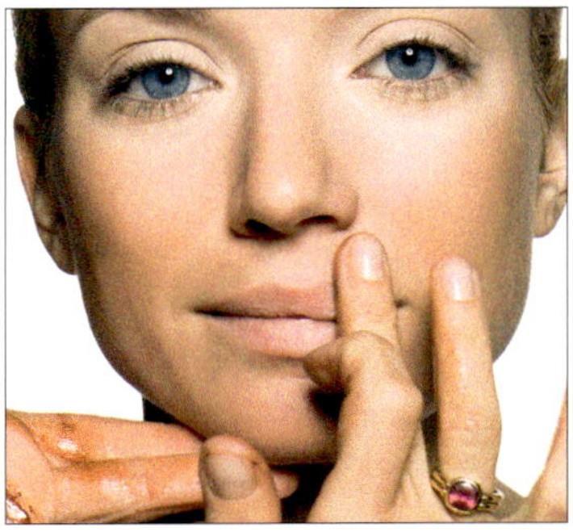

3

Apply bronzer lightly to the areas around the lips, forehead, neck, and ears.

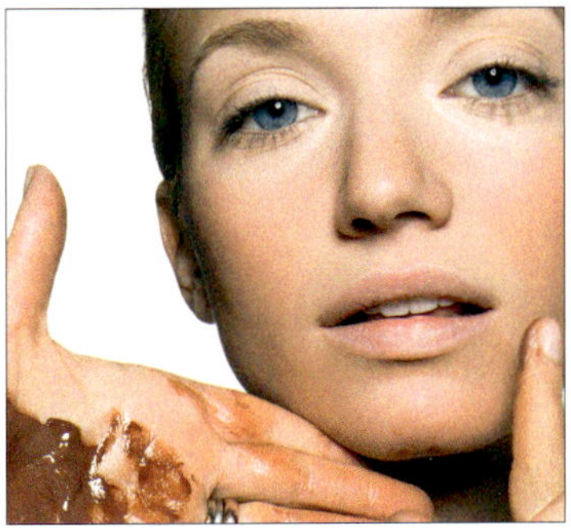

4

Blend with a clean hand. Add more bronzer if necessary.

Tip

Bronzers as Correctors
Some women have more color on their face and chest and less on their neck. Use bronzer to warm up the paler skin on the neck. For those with very red areas, sunspots, or rosacea, bronzers can be used to even out the skin tone.

Self-Tanner

Use self-tanners to add color to any area of the body including the face. It's an easy way to mask cellulite and veins on the legs. On the face, self-tanner can brighten up a tired complexion. It can be difficult to decide which product to use so it's important to test in a hidden spot before applying all over.

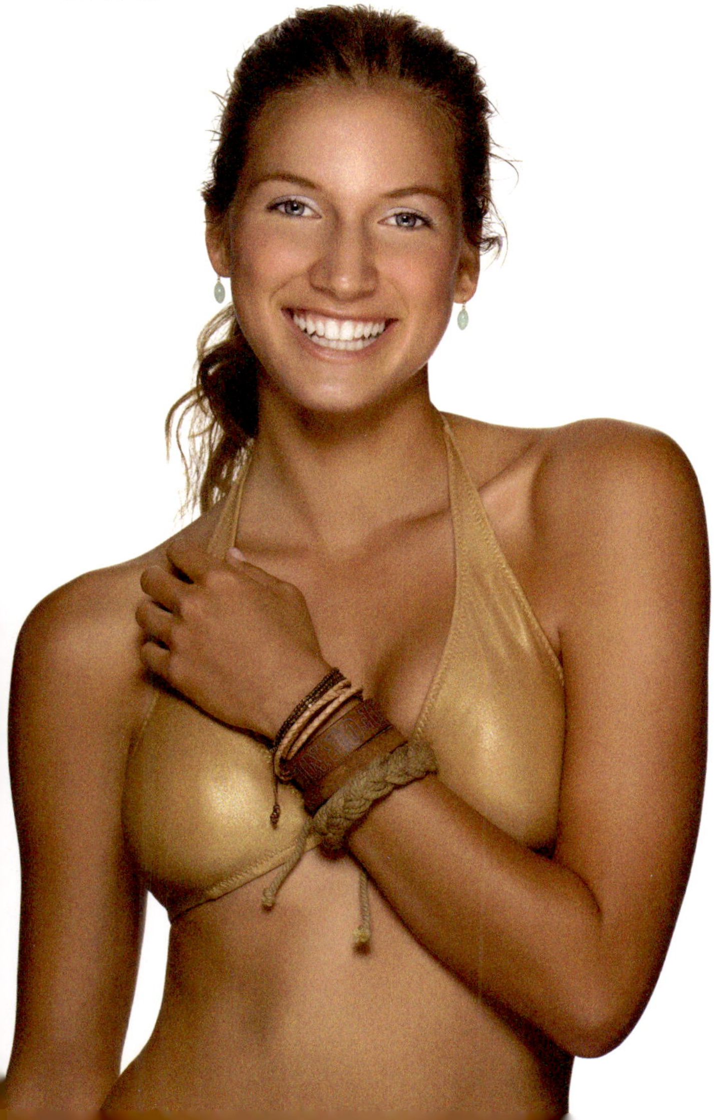

Self-Tanner Application

Prepare the skin. Always apply self-tanner to clean, smooth, makeup-free skin. It is best to exfoliate first if there are any rough patches. Knees, elbows, and heels are often areas with coarse, dry skin.

Apply a light, even layer. Wait for the color to develop, and then apply a light second coat for a deeper tan. It is easier to build color than to fix mistakes.

Do not forget to apply the product to the neck and ears for a natural-looking result.

Wash your hands immediately after using self-tanner. The product will stain palms and the skin between the fingers.

Wait ten minutes after applying self-tanner to the face before applying any other makeup or getting dressed.

Most self-tanners take an hour or more to develop into a "tan," so plan ahead.

Troubleshooting: Dark or Streaky Self-Tanning Results

Fade overly dark color by exfoliating the skin in the shower with a washcloth or loofah. Then, thoroughly clean the skin with cold cream or baby oil. Some self-tanners can be removed with lemon juice. Fix streaks by applying an additional light coat of self-tanner on the lightest parts of the skin.

BLUSH

Blush is used to create a healthy, pretty look. Blush can also be used to create the dramatic contouring sometimes seen in fashion shows and the theater.

Pick a skin-type-appropriate formula that you find easy to use. Different formulas can be used, depending on the desired finish or time of year. For the most natural look, match the blush color to that of the cheeks when flushed from exercise. You can also pinch the cheeks and look at the tone; match that color. By holding several shades of blush next to the cheek, you will see which add a lift and can eliminate those that are too dull or orange. The right shade will add a pretty brightness to the face without looking obvious.

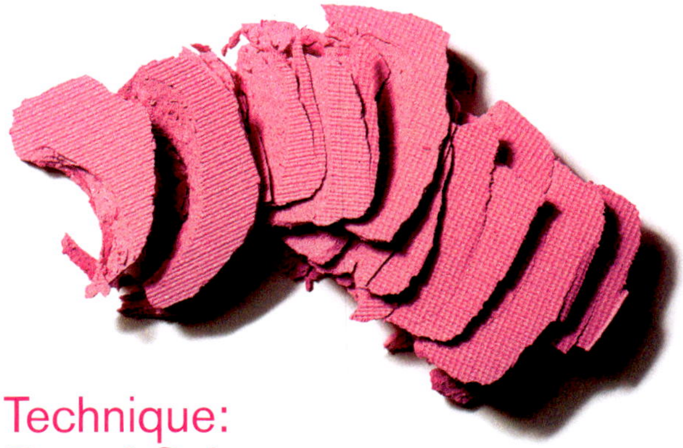

Technique: Pop of Color

Using two shades of blush, apply your natural color and then add a pop of a brighter color on top. The natural shade looks great at first, but often fades easily. The brighter shade alone is often great for evening, but too much of a contrast for every day. This layering technique offers natural brightness. When using a bronzer, skip natural color and layer the pop color on top. Using a natural shade on top of bronzer makes the cheeks look dirty.

Blush Formulas

POWDER is the easiest formula to use. It blends easily and works on all skin types.

GEL delivers sheer color, but blending is a bit more difficult. It works well for smooth skin.

CREAM goes on smoothly and leaves a dewy finish, which is great for dry skin.

CREAM/POWDER goes on as cream and dries to a long-lasting powder finish. It is best for normal skin.

CHUBBY PENCILS are very portable and easy to blend. They are best for normal to dry skin.

CHEEK TINTS are similar to gels. They go on sheer for a stained look and can be difficult to blend. Tints work only for smooth skin.

POT ROUGE provides blendable color for normal to dry skin types. These products are usually creamy in texture and packaged in pots. They provide a sheer stain on the cheeks and medium coverage on the lips.

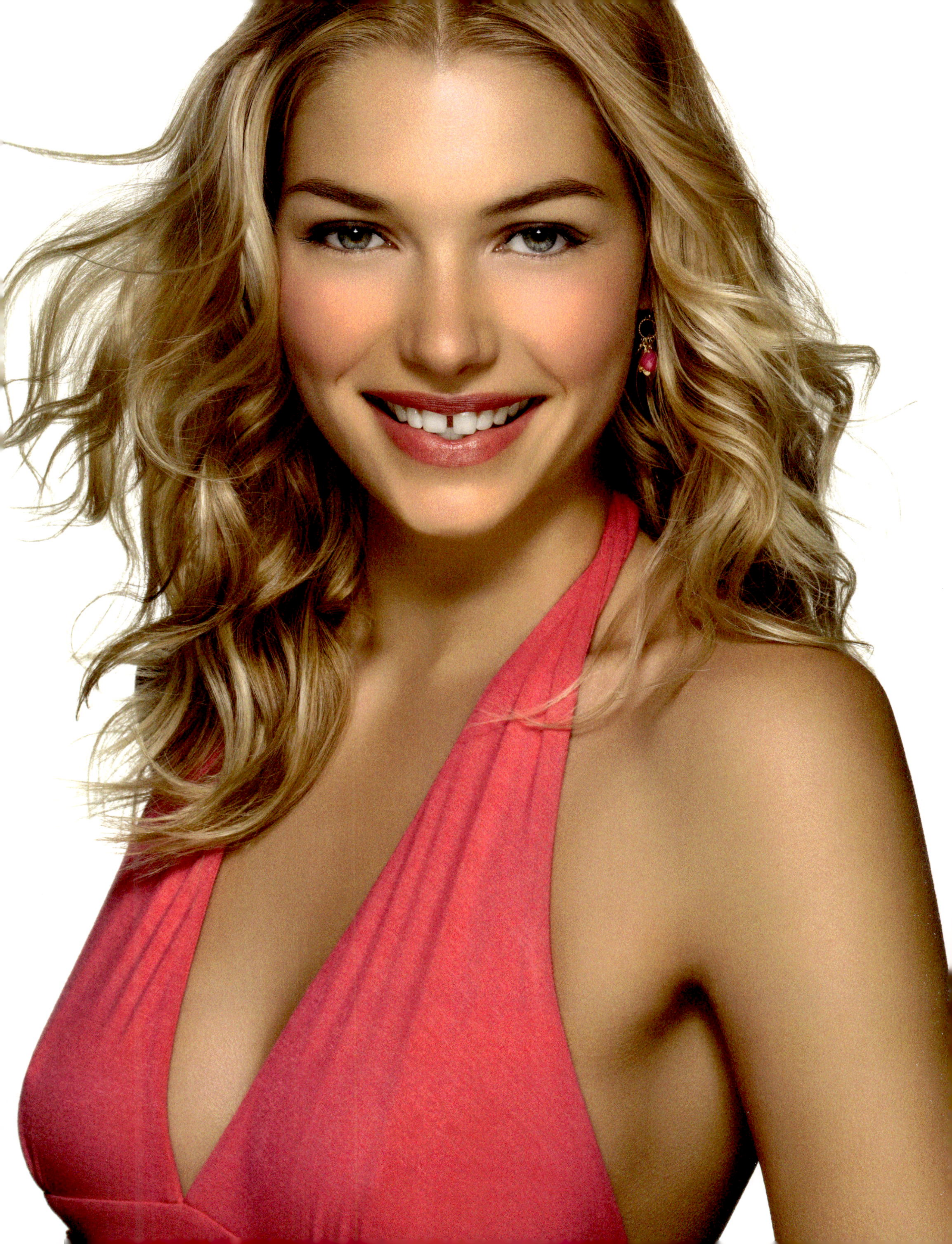

POWDER BLUSH APPLICATION

Powder is the easiest blush formula to use. Make sure your brush is totally clean, or it will affect your color choice.

1 Smile and apply the product to the apple of the cheeks.

2 Blend toward the hairline, then down to soften the edges.

3 Blend thoroughly, keeping the most product on the highest part of the cheekbones.

4 Step back and consider the results. Turn your head to each side. Your face should look absolutely natural and balanced. A powder puff or fingers can be used to soften and correct a heavy application.

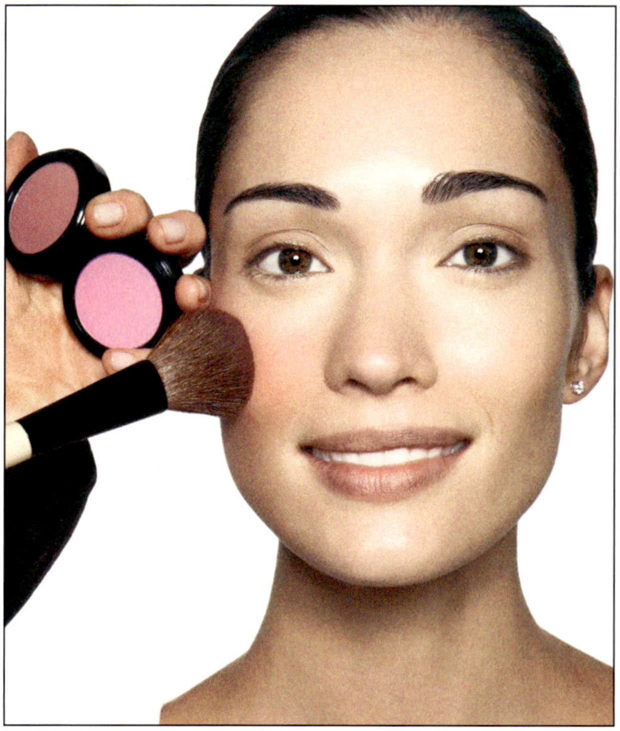

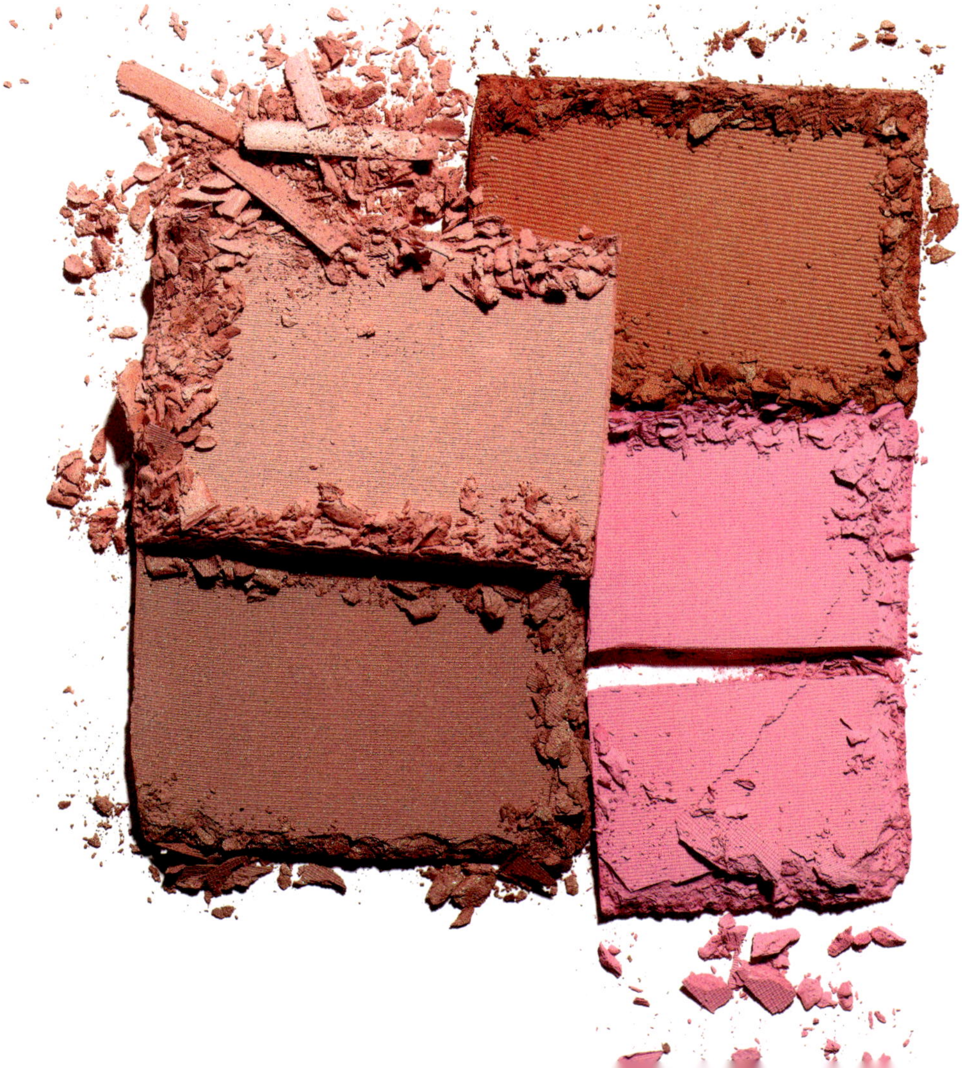

Tip

Never use blush on the eyelids as it is too red and will make the eyes look sore and tired.

CREAM & GEL BLUSH APPLICATION

Cream and gel formulas should be saved for smooth skin. Powder formula is better for textured or blemished skin.

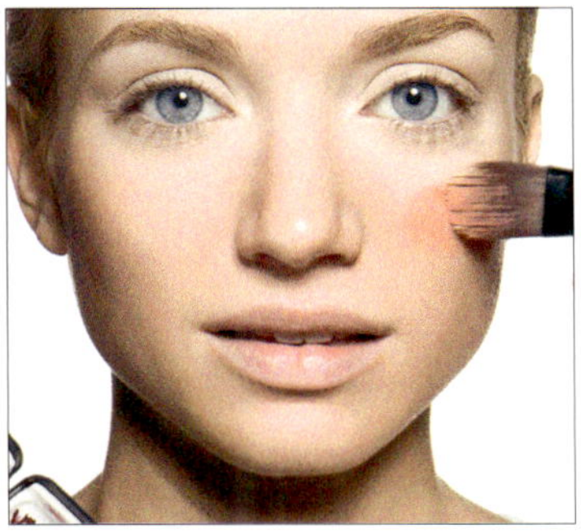

1

Apply over clean skin or foundation. The product can be applied with fingers, a foundation brush, or a sponge.

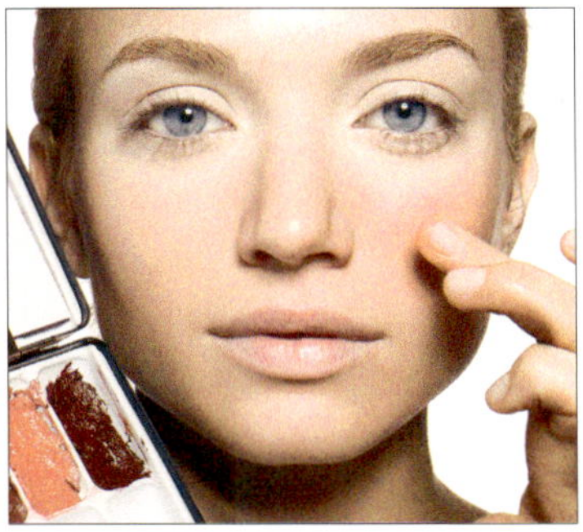

2

Use sparingly at first. You can always add more product if needed.

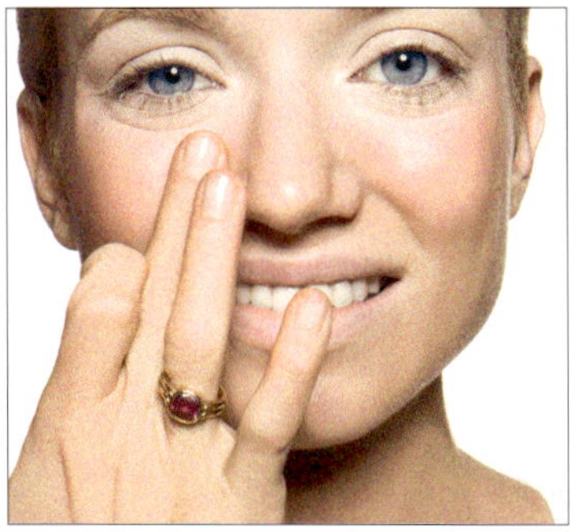

3

Smile, and apply the product to the apples of the cheeks and up toward the hairline, then down to soften the edges.

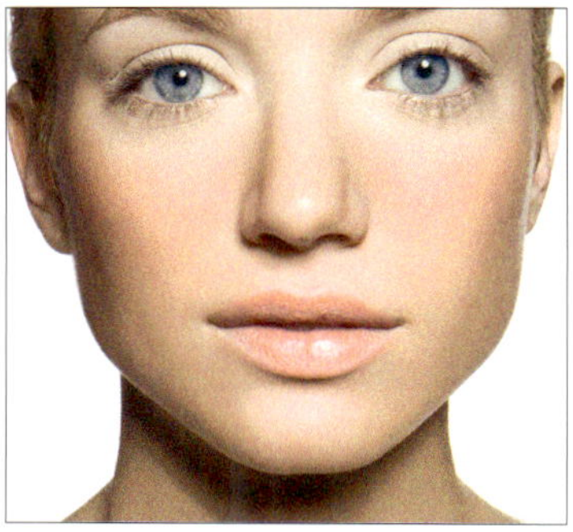

4

Blend thoroughly, keeping the most product on the highest part of the cheekbones.

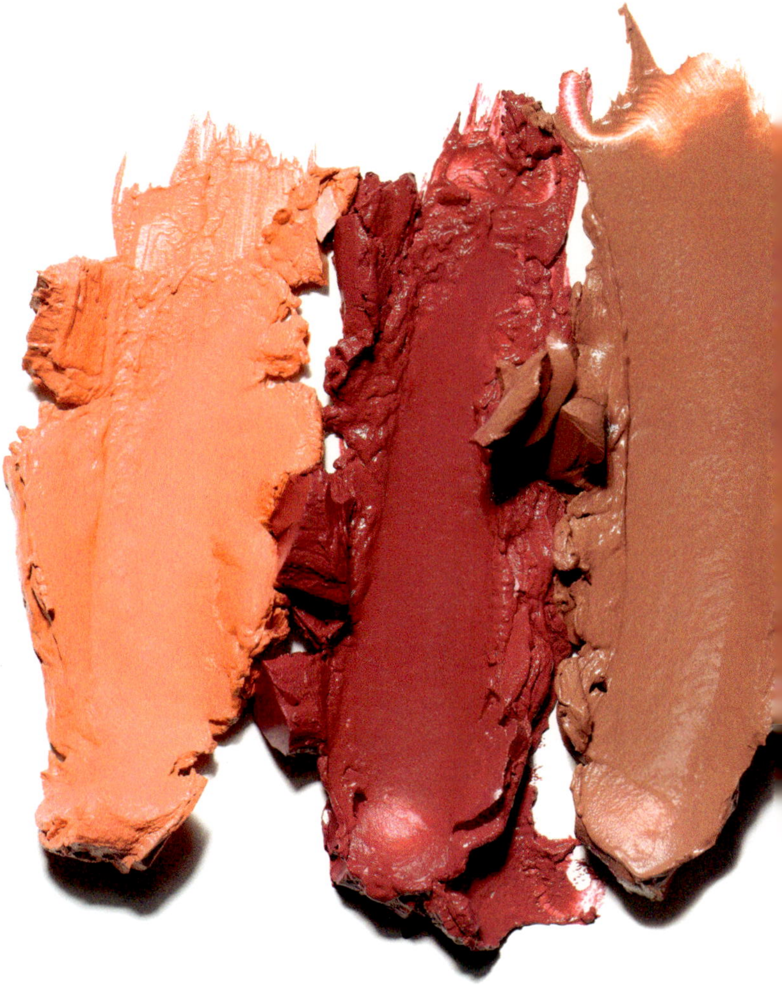

Troubleshooting: Blush

Blush streaks
Your foundation probably wasn't powdered, or you've used too much moisturizer under the foundation.

Looks flat
Layer cream rouge or balm on top of the color for a glow.

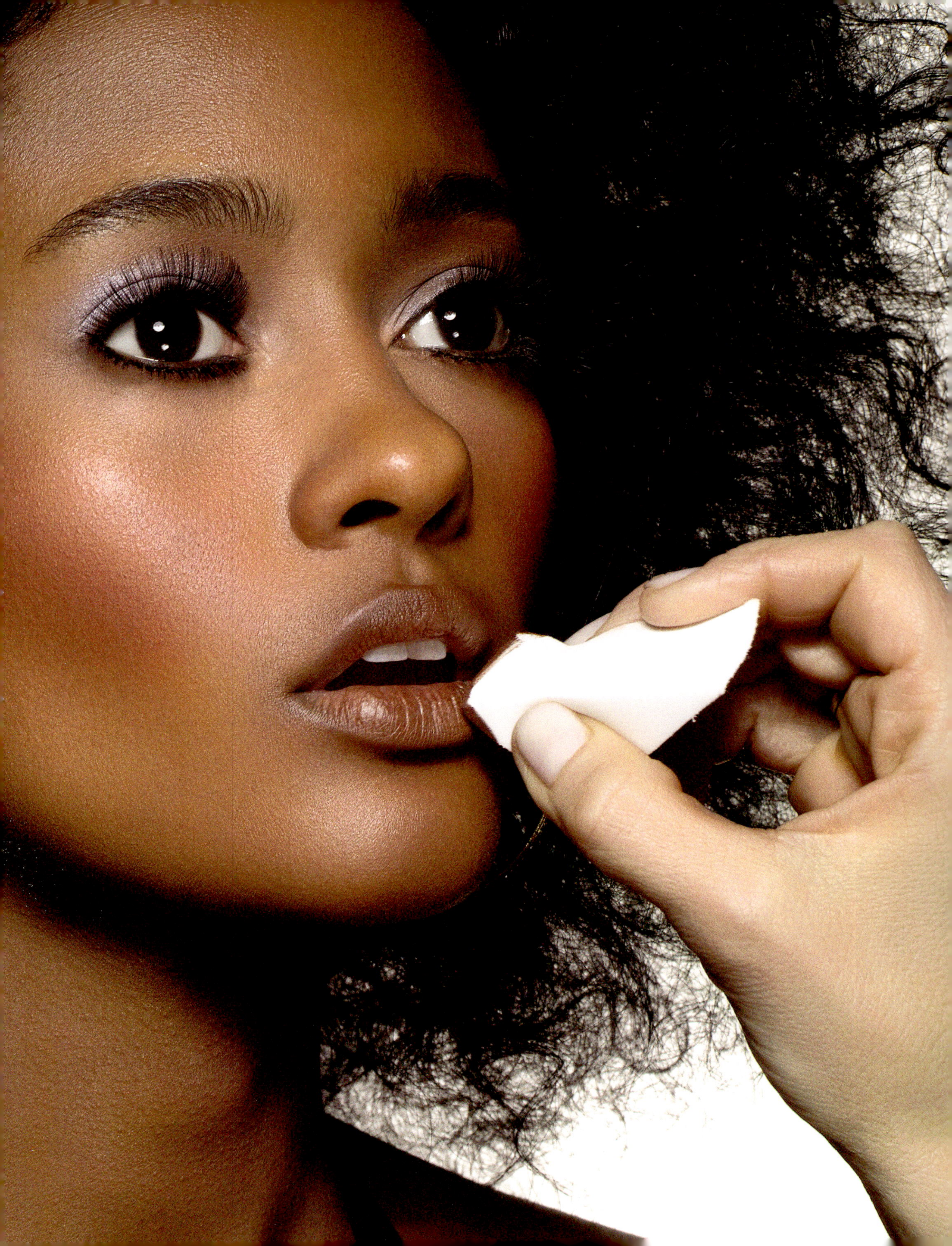

Chapter 5

LIPS

Applying lip color is one of the simplest of all makeup steps and is **a great way to instantly change a look.** Lip color applications range from simple, blotted-on stains to combinations of lip pencil, lipstick, and gloss. The right shade works with the skin tone and complements the natural color of the lips. You can choose from a wide range of product formulas, which include matte, sheer, shimmery, and creamy lipsticks and glosses.

COLOR & APPLICATION

Finding the Perfect Shade

To identify the best basic lip color, remove all makeup. The perfect neutral shade—pinky brown, nude, beige pink, rosy brown, pink, chocolate, or blackberry—will generally be close in tone to the natural lip color. The one that looks good on the naked face is the right neutral, everyday, mistake-proof color. It should not look ashy, orange, or pink but like an enhanced version of the natural lip color. Some women might need more color, and the shade that works best without makeup could be bright or dark rather than neutral. You know you have found the right shade when it enhances the skin tone, makes the eyes look brighter, and gives the face a lift.

Once you have identified the right neutral or everyday shade of lip color, you have the basis for selecting more dramatic colors. Most lip colors with the same undertone as the natural shade will look flattering.

Guide for Selecting Lip Color

NATURAL COLOR OF LIPS	LIPSTICK SHADE				
Pale Lips	beige	sandy pink	light coral	pale pink	bright red
Medium Lips	brown	rose	pink	orange	warm red
Dark Lips	brown	deep red	plum	deep chocolate	deep raisin/ berries
Two-toned Lips	chocolate	blackberry	deep plum	deep raisin	deep red

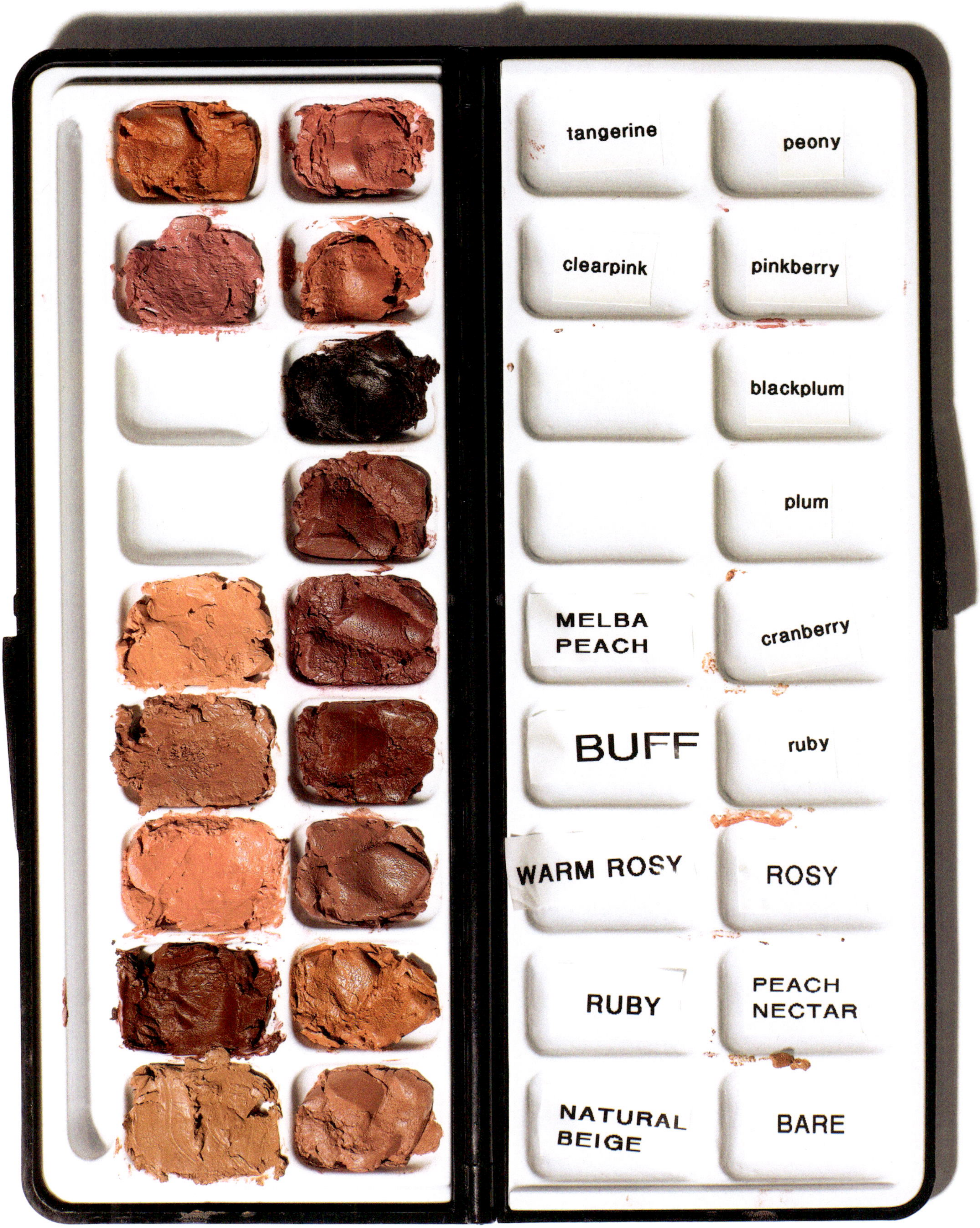
tangerine
peony
clearpink
pinkberry
blackplum
plum
MELBA PEACH
cranberry
BUFF
ruby
WARM ROSY
ROSY
RUBY
PEACH NECTAR
NATURAL BEIGE
BARE

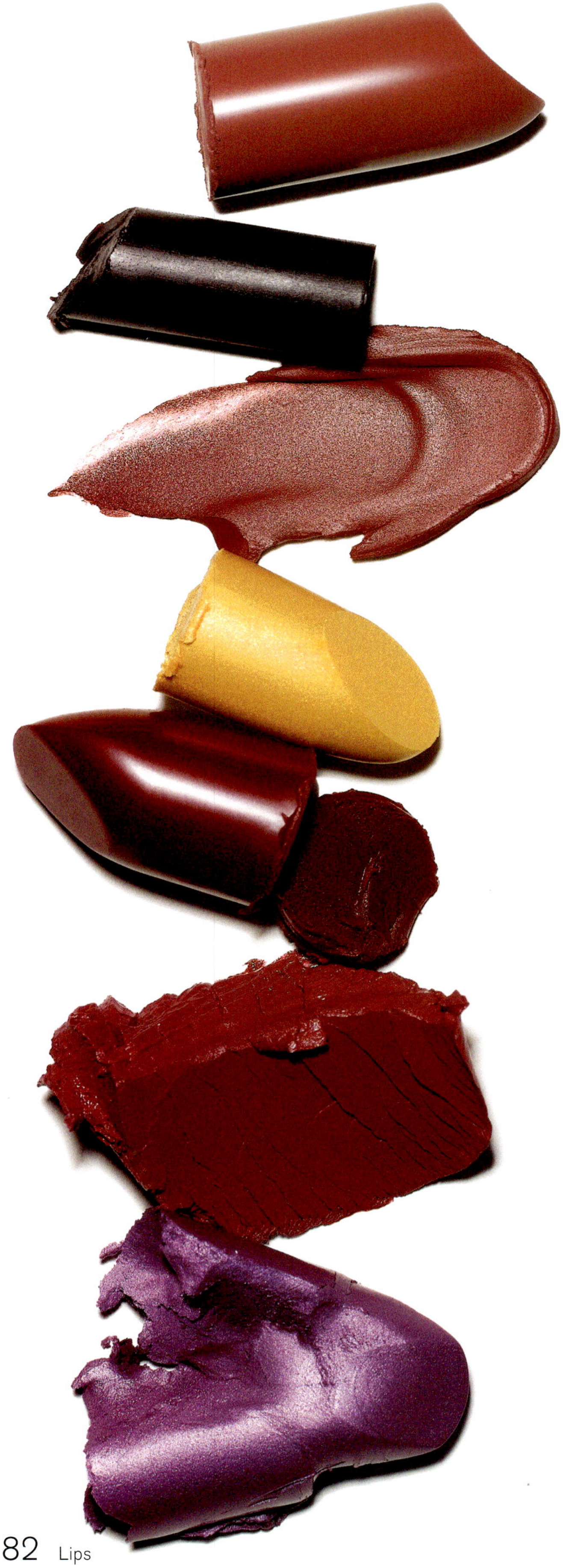

Formula

MATTE PRODUCTS are dense and last longest. They contain less moisture than other products, so they adhere to the lips and don't fade as quickly. They are not appropriate for very dry lips.

SEMIMATTE PRODUCTS are less dry than matte products and don't last as long. They work best on textured or dry lips and give off a soft sheen.

SHEER COLORS are see-through, forgiving, and easy to use.

STAINS provide long-lasting, highly pigmented color.

TINTS, like sheer glosses or balms, protect the lips with moisturizing formulas that usually contain sunscreen.

BALMS are tinted or clear formulas and help soften the lips.

GLOSS STICKS are hybrids, between sheer lipstick and gloss. They add a bit more pigment than lip gloss does but both are see-through and moist.

LIP GLOSSES provide hydration, sun protection, and sheen. This formula is great for making the lips look fuller and for layering on top of other lip colors.

CHUBBY LIP PENCILS will both define lips and provide a creamy matte texture. They are long lasting but can be a bit dry.

LIP LINERS define the lips and keep lipstick on longer when used on the entire lip area.

LIP COLOR APPLICATION

Mixing and blending are fun but it's always great to find a color that works directly out of the tube. Never buy a color that the makeup artist has to "fix" to work on you.

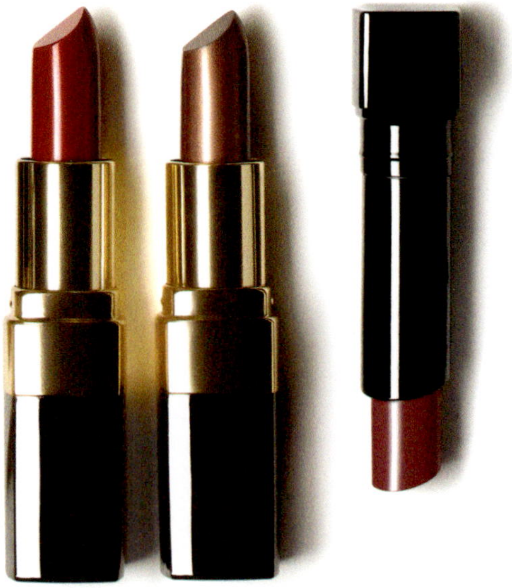

Troubleshooting: Lip Color

For pale lips use pastel shades, such as pale pink or light beige. Deep tones appear very dark on pale lips, so apply them with a light hand.

Very dark lips look best with blue-toned and deep, saturated lip color. Very pale shades of lipstick can appear gray or ashy on dark lips.

For uneven colored lips that are either dark with pink inside the lower lip or one darker and one lighter lip, you can choose to enhance or conceal the natural colors. Use a light shade that corresponds to the lighter lip color to enhance and bring out the paler lip, or use a deeper shade for a dramatic, full-coverage look. To even out tone, use a sheer, dark lipstick as a base on the lighter area, and then apply regular lipstick.

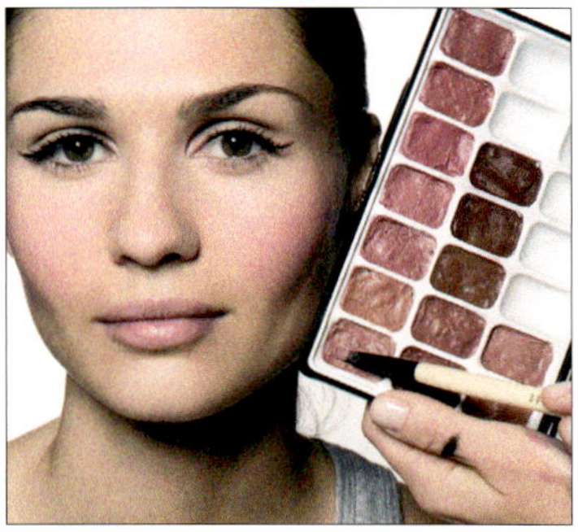

1

Choose the color and apply it using a lip brush or directly out of the tube.

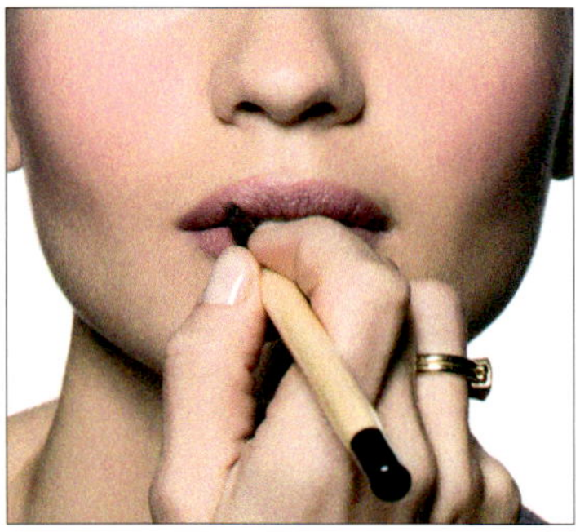

2

Beginning at one corner of the mouth, apply an even layer of color over the entire lip area.

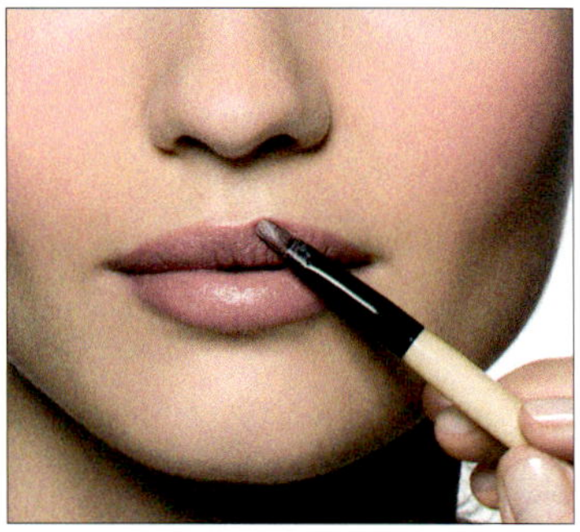

3

Keep the color within the natural lines of the lips. Use the brush to accurately line the lips.

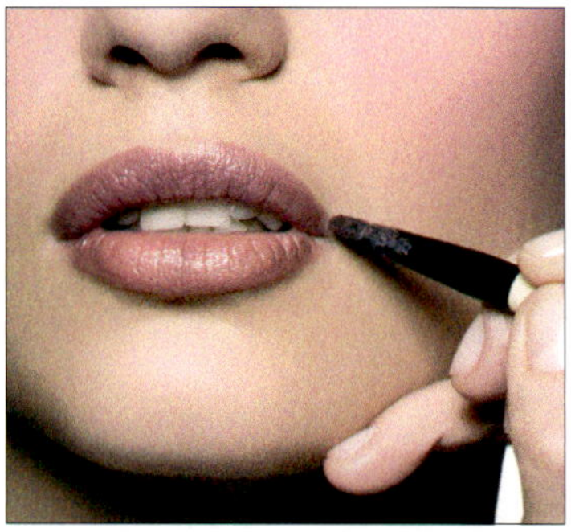

4

Continue the application to the other corner of the mouth. Always apply the color into the corners on both top and bottom lips.

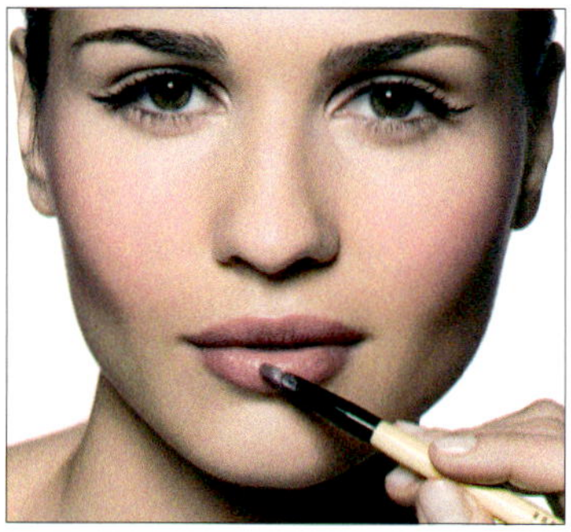

5

Fill in the bottom lip and any missed areas. Press your lips together to evenly distribute the color.

LIP PENCIL APPLICATION

It's so much easier to match the lip color than to use a dark color that has to be blended.

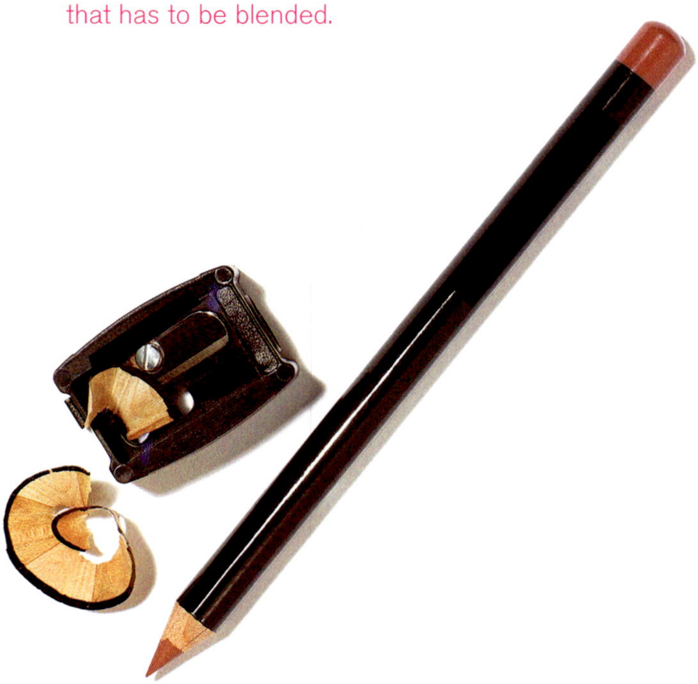

Tips for Long-Lasting Color

Some lip color products are long-lasting, but often those formulas are far too dry. Here are some techniques that provide extended wear to regular lipstick formulas.

Use a lip pencil that matches the natural color of the lips to line and completely fill in the lips. This base helps hold lip color in place. Layer lipstick on top.

Use pencil on top of lipstick to create a waxy barrier.

Blotting lipstick with your finger presses color into the lips and will create a stain that will last.

A bit of powder or blush patted on top of lipstick will keep it on longer.

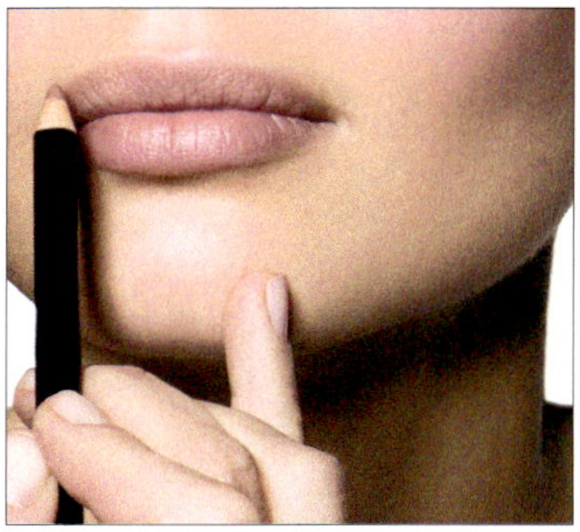

1

Begin by choosing color that matches the lips or lipstick. Begin lining the top lip.

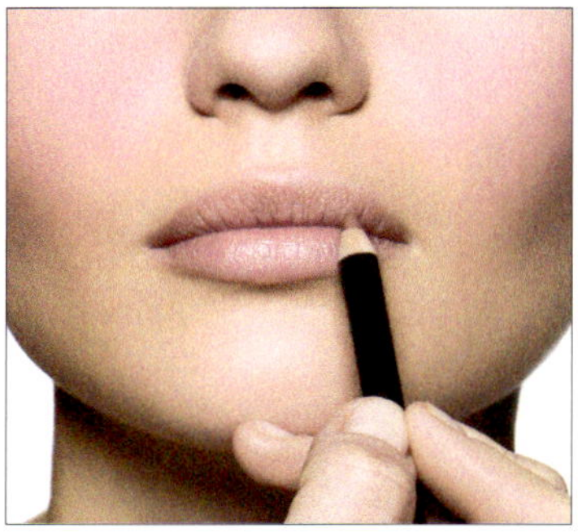

2

Extend the line across the top lip.

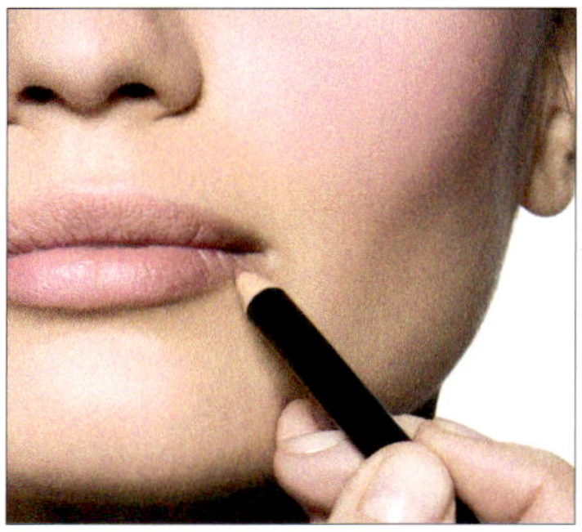

3

Define the line across the bottom lip.

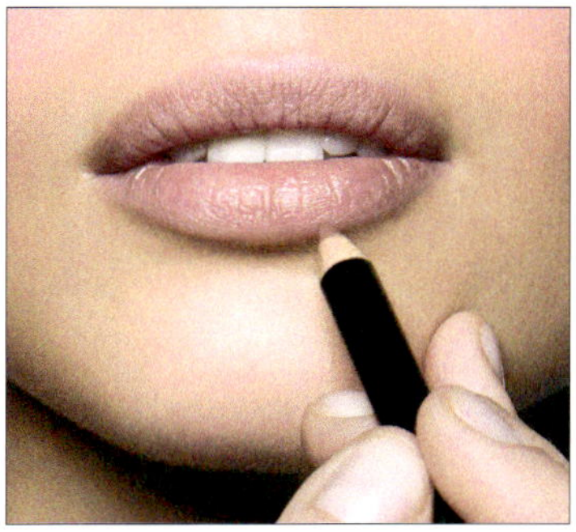

4

Line underneath the lower lip.

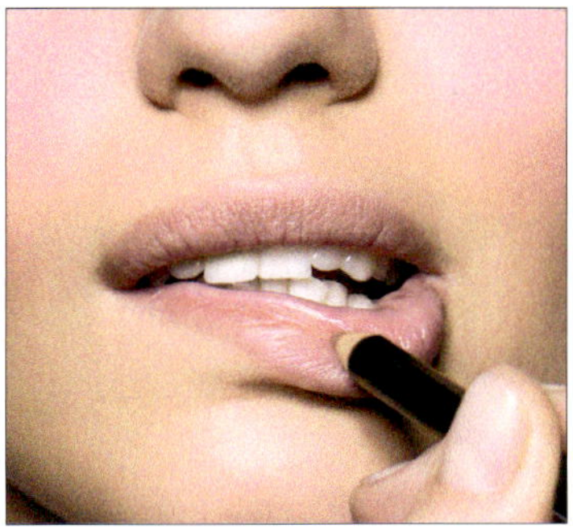

5

Fill in any missed areas and blend.

LIP GLOSS APPLICATION

Lip gloss gives a nice shine and can make the lips look a bit fuller. Don't overdo it by applying too much.

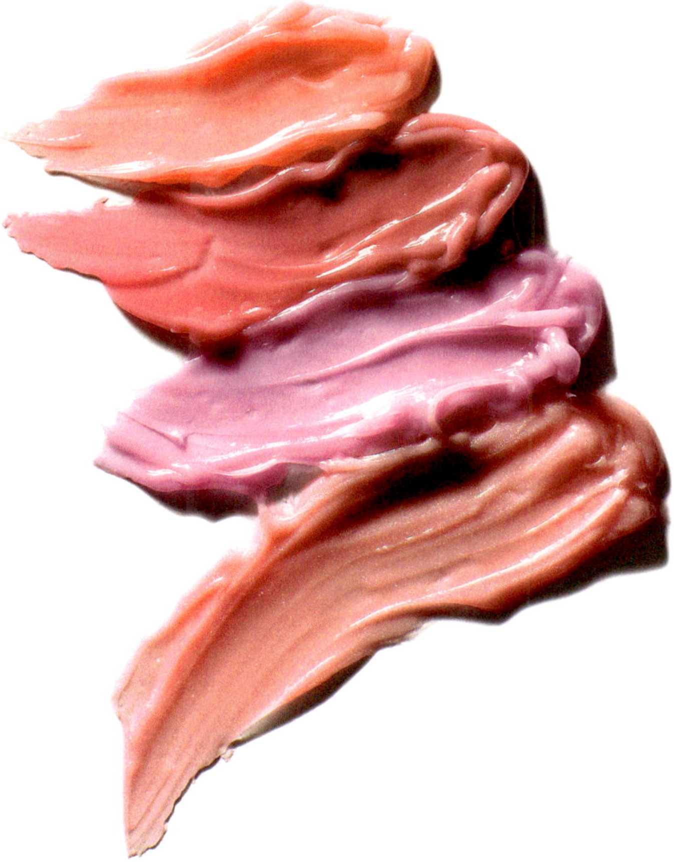

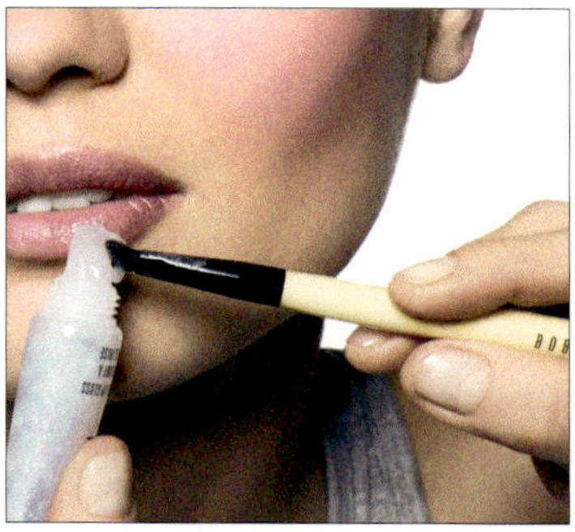

1

Apply gloss to a lip brush or directly to the lips.

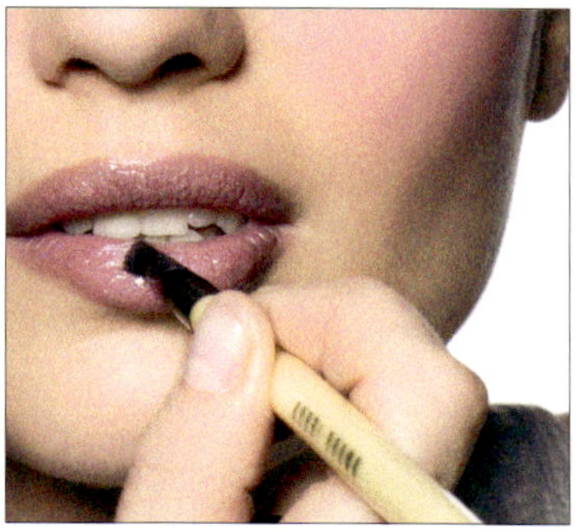

2

Using the brush or your finger, begin at the middle of the lips.

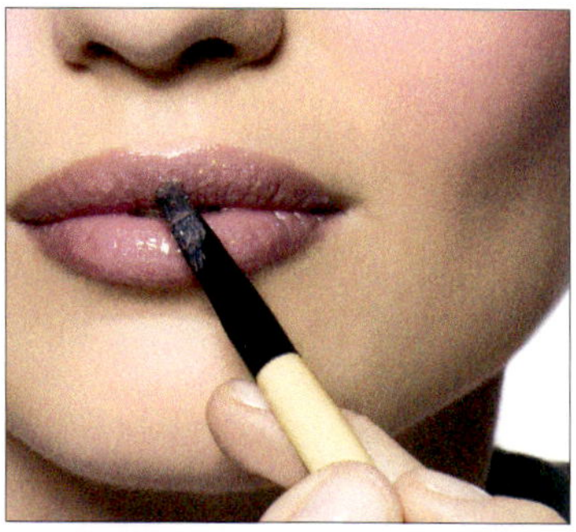

3

Apply gloss to both the top and bottom lips.

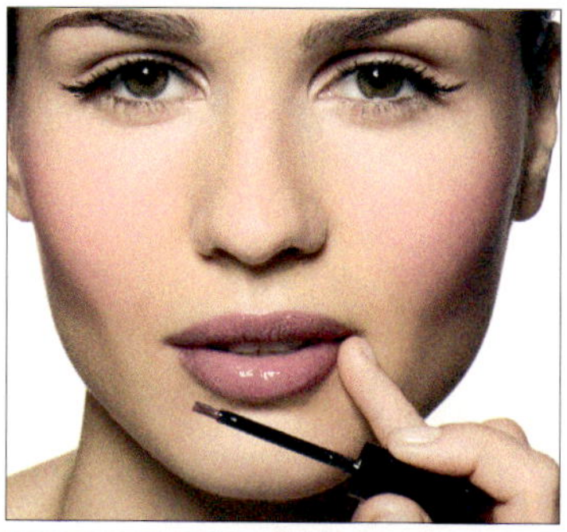

4

Wipe the edges of the lips when finished.

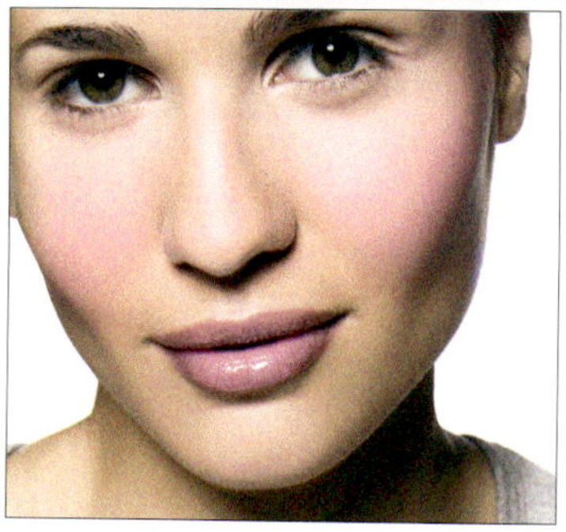

5

The lips look fuller and hydrated.

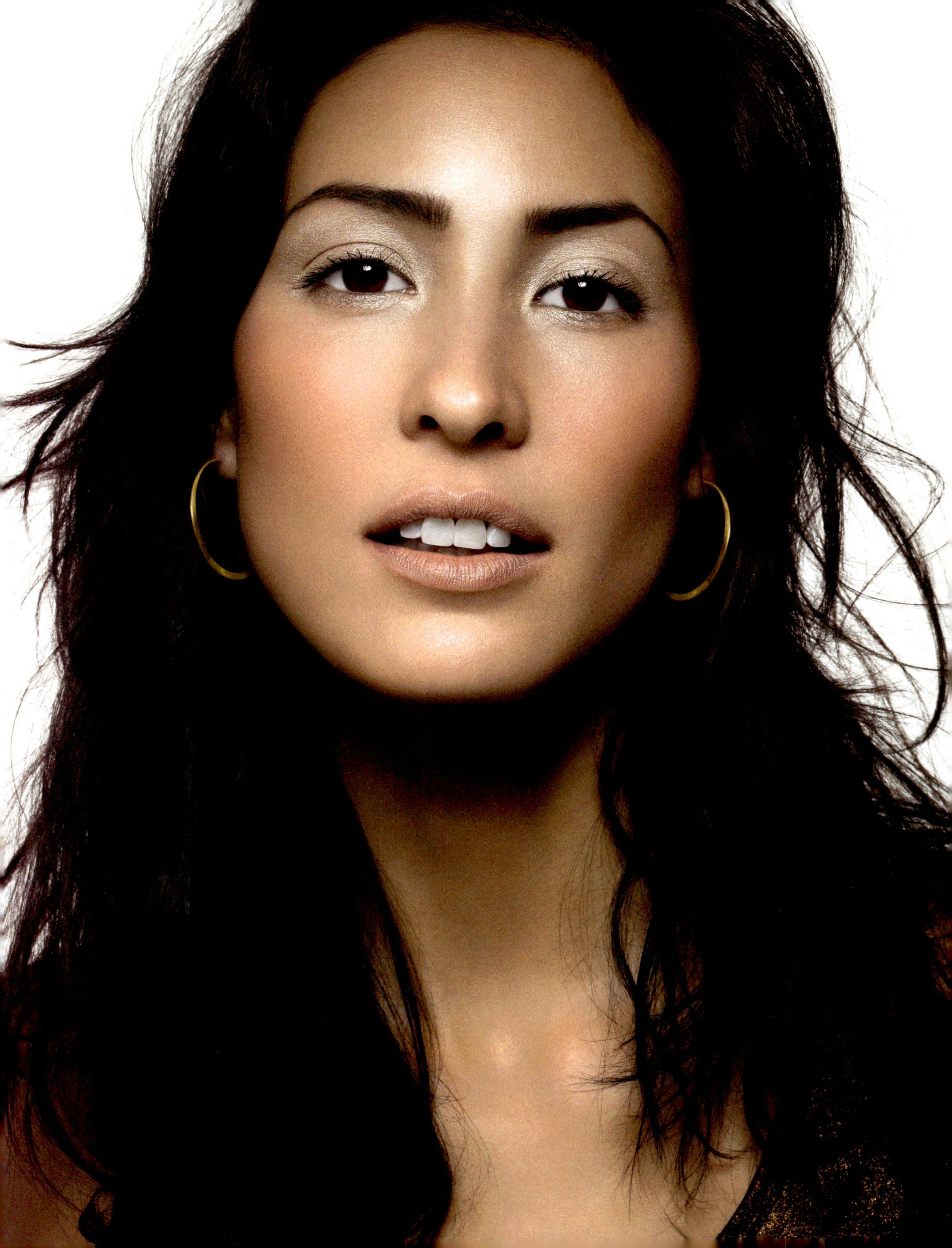

Chapter 6

EYES

The purpose of eye makeup—whether it's simple black mascara or dramatic contouring shadow—**is to make the eyes stand out.** When it's done right, eye makeup can give the appearance of **brighter, more beautiful eyes.** Here I cover the basics, like choosing flattering shades and lining the eyes, as well as advanced techniques, like creating a smoky eye and applying false lashes.

EYEBROW SHAPE & DEFINITION

You have seen what a difference a great frame can make to a painting. It is the eyebrows that form a frame for your eyes. Beautifully groomed eyebrows make a huge difference. It is possible to transform a face with just tweezers, shadow, a brow brush, and brow gel. A professional will help you find your ideal shape. Once the brows have been groomed, it is easy to do your own upkeep.

All brows benefit from added definition. Brow brushes and combs quickly tame and shape the brow hair. Brow shapers define, control, and shape the brows quickly and easily while adding just a bit of color.

Brow-Grooming Supplies

Brow brush

Brow pencil

Clear brow gel

Tinted brow gel

Brow shadow

Tweezers

Baby scissors for trimming extra-long or curly hair

Color Chart for Eyebrows

HAIR COLOR	PENCIL, SHADOW, & SHAPER TONES	
Blond	ash blond	soft gray
Light Brown	sable	light brown
Red	ash blond	camel
Brunette	mahogany	warm brown
Black	darkest brown	dark gray (do not use black)
Gray	slate	gray
White	gray	ash blond

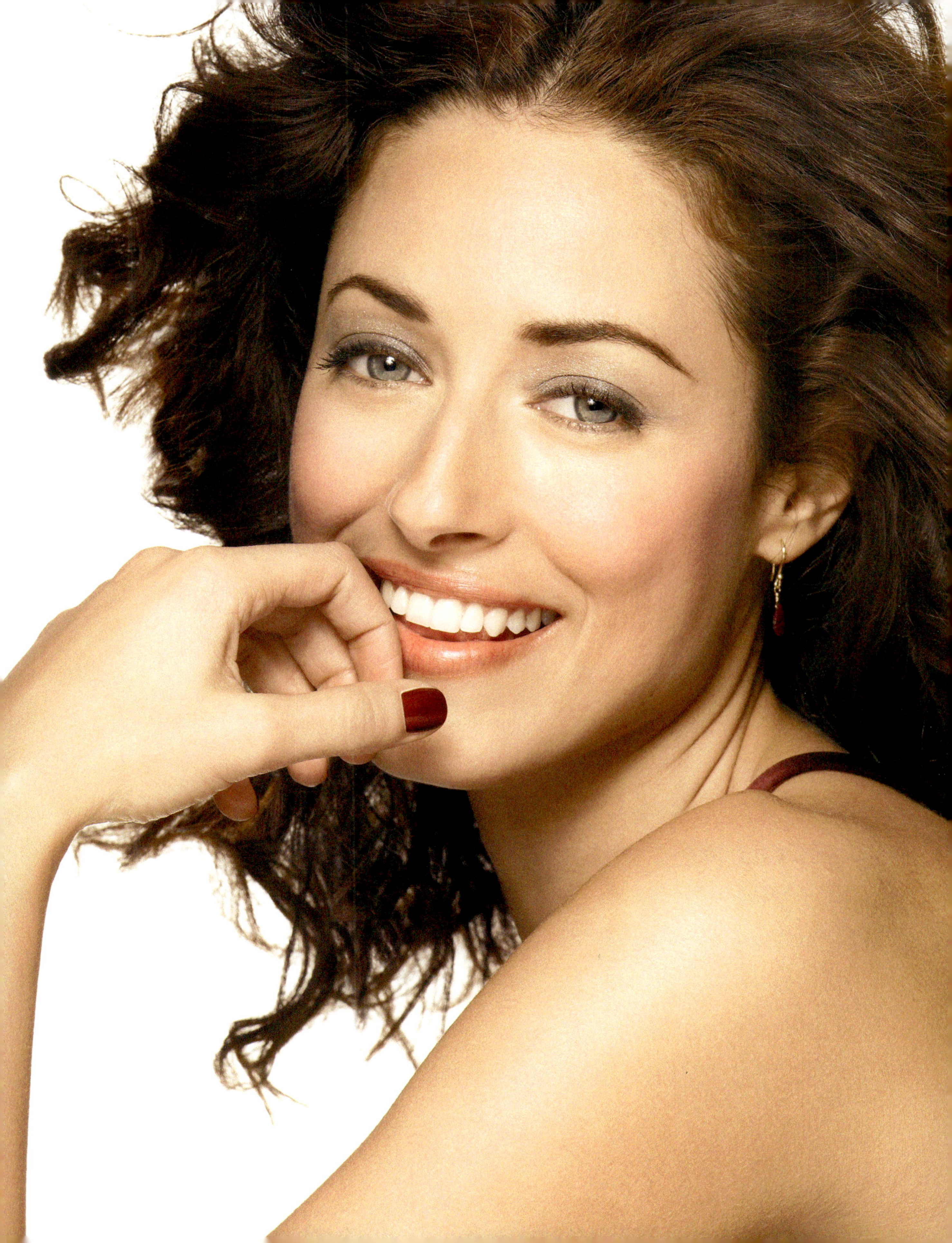

HOW TO SHAPE BROWS

The start of the brow should follow an imaginary line drawn from the outside of the nose to the inside corner of the eye.

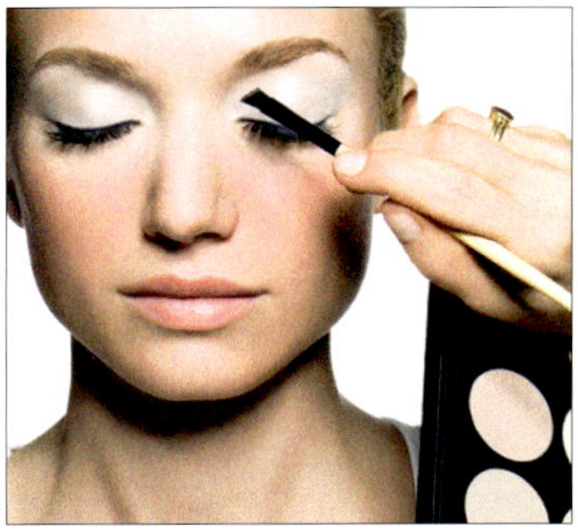

1

Choose the color that matches your eyebrows and hair.

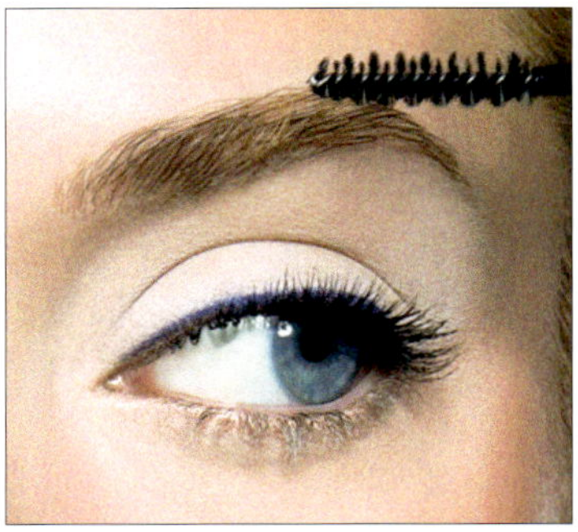

2

For a natural option, use eyebrow mascara to create the look of a natural brow.

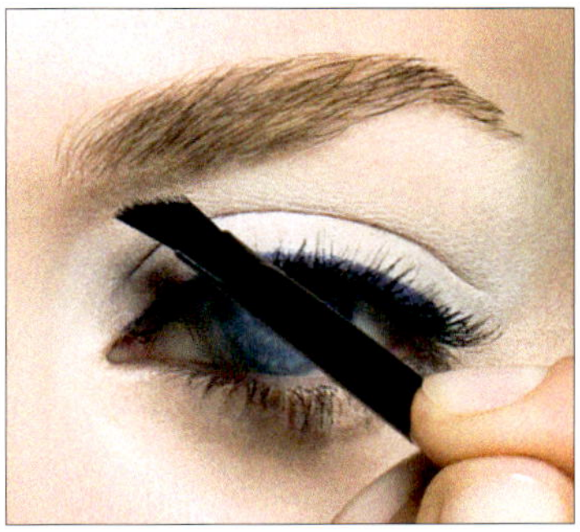

3

For more definition, use powder shadow. Start at the inner corner of the brow. Make sure you fill in all the gaps in the brow hair.

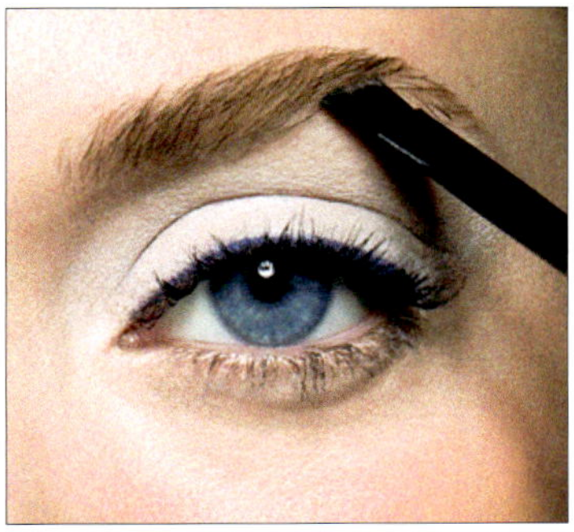

4

Bring the brush to the center, creating an arch, and then turn the brush and go down.

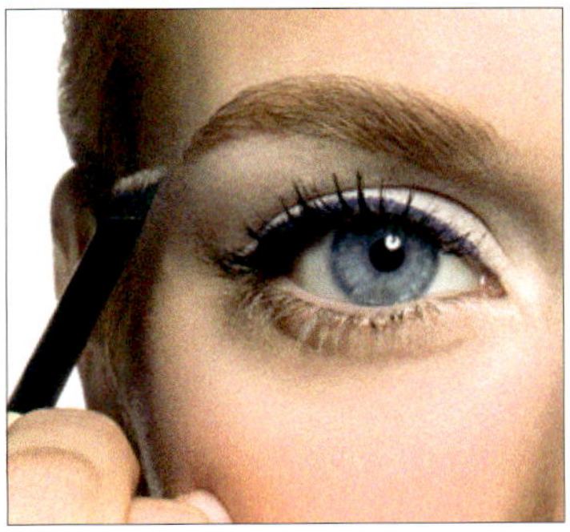

5

Make sure the brow is long enough.

Special Cases

Nonexistent brows
Brows damaged by overtweezing, age, or chemotherapy can be drawn in to look quite natural. Use a pencil the color of original brows, and softly draw in the shape. Layer a complementary color of powder shadow with a brow brush to fill in and soften.

Bare spots
Bare spots can be filled in with light strokes of pencil or with powder shadow. If neither works, try layering both.

Brows too far apart
Brows too far apart can be corrected by filling in missing brow areas with light pencil strokes. Balance the brows carefully. Layer powder shadow on top.

Tadpole brows
Tadpole brows can be reshaped with shadow. Fill them in to create a straight line.

ASIAN BROWS

Asian women often have sparse brows and need to fill in the brows to match a full head of hair.

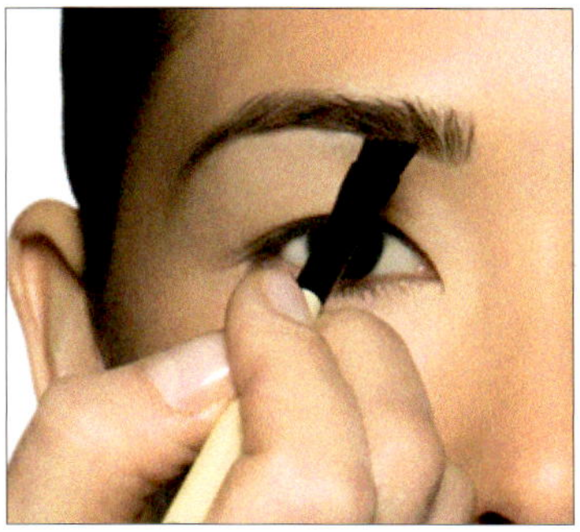

1

Begin at the inside of the brow.

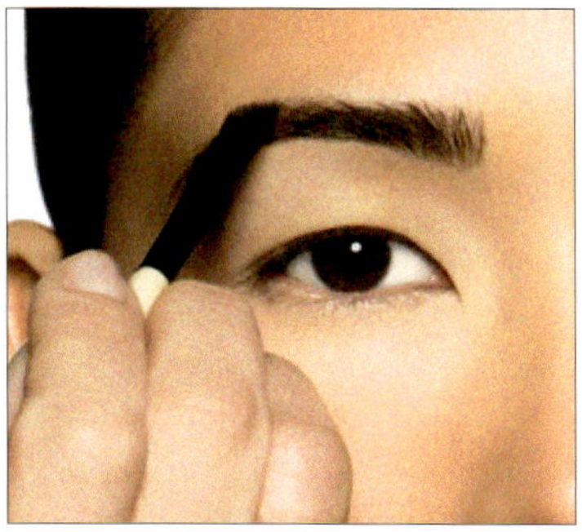

2

Fill in the brow using a shade that matches it. Use the powder to add density so it matches the hair on your head.

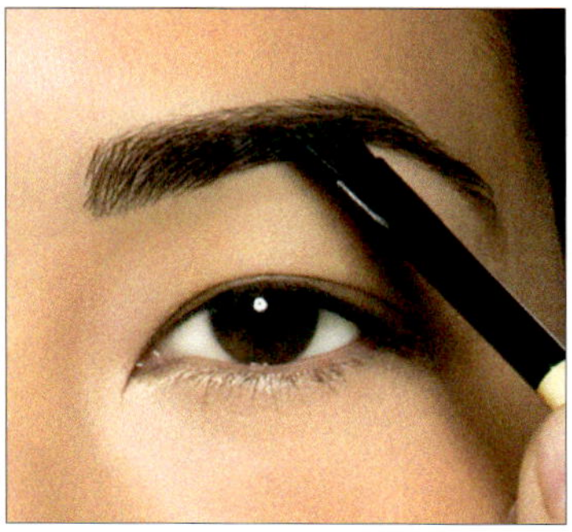

3

Lightly stroke along the length of the brow.

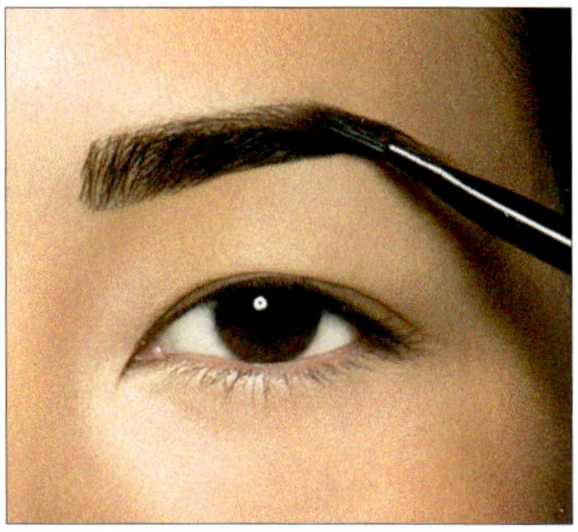

4

Continue all the way up the arch, turning the brush as it goes down.

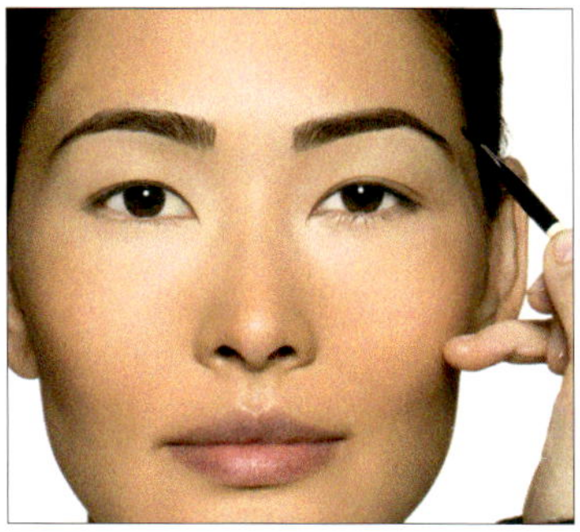

5

Make sure the brow is long enough.

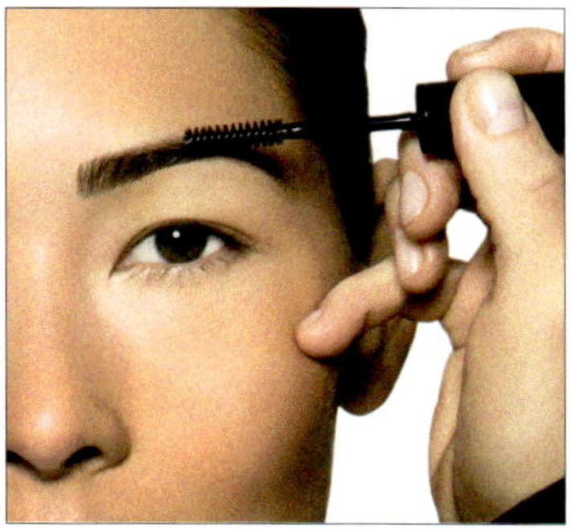

6

Use a clear eyebrow mascara to brush up an unruly brow.

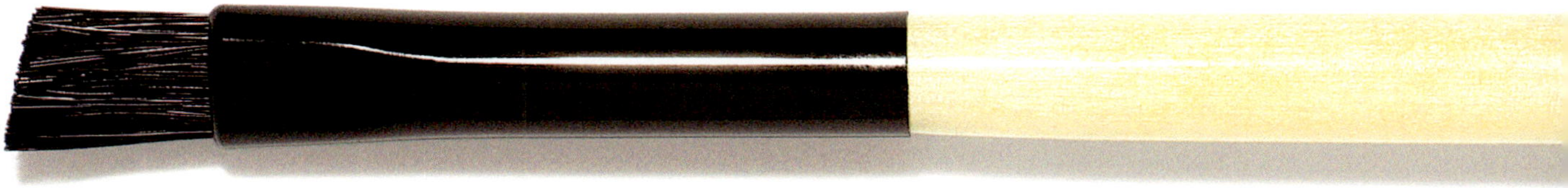

TWEEZING

It's best to get a professional shaping to begin. It's easier for upkeep. Tweezing after the shower is less painful than at other times.

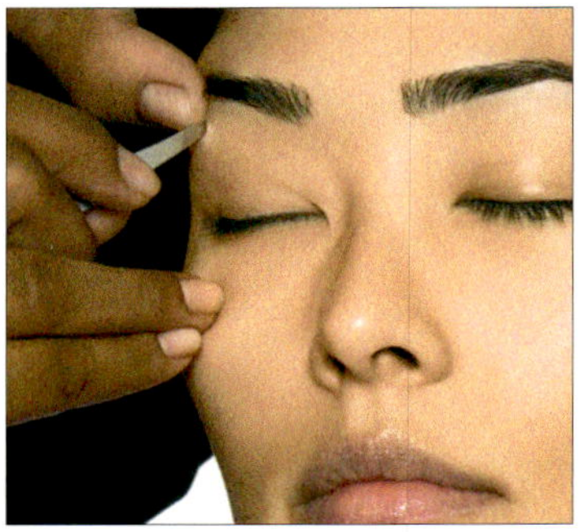

1

Begin by cleaning under the arch of the eyebrow. Remove a few hairs at a time, checking the results as you go.

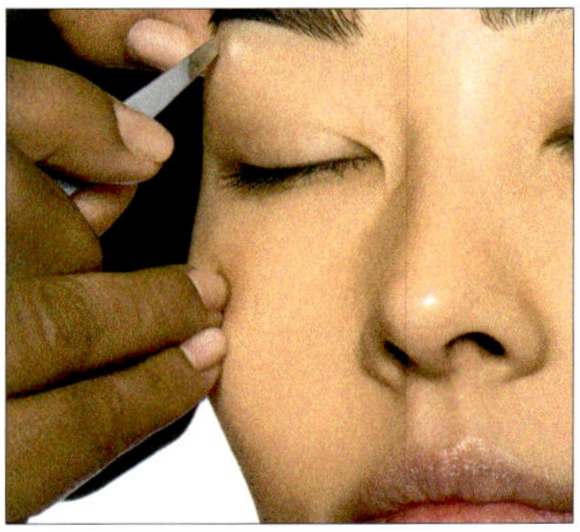

2

Slowly tweeze, moving inward toward the thickest part of the brow.

Tip

Some unruly brows will benefit from trimming long hairs with baby scissors.

Grooming Brows

To fill obvious holes or lengthen overplucked brows, use either pencil alone or a pencil-to-powder method. Using an eyebrow pencil in a shade that matches the brow color, fill with a light, feathery stroke, mimicking the look of hair. If using a powdered eye shadow, choose one that closely matches the hair and brow color. Using a stiff, flat, angled brow brush, pick up a small amount of color, and tap off the excess. Lightly stroke the shadow from the inner corner of the brow along the entire length to fill it in. Stroke color along the upper edge of the brow to accentuate the arch and give a "lift" to the eye area.

Apply shadow color only to the hair of the brows.

Finish with a coat of clear brow gel to set and tame any unruly brow hairs.

Look at your brows. Does the shape and intensity of color look natural and balance the face? A dusting of powder can soften the color if needed. Use a brow shaper to tame unruly brow hairs.

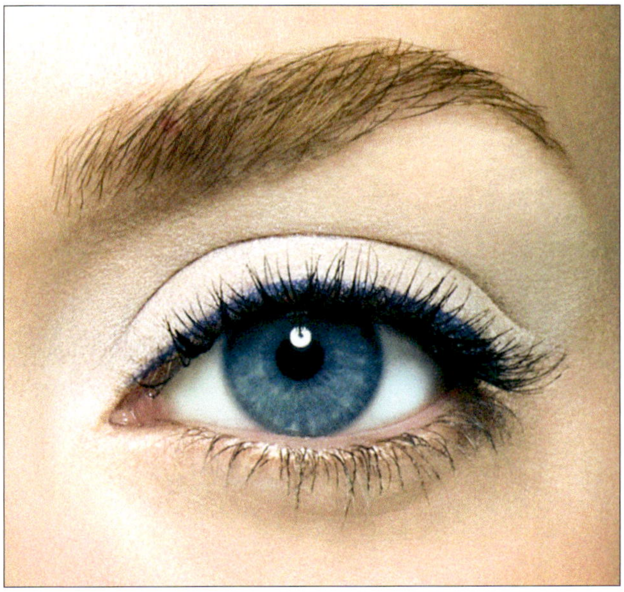

The Perfect Brow
The start of the brow should be aligned with the inner corner of the eye. The arch is three-quarters of the way across the brow from there.

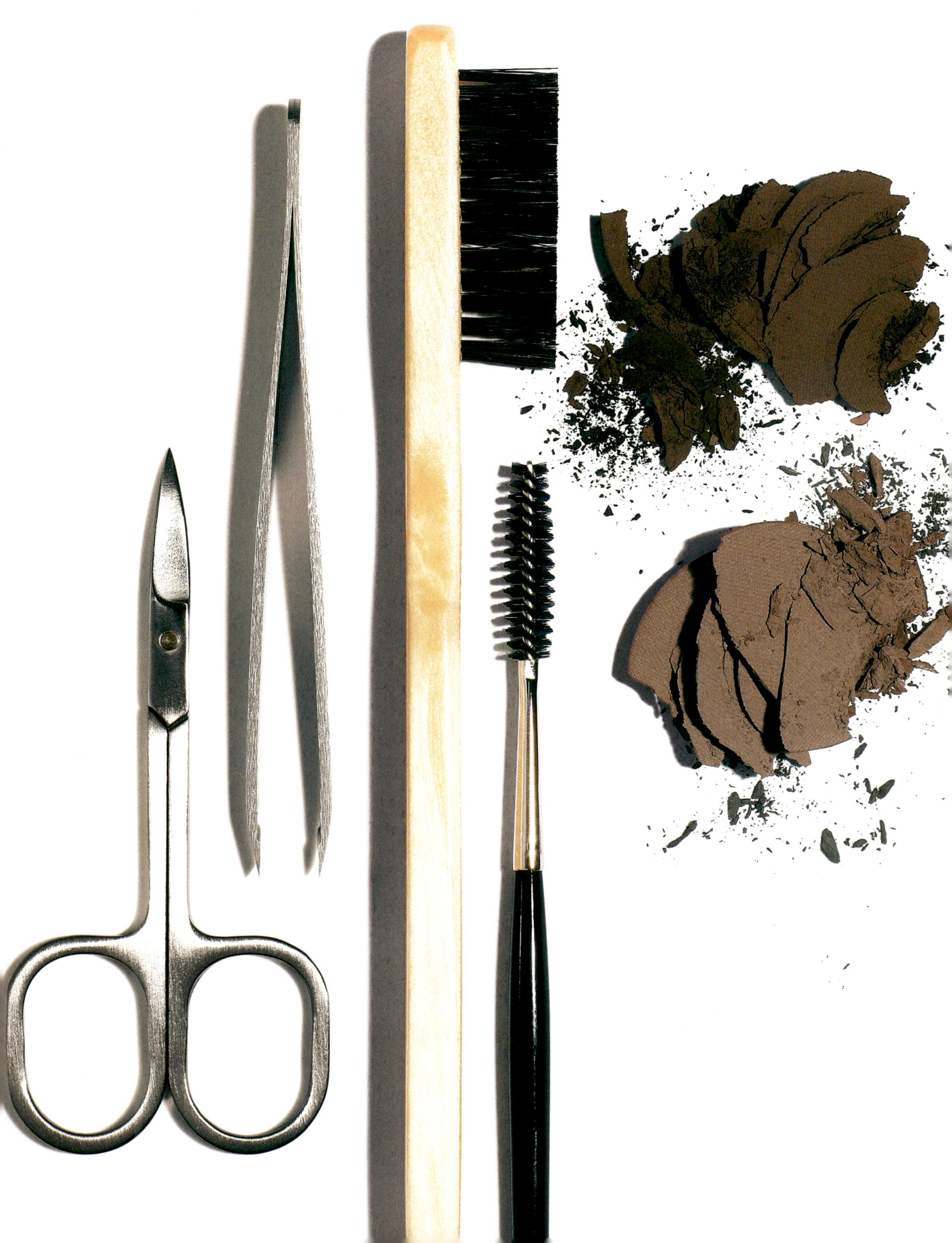

EYE SHADOW

Eye shadow helps accentuate the eye and makes eye color stand out. It is also used to correct eye shape.

Formula and Texture

Eye shadow is available in many formulas and textures: powder, cream, and pencil, matte, sheer, shimmery, glittery, creamy, glossy, etc.

The Basic Eye

Most of the time, a simple, natural look works best. For everyday application, pick shades of shadow that bring out the eye color rather than shadows that make a statement. The basic application is a simple, three-step process.

Crease Color or Contour

If you want to create depth or contour, choose a slightly deeper medium-toned shadow to sweep in the crease of the eye. Crease contour creates definition for puffy or deep-set eyes and can make a stronger eye statement for evening. Begin the shadow at the outside edge of the crease, and move inward with your brush. Softly layer the shadow, repeating and blending until you achieve the desired effect. Always use a blending brush or finger to create a smooth look.

Eye Shadow Color Chart

EYE COLOR	SHADOW COLOR FOR EYELID					
Blue	ash	taupe	gray	heather	slate	lilac
Green	yellow-toned beige	camel	heather	moss	slate	taupe
Brown	cement	sable	mocha	khaki	stone	bark

BASE EYE SHADOW APPLICATION

Use a light shadow color as a base on the lids; apply it with a full shadow brush that covers the entire lid from lash line to browbone. This step creates a clean slate for the other shadows. It also keeps moisture away from the lid and takes away any discoloration. For some women who prefer a clean eye look, this may be the only shadow that's needed.

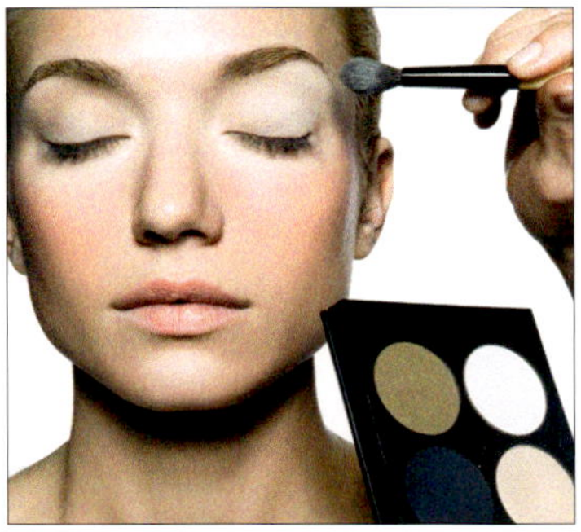

1

With a full shadow brush, apply a light shade (also known as your base color).

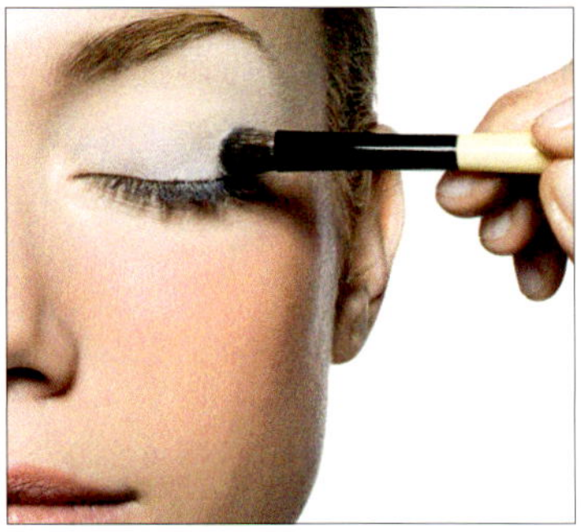

2

Apply color from the brow bone down to the lash line.

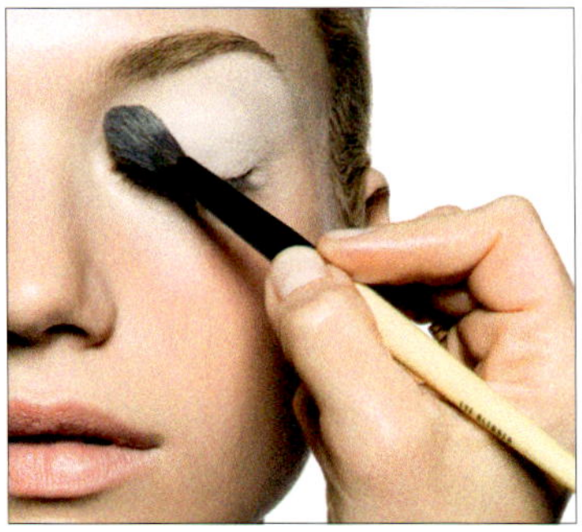

3

Don't forget to cover the inner corner of the eye.

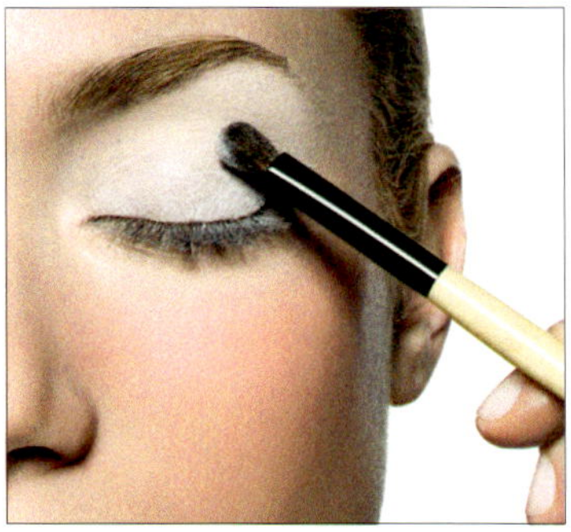

4

Brush all the way up to the brow.

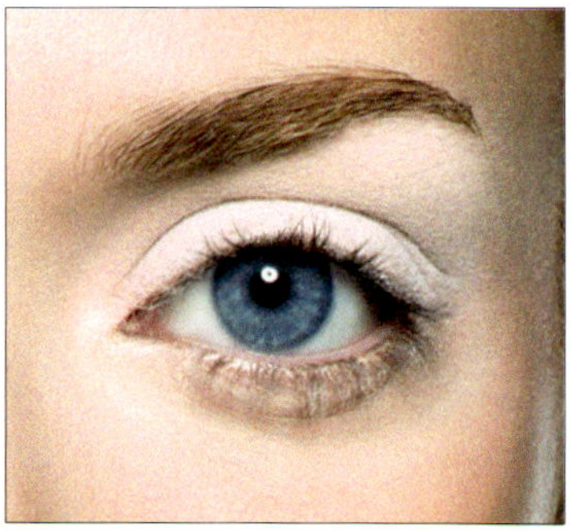

5

Make sure the eyelid is covered and the shadow is dense enough.

Tip

Avoid eye shadows with red and purple undertones if you have redness around the eyes, as these colors will make your eyes look tired. Stick with neutral, brown, or gray colors, but beware that some browns and grays have so much red in them that they should not be used.

MEDIUM SHADOW & CONTOUR APPLICATION

This step starts with a color that doesn't need to be blended to deepen the lid. Next, a deeper color is layered as a contour.

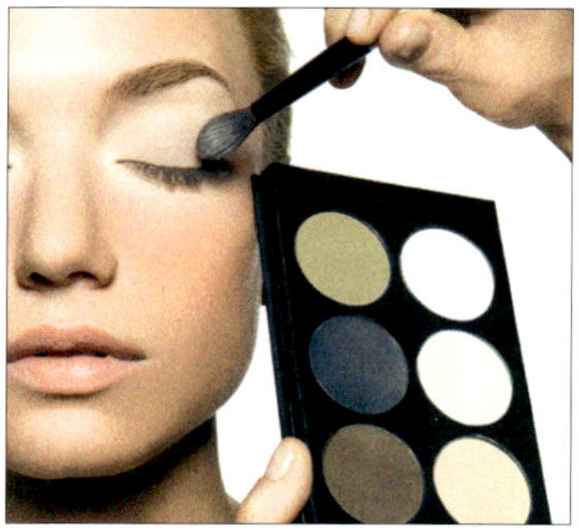

1

Choose a medium-tone shadow for the lid.

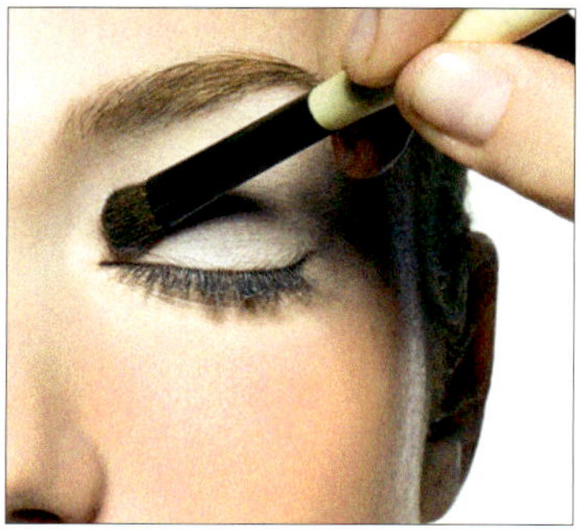

2

With a medium fluffy shadow brush, apply color to the lid.

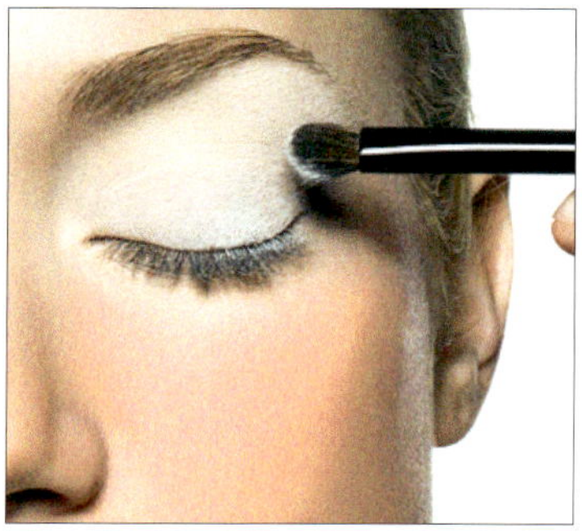

3

Continue applying from the lash line to the crease.

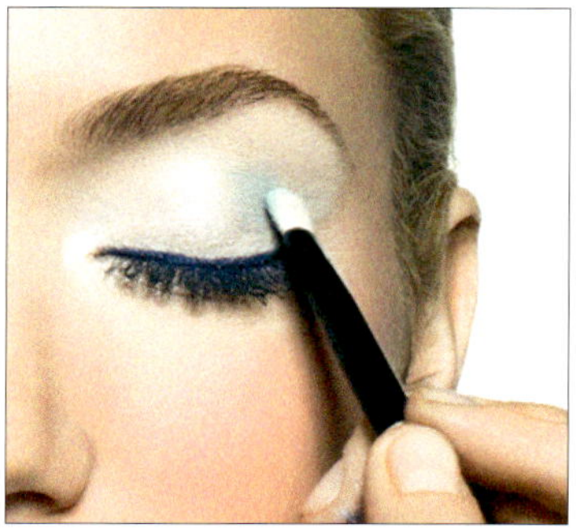

4

Layer a deeper medium shade on the outer corner and blend as you apply it. The correct shade will require little blending.

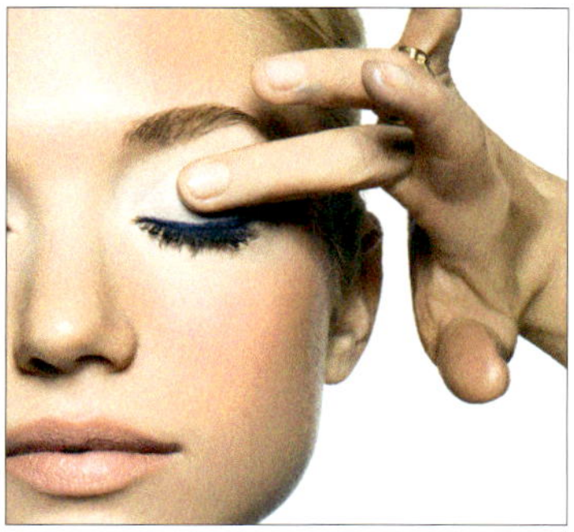

5

Continue blending with your fingers.

Contouring for Eyes

These tips can help change the look of your eyes, making them stand out or correcting a full, puffy eyelid.

Deep-set eyes need to be brought out with light and medium to deep medium shades of shadow. Colors that are too dark recede and will make the eyes look even more deep set.

Wide-set eyes will appear closer together with a sweep of shadow one to two shades darker than the foundation tone at the inner corner of the eye. When applying liner, thicken the line a bit at the inner corner, and do not extend it past the outer corner of the eye.

To make eyes look bigger, line your eyes all the way around.

To make eyes look more oval, top and bottom liner should meet at the outer corners. Then contour shadow from the lash line along the eyeliner outward and into the crease.

To make large eyes look smaller, use a soft shadow color as a liner at the lower lash line. The shadow should be several shades lighter than the top liner.

To make eyes look less puffy, apply contour shadow at the outer corners and blend it as you move in toward the nose.

PLAYING WITH COLOR

Neutrals work for most applications but color is fun to play with.

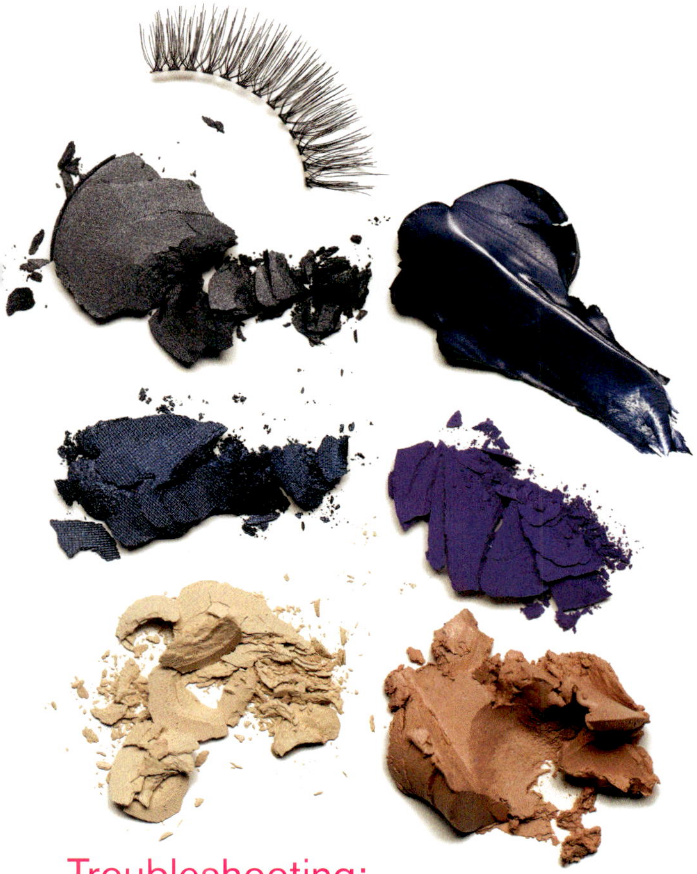

Troubleshooting: Eyes

Eye shadow flakes on the face.
First try a clean powder brush to sweep it off. If this doesn't work, use a nonoily makeup remover on a cotton swab or makeup sponge to gently clean the flakes off the skin. When creating a smoky eye, be sure to do the eyes first, clear the area of flakes, and then apply concealer and foundation.

You've made wings when trying to contour.
Using your finger or a cotton swab, wipe away, going up, and then blend toward the eye.

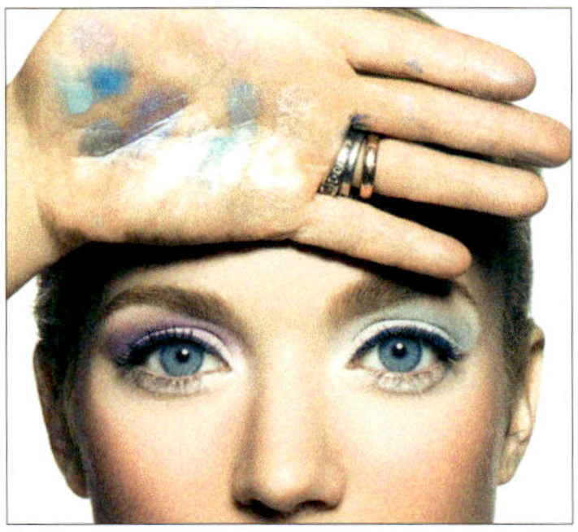

1
Choose a shade that you like.

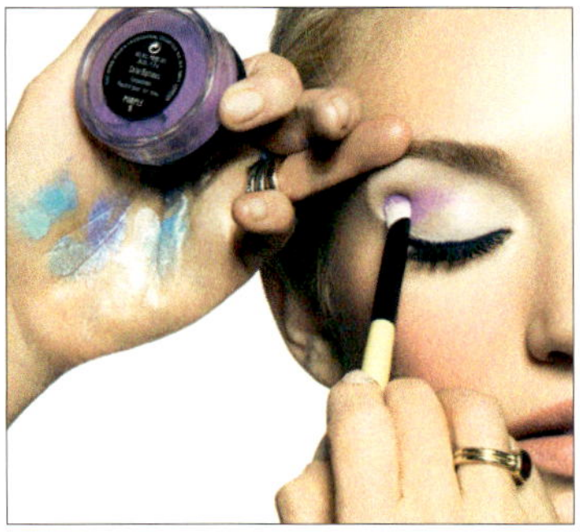

2
Cover the entire lid three-quarters of the way to the brow bone, blending as you go.

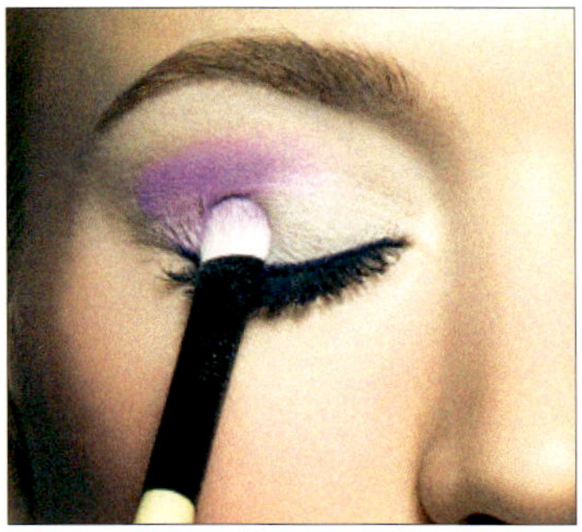

3
Layer with bold color.

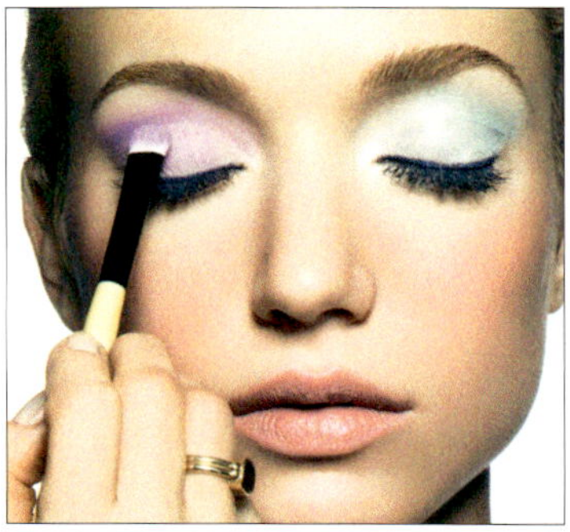

4
Blend the color with your fingers or a clean brush.

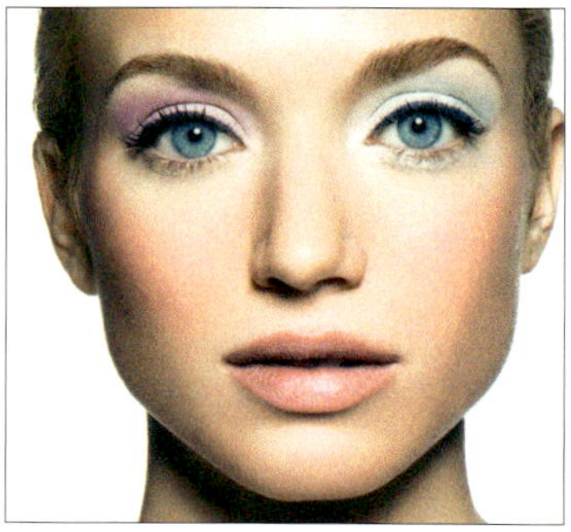

5
Experiment with different colors to find the shades you like most.

CREAM SHADOW APPLICATION

Choose a formula with or without powder in it. If it doesn't contain powder, be sure to apply it over powder.

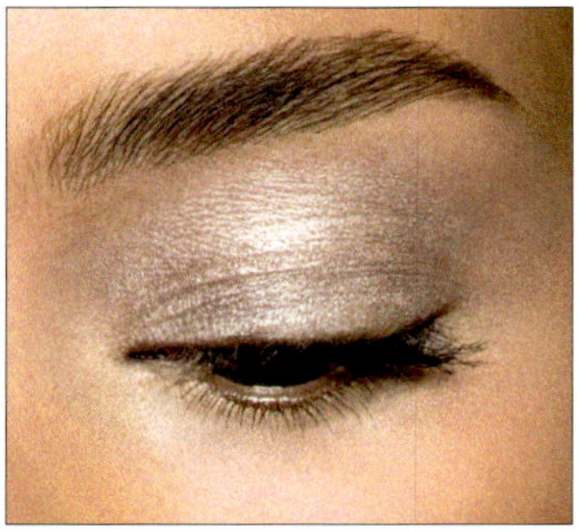

1

Apply cream shadow base or base powder color to hold the color on the eyelid.

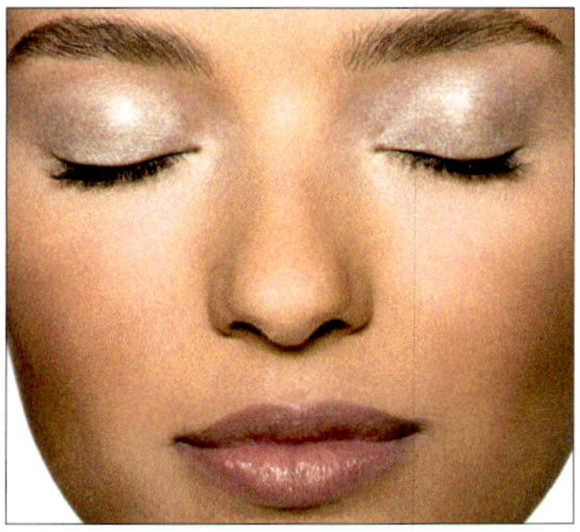

2

Apply cream shadow across the whole lid to three-quarters of the way up.

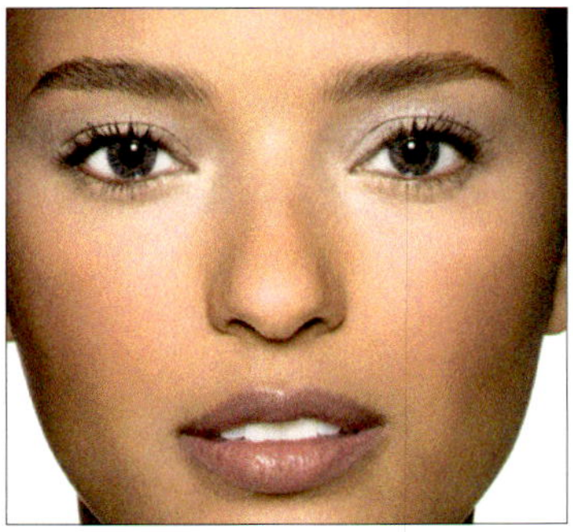

3

Make sure you apply shadow high enough on the lid and layer a second coat to be sure it's dense enough.

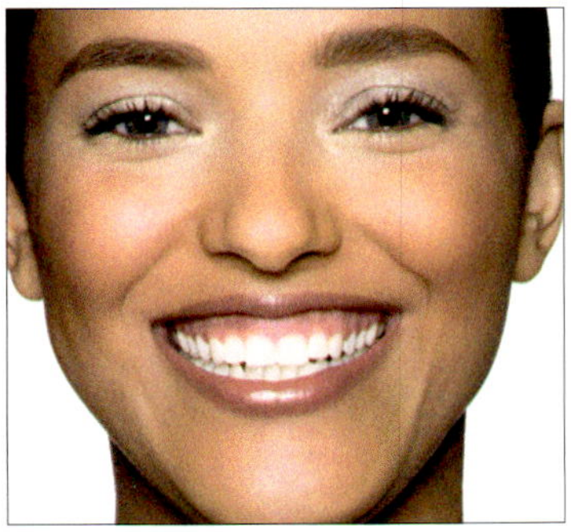

4

Check how the shadow looks. Add more as needed. You can use one or multiple colors.

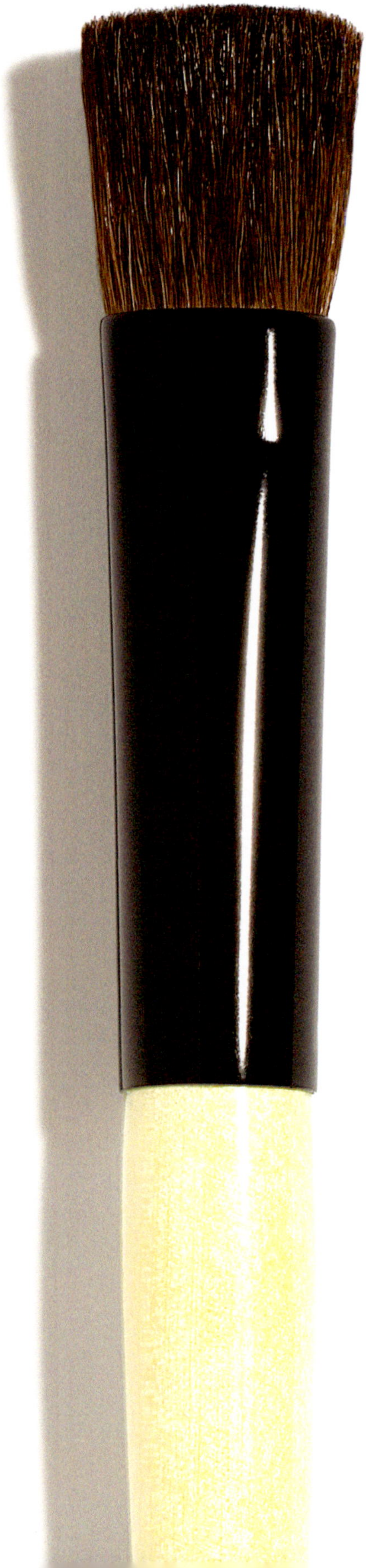

ASIAN EYE SHADOW APPLICATION

Always enhance the eye's natural shape and don't try to change it. It's never appropriate to use a dark color in the crease.

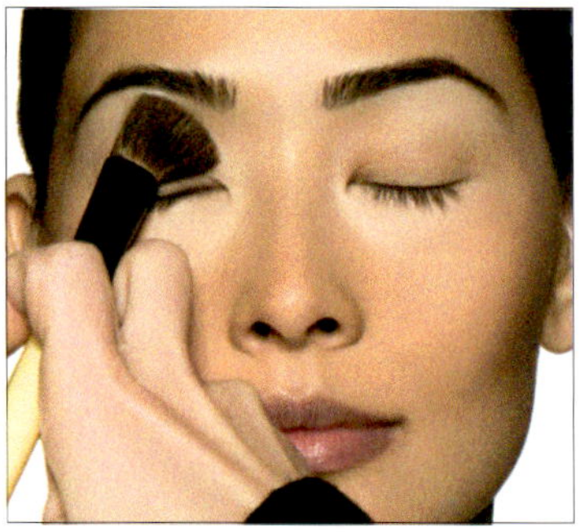

1

With a full shadow brush, apply a light shade (also known as your base color).

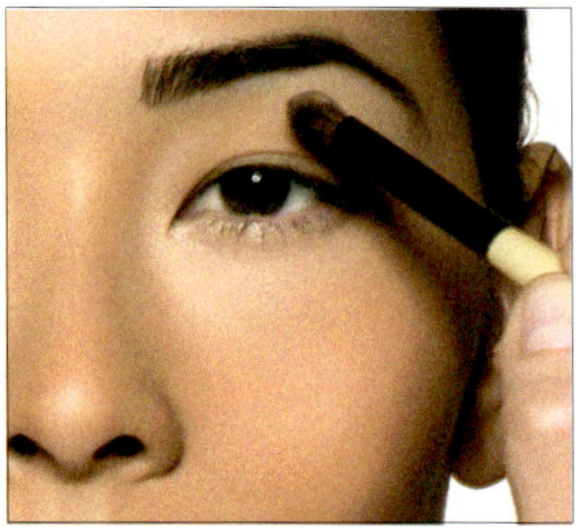

2

Choose medium-tone shadow for the lid and apply it three-quarters of the way up to the brow.

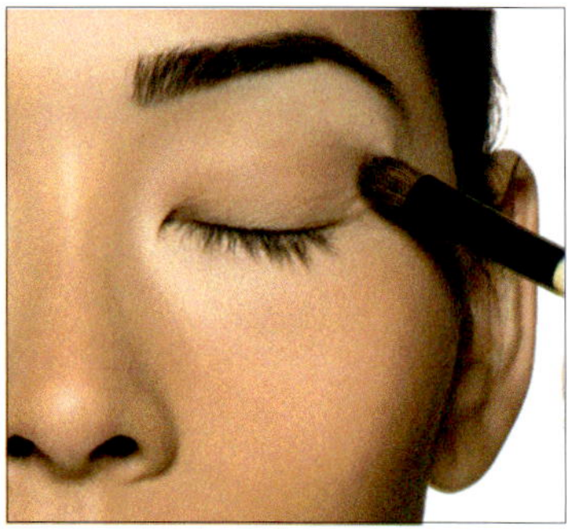

3

Sweep color all the way to the crease, blending as you go up.

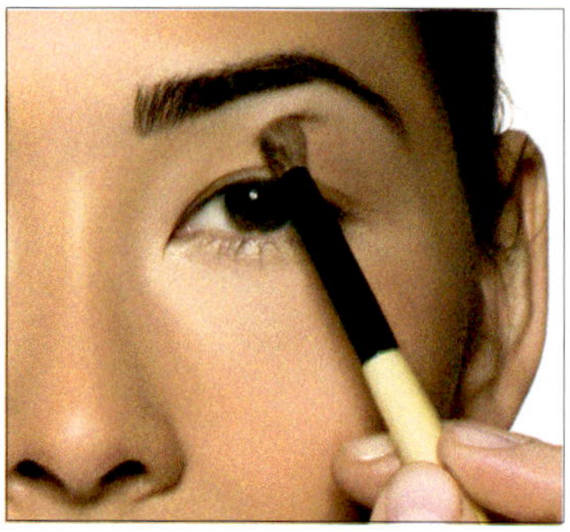

4

Apply a deeper color on top of the first color for density. Blend.

EYELINER

Eyeliner is the ultimate way to define and enhance the eyes. It frames the eyes, makes them appear larger, and really makes them stand out. Liner can also be used to improve the shape of the eyes. Its application needs to be generous enough to be visible when the eyes are open to make the most impact. Many women achieve a beautiful, defined look using liner only on the top lash line. For those who use liner on both top and bottom lash lines, it is important to keep the top thicker than the bottom. To avoid the appearance of tiredness and darkness under the eye, apply a relatively thin or smudged line as close as possible to the lower lash line.

Liner Formulas

There are several eyeliner formulations: powdered shadow, eye pencil, and liquid or gel liner. Each has its advantages and specific application techniques.

SHADOW LINERS are easy to apply, dry or damp, and can be long-lasting if applied correctly. Using shadow liner requires a good eyeliner brush—one that is thin, stiff, and flat, with either a straight or a slightly rounded tip.

EYELINER PENCILS are easy to apply but may smudge. Pencil liners have a creamy consistency that smears if they are not set with either eyeshadow or face powder.

LIQUID, CAKE, AND GEL LINERS are the most difficult to apply, but with practice, you can achieve incredible results. These liners are extremely long-wearing, very precise, and a good choice for creating dramatic looks.

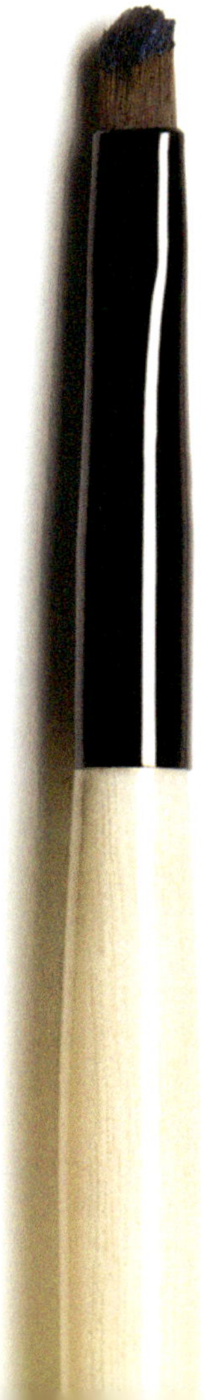

Special Techniques

Dark circles look darker when liner is applied on the lower lash line. Bring concealer up to the lash line, and use only mascara on the lower lashes.

Make eyes look more intense by double lining. Use a dark shadow with a dry eyeliner brush, then repeat with a liquid liner or wet brush using a slightly thinner line. The gradation in depth from the lash line will give a dense look to the lashes. The technique can also be reversed—gel can be softened with shadow.

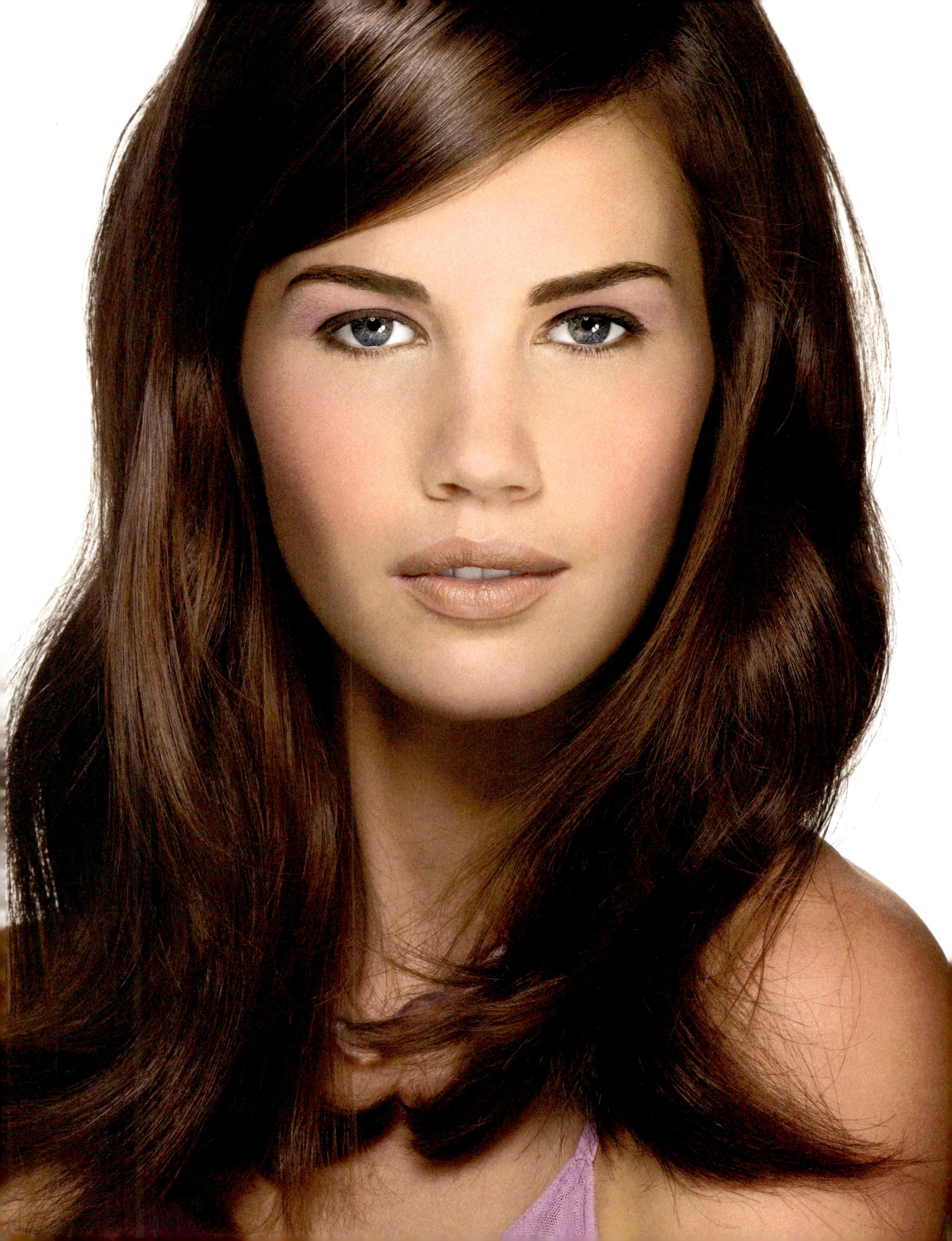

GEL, LIQUID & CAKE LINER APPLICATION

These formulas are the longest lasting. Mastering the techniques for using them will be worthwhile. Always line the whole lid across, with a thicker line at the outer corner, gradually thinning the line toward the inner corner.

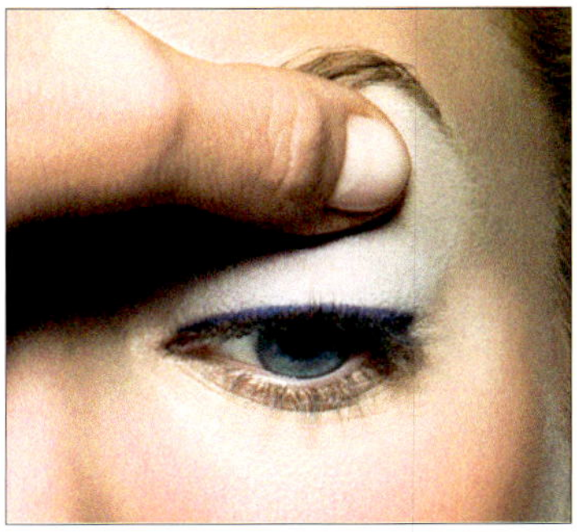

1

Begin lining in the middle of the lash line and move to the outside corner of the eye. Gently lift the lid to get close to the eye.

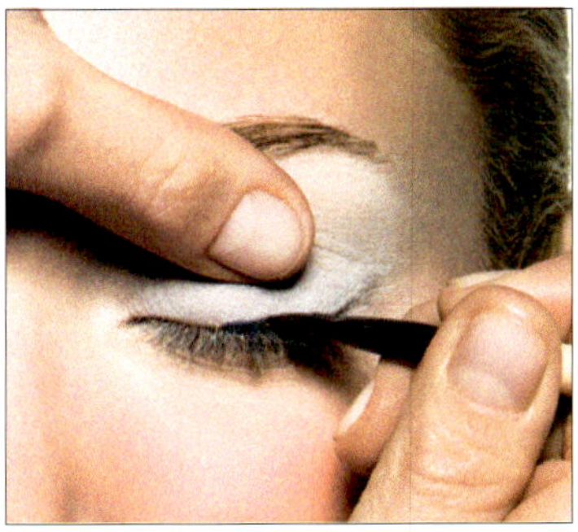

2

Apply the liner in smooth strokes.

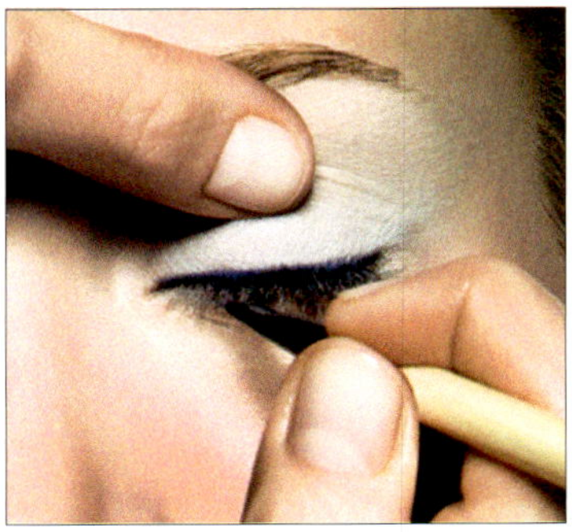

3

Next, apply the liner all the way to the inner corner of eye.

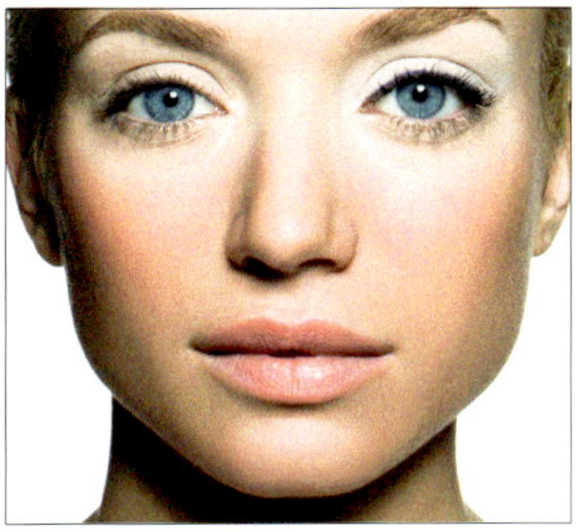

4

See the difference with one eye lined.

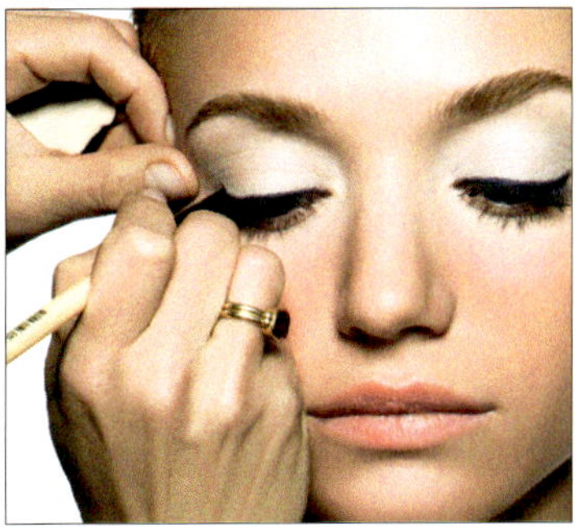

5

Repeat with the other eye.

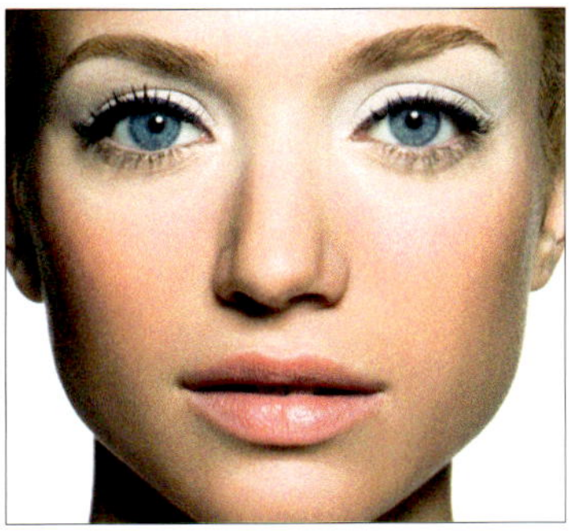

6

Note the difference when both eyes are lined.

Tip

Do not leave space between the eyeliner and the lash line. If, after application, there is a small space, fill it in with the same shade of powdered eye shadow.

PENCIL LINER APPLICATION

Pencils are easy to use but are not long lasting and can smear. Layering powder shadow on top will help with these drawbacks.

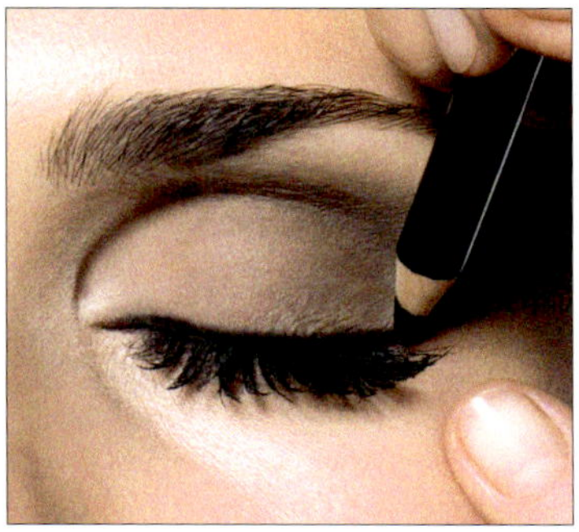

1

Draw the pencil across the lash line and blend gently using a clean finger or brush.

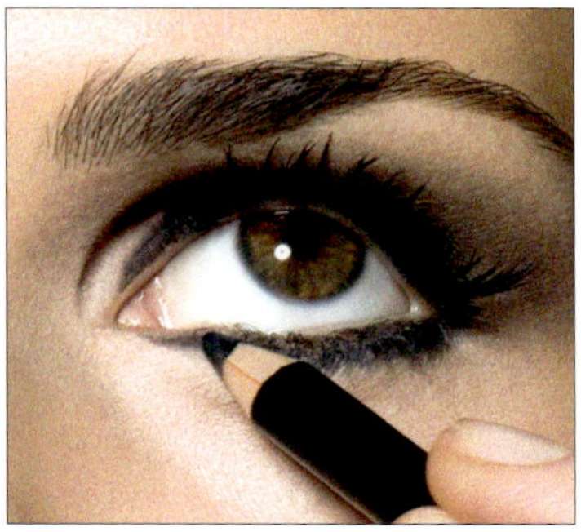

2

Using short feathery strokes can result in a more natural effect.

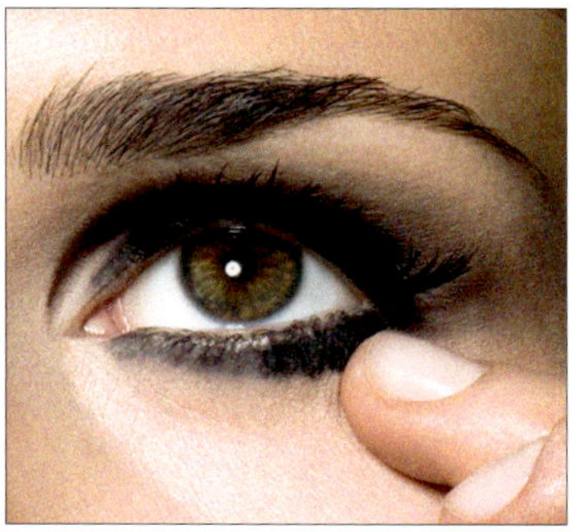

3

To soften, smudge the line using your finger or a brush.

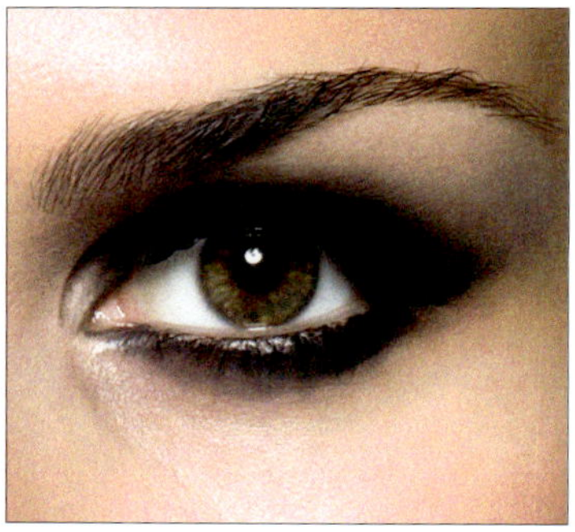

4

To give a pencil line staying power, use a liner brush to sweep a layer of powdered eye shadow in a corresponding shade over the pencil.

Eyeliner Dos & Don'ts

Don't apply liner to the inside rim of the eyelids, except for a theatrical effect or a fashion shoot. You risk infection and injury. And, rather than making the eyes stand out, lining inside the rim actually makes the eyes appear smaller.

Don't line just the bottom of the eye.

Do line all the way across the lids! You can line just the top and not the bottom, but don't line either lid halfway. Lining from the inner corner to the outer corner will help open up the eye.

Do apply liner as close as possible to the lash line, making sure there is no gap. This has the added benefit of making the lashes look fuller and lush.

Do apply liner thinnest at the inner corner of the eye, and thicken it as you move outward. This accentuates the eye's shape and gives the eyes a lift.

Do make the top and bottom lines of liner meet at the inside and outside corners to make the eyes appear larger. Not connecting the lines makes the eyelids appear too round and small.

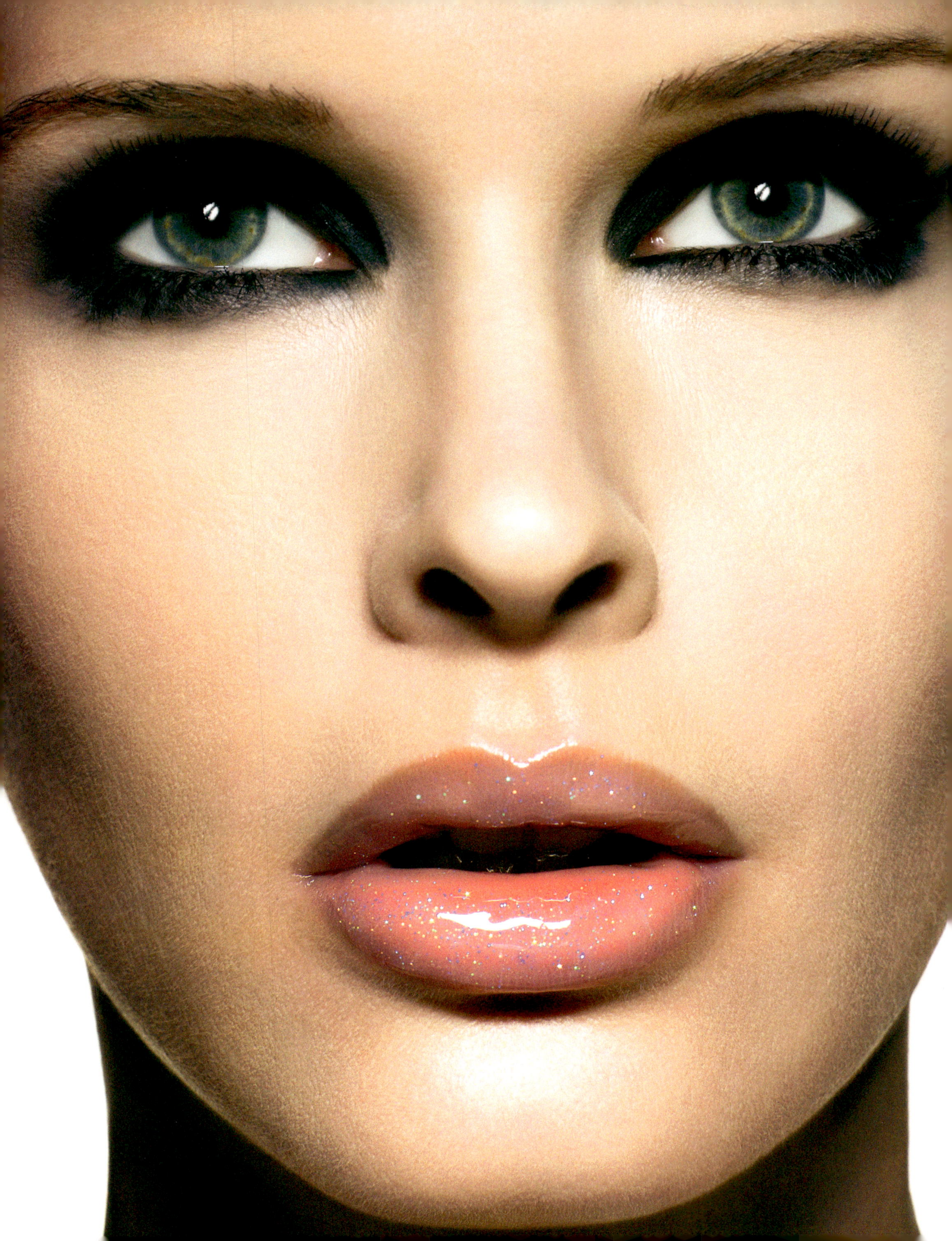

Special Effects

For evening or other special occasions, you may want to use bolder, more dramatic eye-makeup techniques.

Smoky Eyes

Prime the eye area with an all-over white base that will allow the darker colors to blend. Apply a slightly darker shadow on the lower lid, from the lash line up to the crease and use a deeper one in the same color family layered on top. The standard technique described above can be used to line the lower lashes, keeping the application lighter and balanced with the upper eye. Apply a double layer of liner, first using a dry brush and then a gel or pencil. Extend the liner line slightly beyond the outer corners of the eyes. Then reapply the liner a bit heavier and repeat two more times if desired. Always add multiple coats of mascara. Smudge and blend.

Glam Eyes

This look is great for New Year's Eve or the Oscars. Over a white base, layer cool colors, such as gray and slate. Build the depth of the color gradually, from the lash line to the crease. Finish with a strong liner application along the top lash line only, ending in an upward-sweeping point. Sweep a metallic or shimmery color over the lid layered from medium to dark. Finish with false lashes or three to four coats of black mascara.

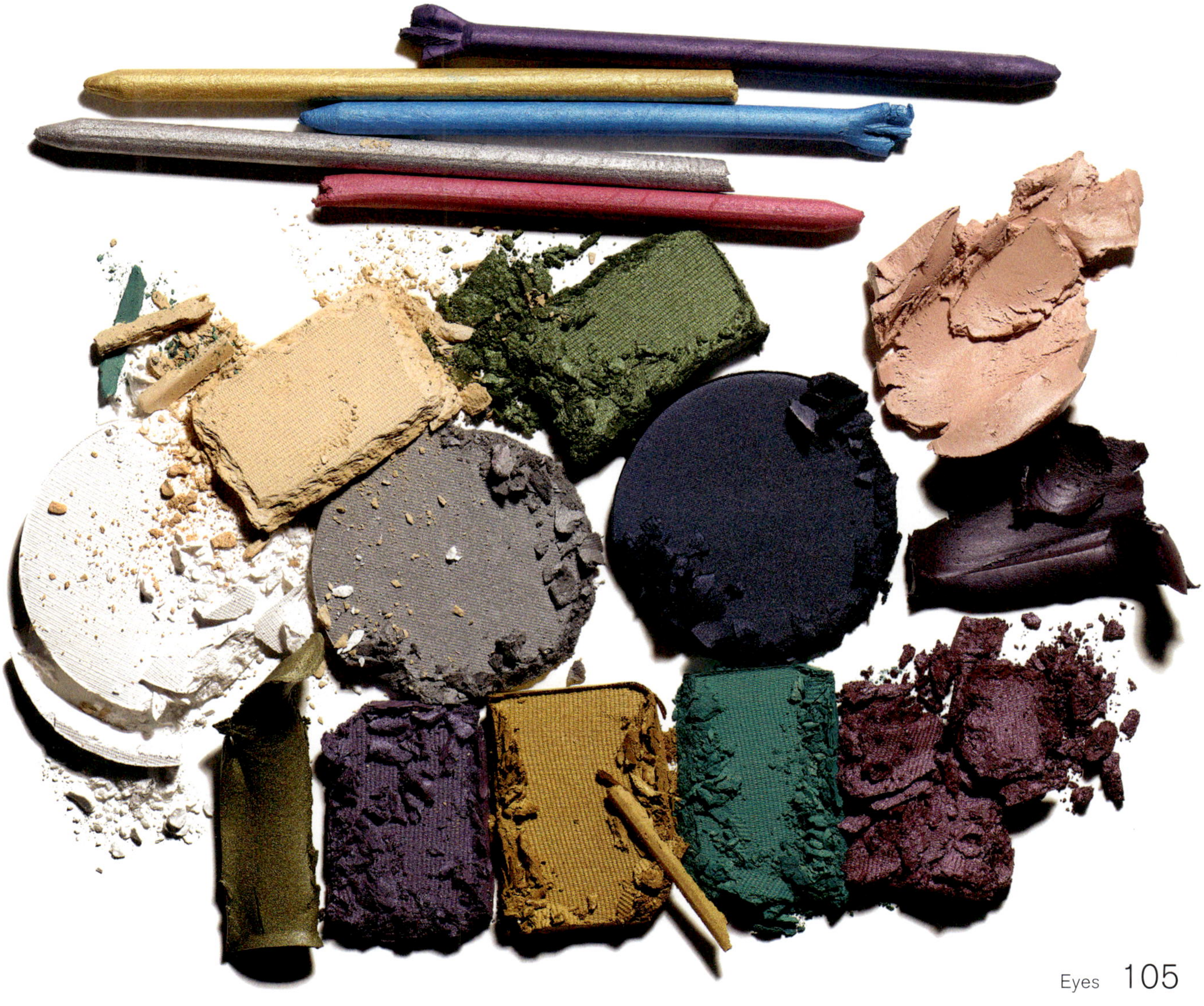

SMOKY EYE APPLICATION

A smoky eye is the most dramatic look for evening—it's pretty and sexy. Remember to keep layering the color and continue to check until you like the look.

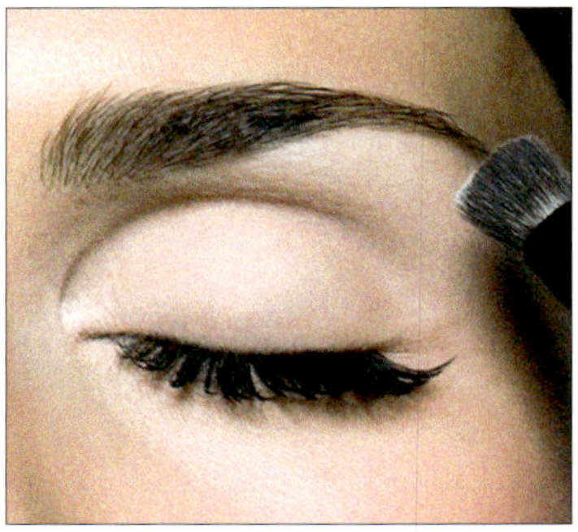

1

Start with white shadow on the entire lid.

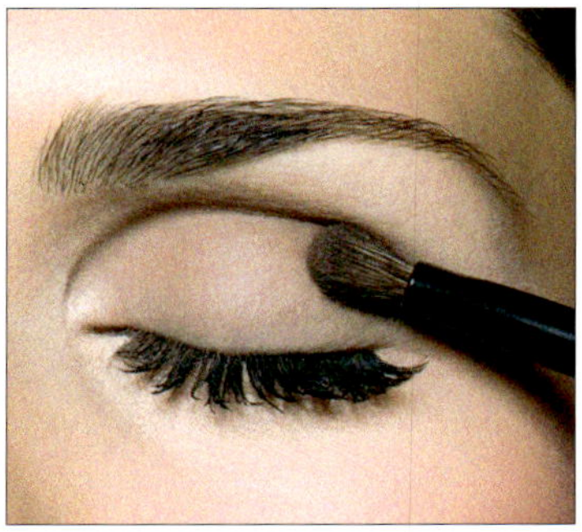

2

Choose a medium, smoky color for the lower lid. Apply it three-quarters of the way up.

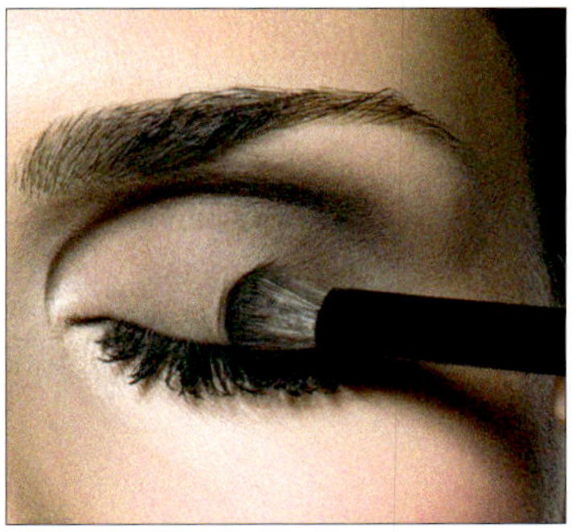

3

Continue to layer the color to make it darker. Add a deeper color on top and in the crease to intensify the look.

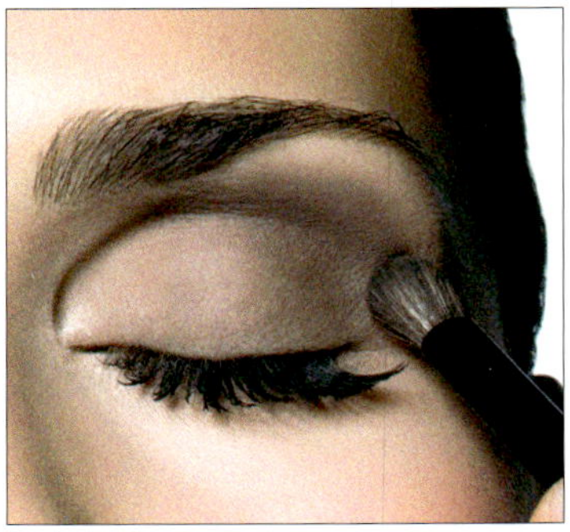

4

Concentrate on the crease. Continue to layer the shadow deeply enough to create a dramatic effect.

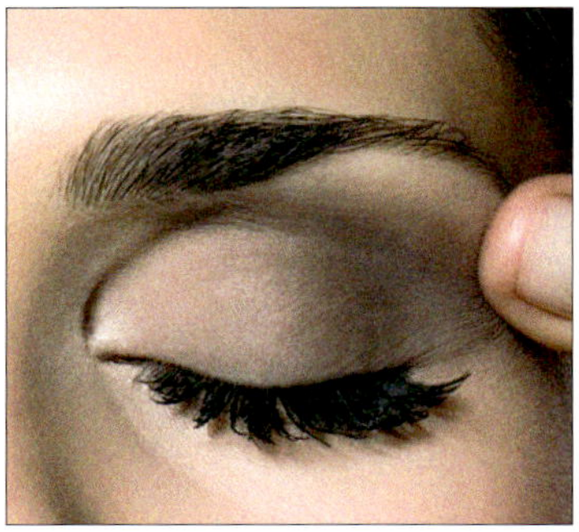

5

Use your finger to soften the shadow.

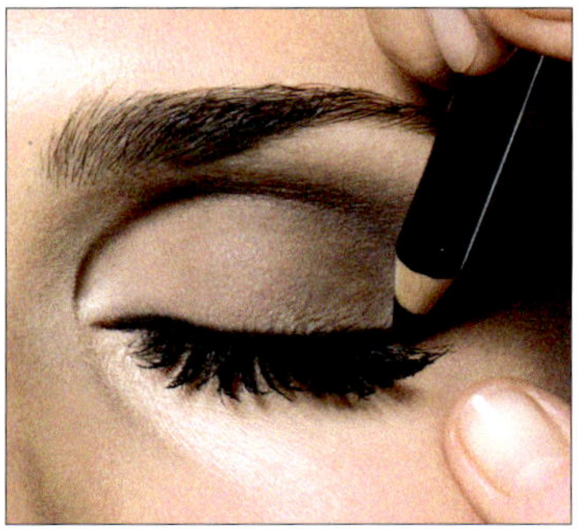

6

Start at the outside corner, using pencil or dark shadow or liner.

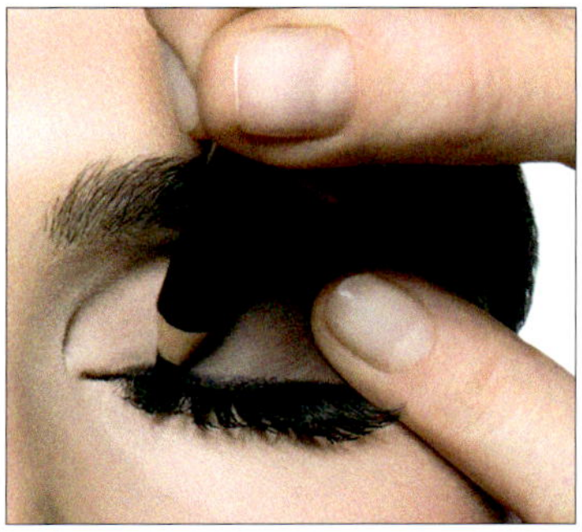

7

Apply in smooth strokes to the inner corner of the eyelid.

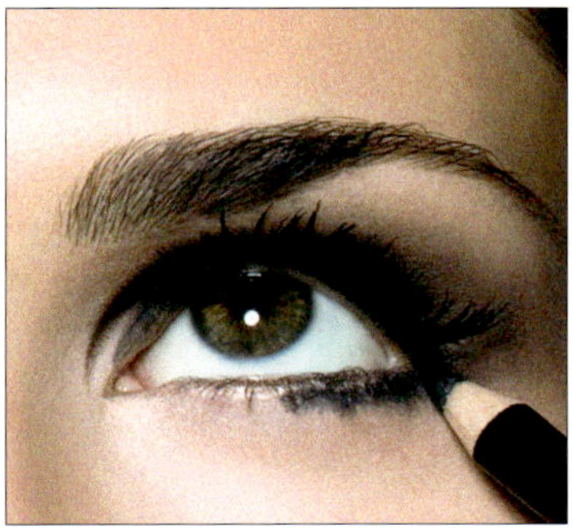

8

Line underneath the eye beginning at the outside corner, moving toward the inner corner.

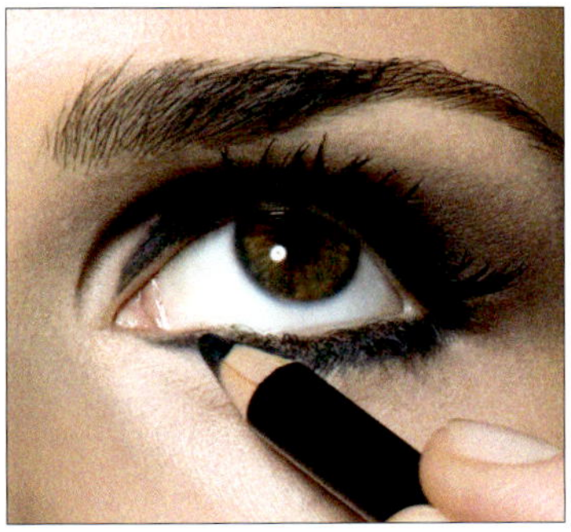

9

Line as close to the lashes as possible.

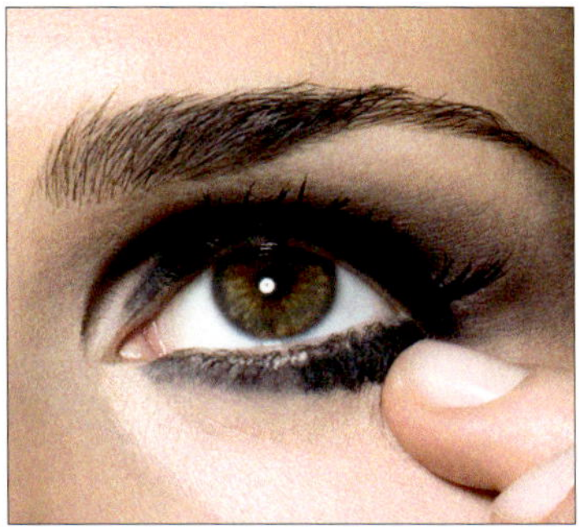

10

Soften the line using a clean finger or Q-tip.

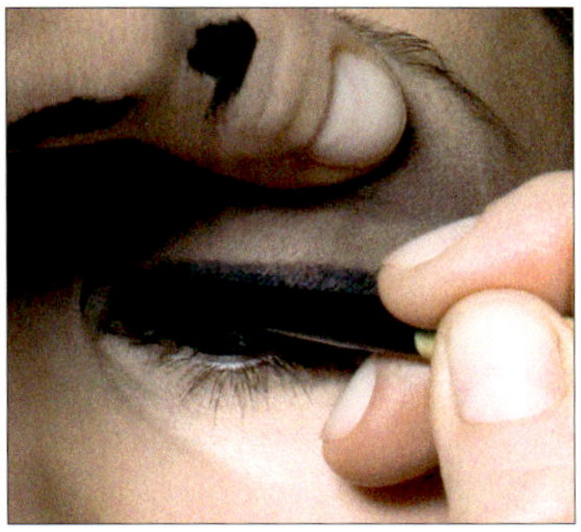

11

To give the pencil line staying power, use a liner brush to sweep a layer of eye shadow over the pencil.

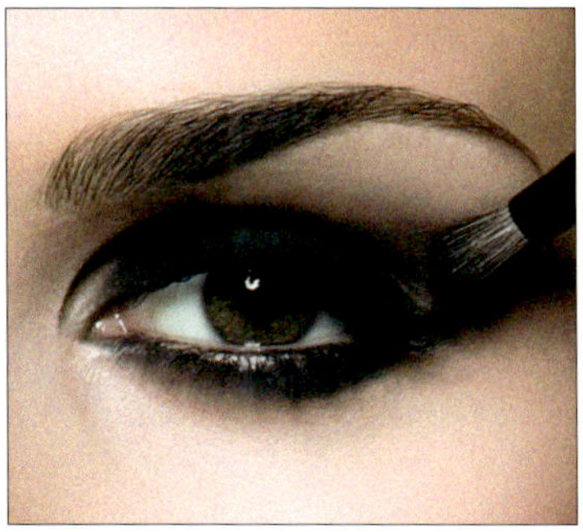

12

Smudge the line to create a smoky look, somewhere between liner and shadow. The liner can be thickened.

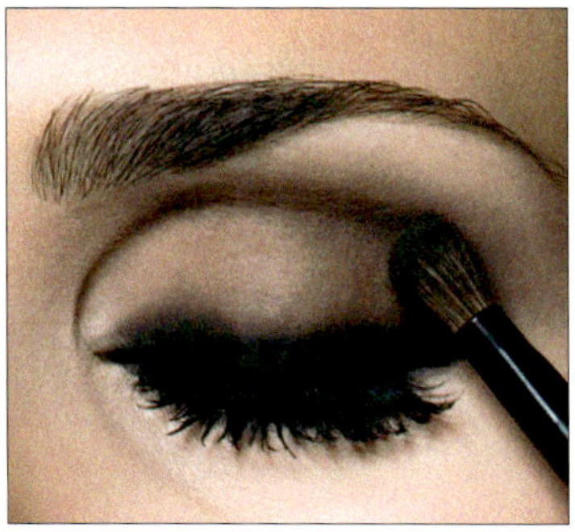

13

Reapply to add more definition. Continue layering and checking for the effect you desire.

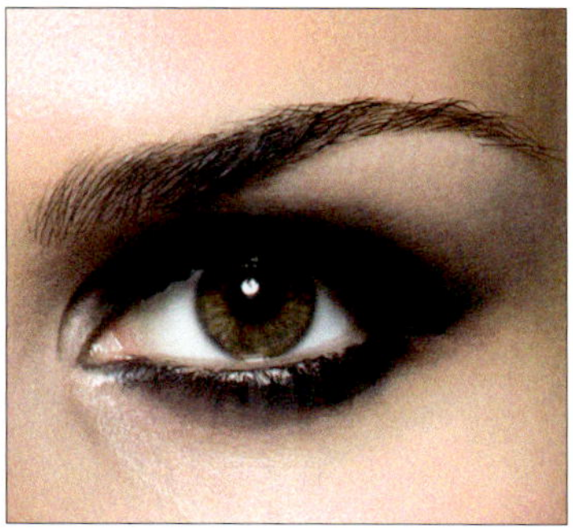

14

Final smoky eye.

For a more dramatic look, adjust your lip color.

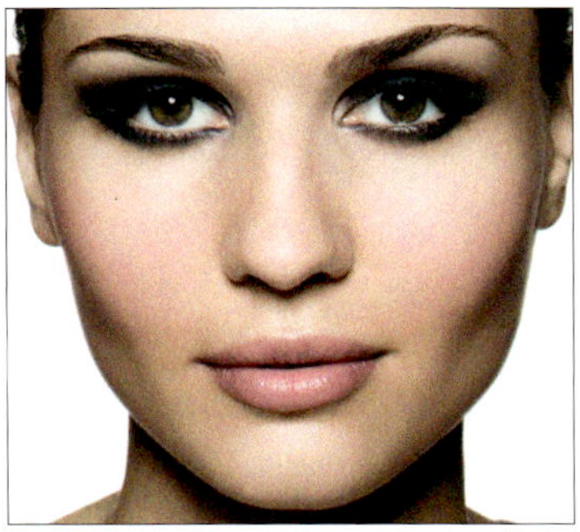

Smoky eyes with pale lip color.

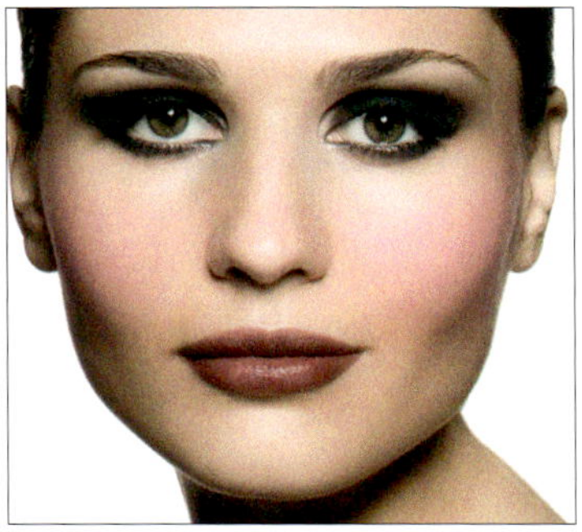

Smoky eyes with medium lip color.

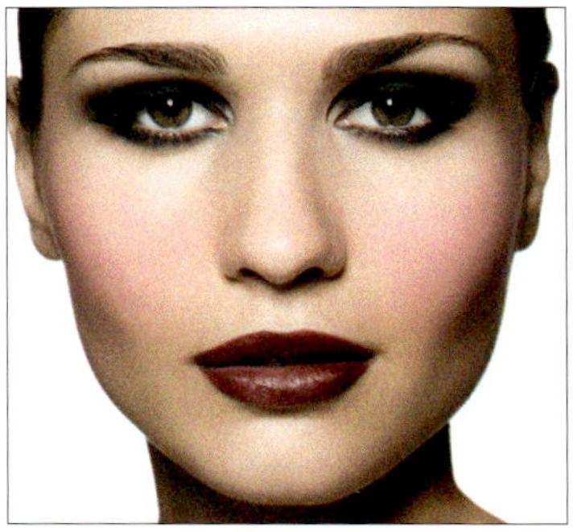

Dramatic look with smoky eyes and dark lipstick.

ASIAN LINER APPLICATION

For Asian women, lining the eyes is a very important step in making the eyes stand out.

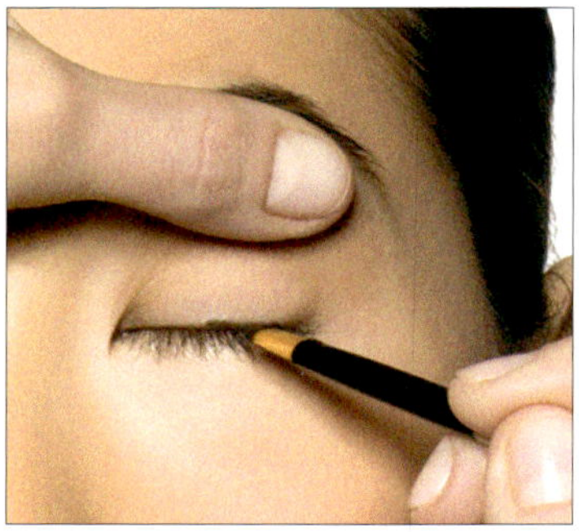

1

Gently pull the eyelid and start in the middle.

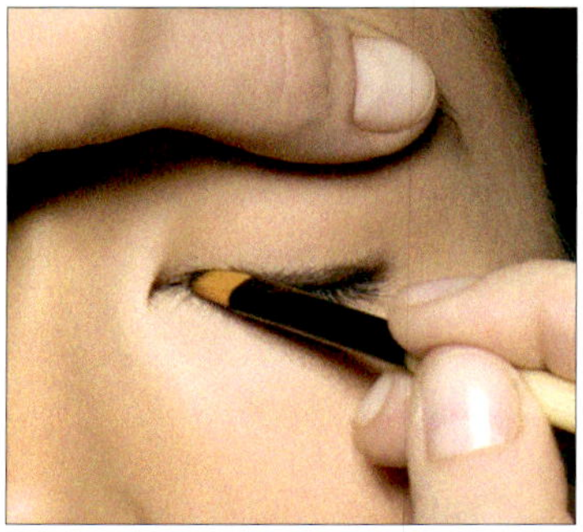

2

Go in close to the lashes.

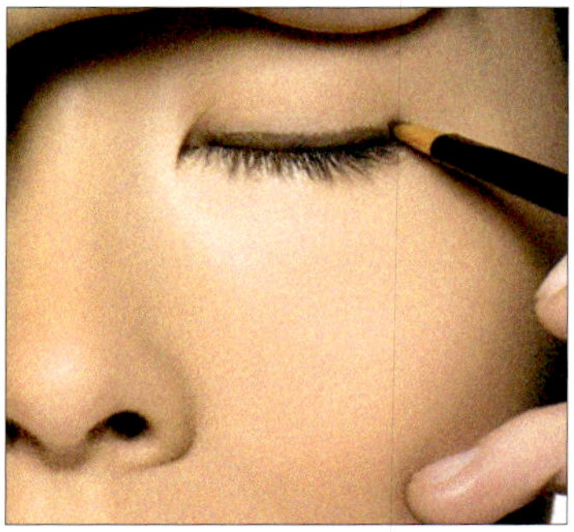

3

Extend the line all the way across.

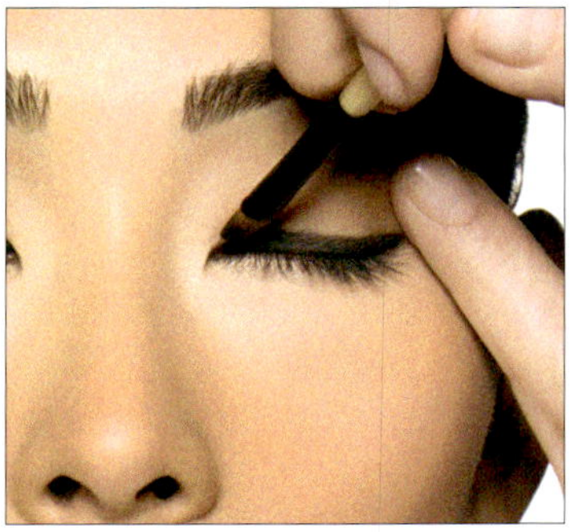

4

Reapply to make the line thicker.

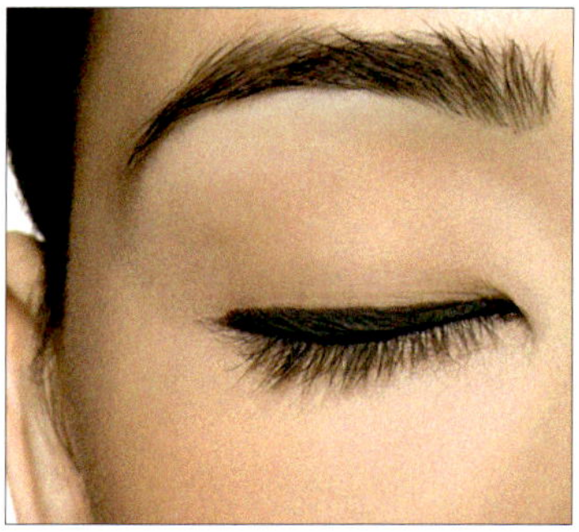

5

Repeat the steps on the other eye.

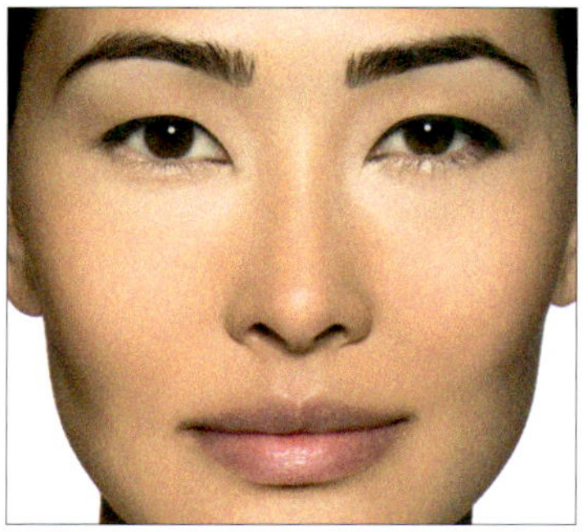

6

Lined eyes.

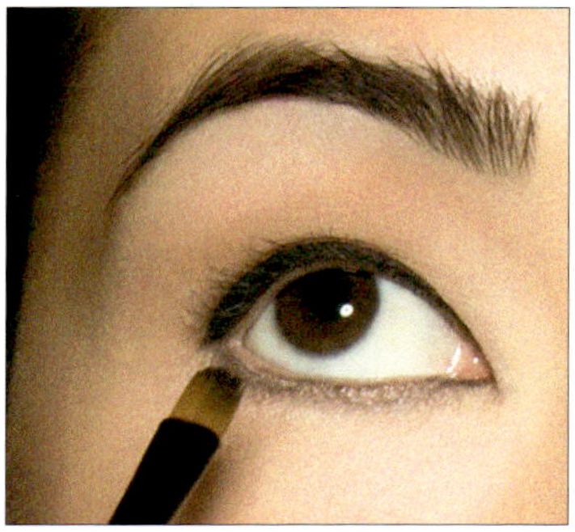

Optional:

If you choose to, line under the eye. Asian eyes look best with a very soft shadow line.

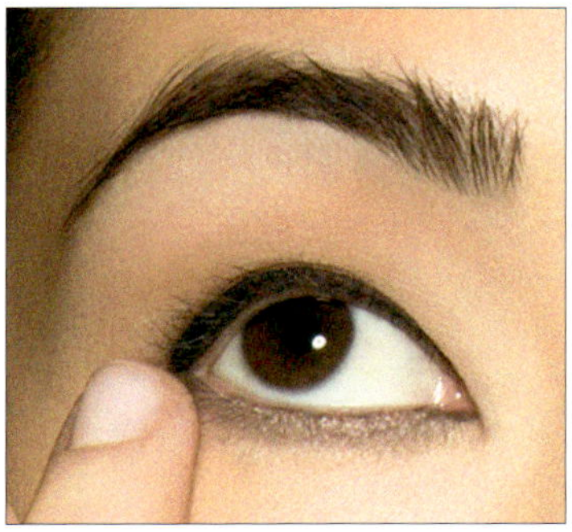

Blend the liner with your fingers.

ASIAN DRAMATIC LINER APPLICATION

It's important to check the result of the eyelining when the eyes are open. You need to make the lines thick enough to show.

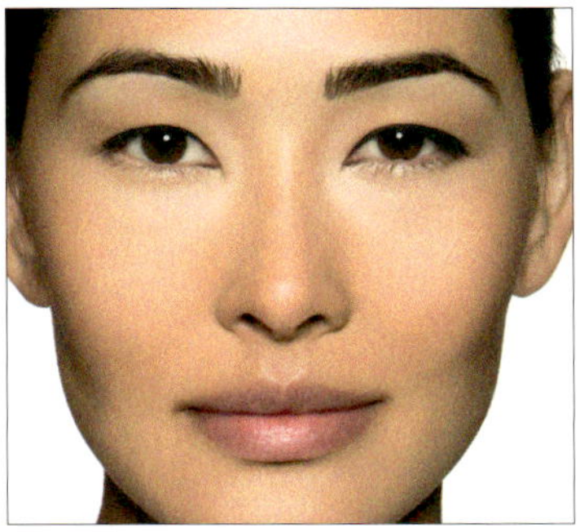

1

Simple eyeliner.

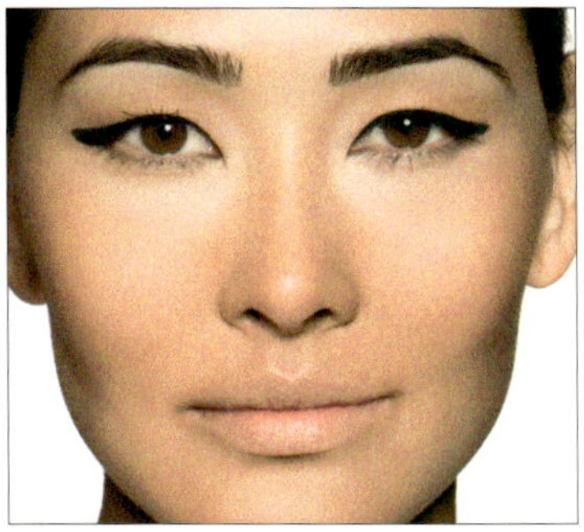

2

For more drama, make the line thicker.

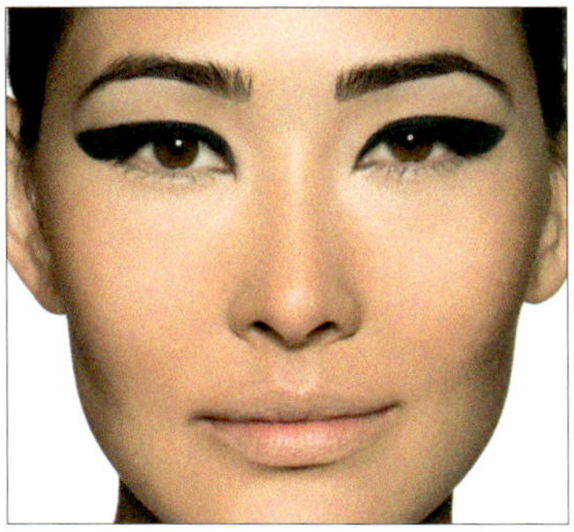

3

And thicker.

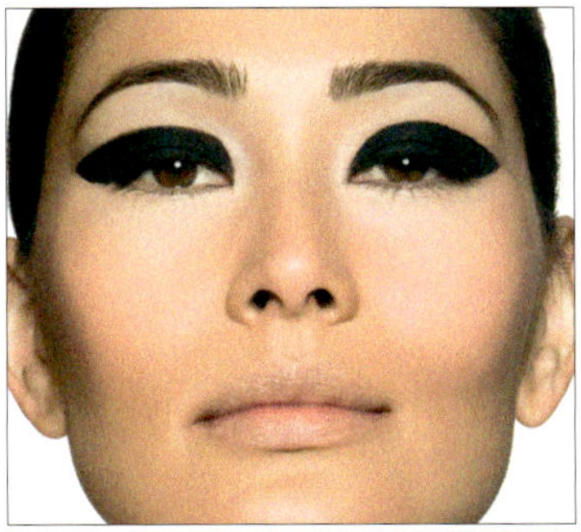

4

Or go way out.

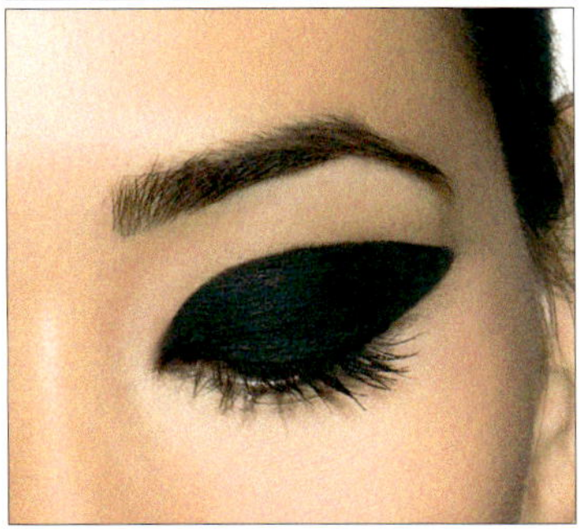

5

Make the line thicker along the lash line and see how far you want to go.

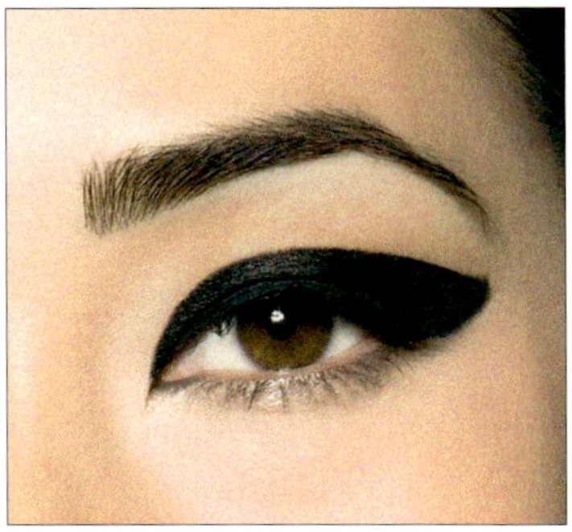

6

If you use strong eyeliner, skip the eye shadow in the crease.

Permanent Solution?

Just say no to tattooed liner. It never looks natural, and the color usually fades to an ashy gray or blue color over time. Deep brown eyeliner can freshen and help the line look natural again.

EYELASHES

Lashes open up and emphasize the eyes. Most lashes are transformed with a sweep of mascara and the use of an eyelash curler. Black mascara is always my first choice. For women with very fair coloring or those who have naturally blond lashes, mascara is a must. Product choices include mascara, curlers, and false lashes.

Formulas

THICKENING MASCARA is designed to make lashes appear fuller. To avoid clumping, wipe the wand before use; following application, the lashes can be separated with a lash comb, or separate them as you go.

LENGTHENING MASCARA is a thinner formula than the thickening product, so it lengthens lashes in a way that looks natural.

WATERPROOF MASCARA is great to use on those occasions when you anticipate tears or sweat, or in humid climates. The product can be removed only with an eye makeup remover specially formulated for waterproof products.

COLORED MASCARAS are fun for the very young and for making theatrical or fashion statements. Henna-colored mascara can work for those with light red hair.

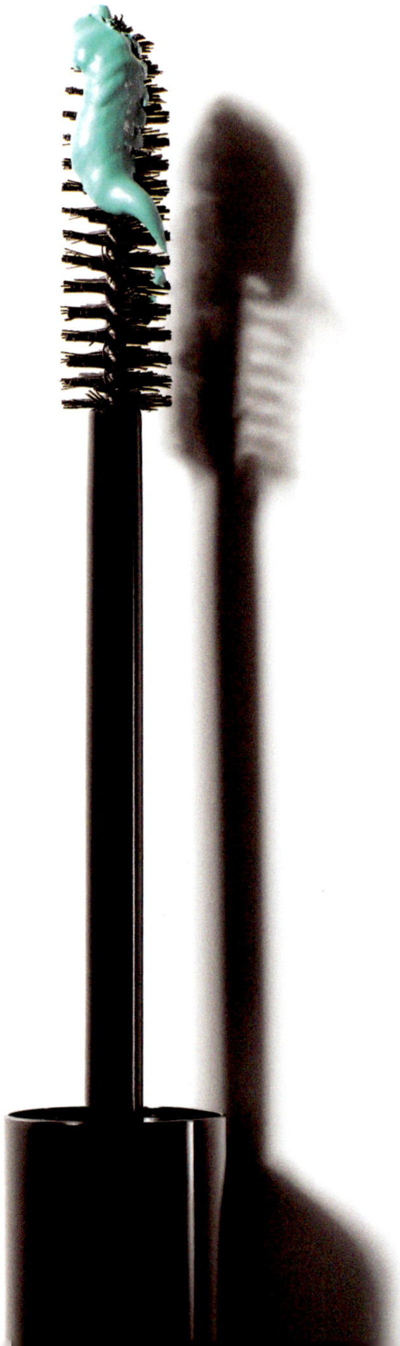

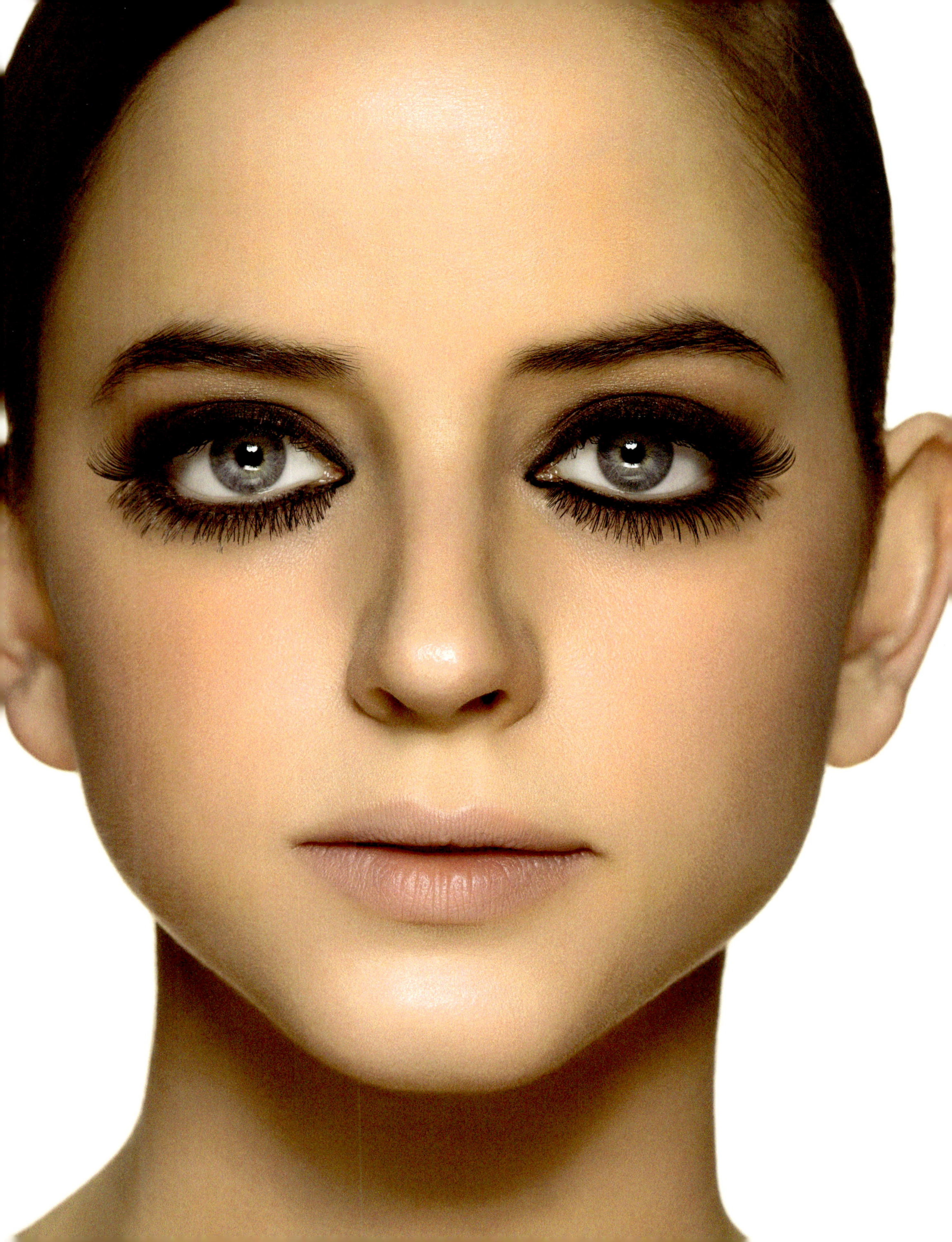

EYELASH CURLING

Start with clean lashes. Gently lift the lid, hold the curler in front, and move the arm up to curl lashes. Hold for five to ten seconds.

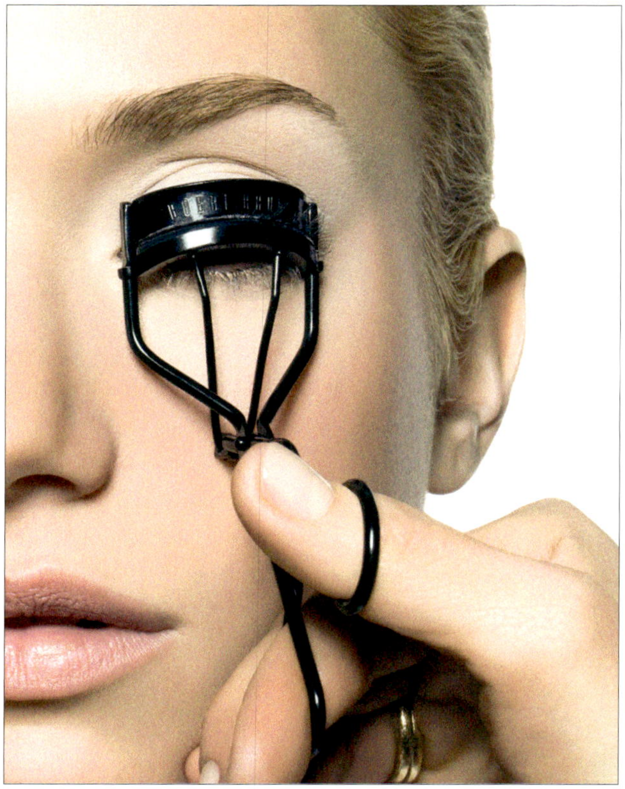

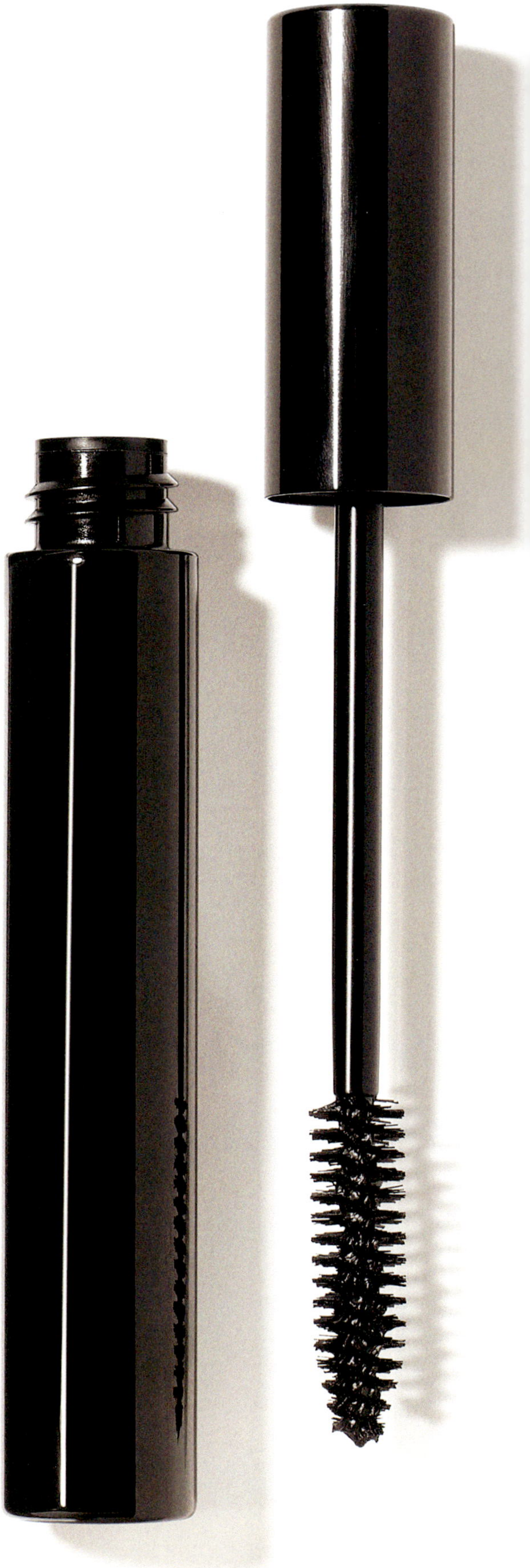

Tips

You can also curl lashes by gently pressing them up with your fingers as the mascara dries.

The blackest of black mascara makes eyes stand out the most.

MASCARA APPLICATION

When applied properly, mascara will both define your eyes and make them stand out. Remember, you'll need two to three coats for impact.

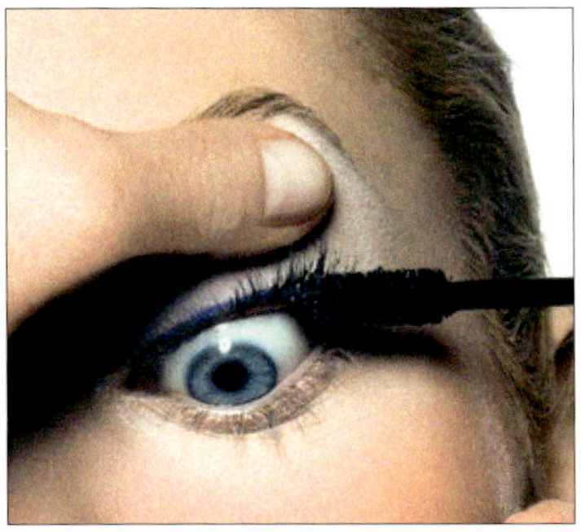

1

Wipe the tip of the wand. Gently lift the lid. Looking down, begin at the outside of the eye.

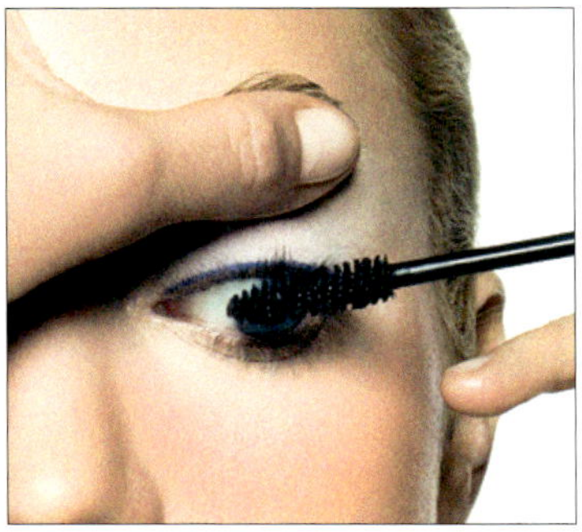

2

Move the wand in close to the nose.

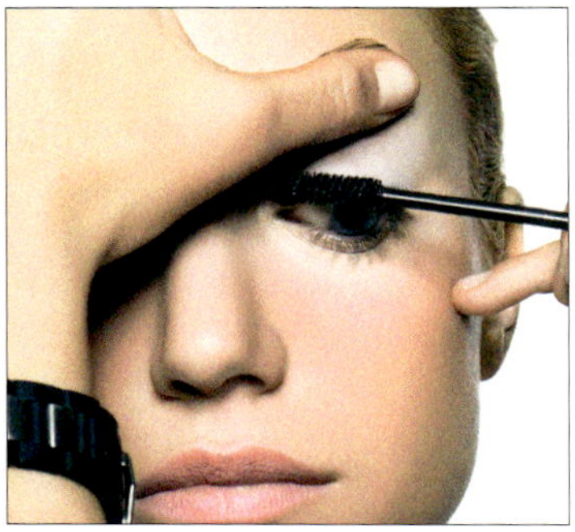

3

Be sure to apply mascara close to the base of the lashes.

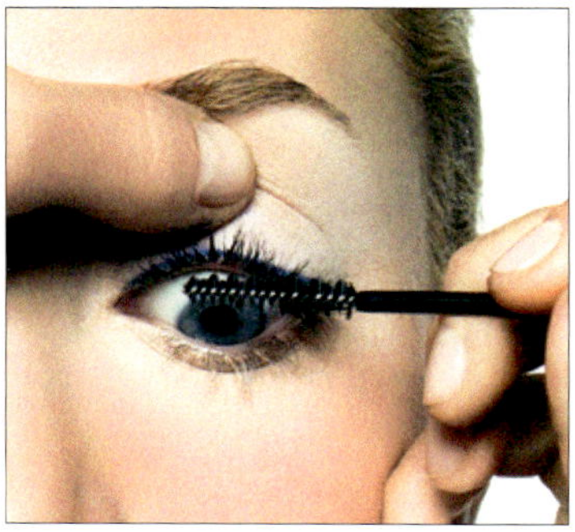

4

Separate the lashes as you go along.

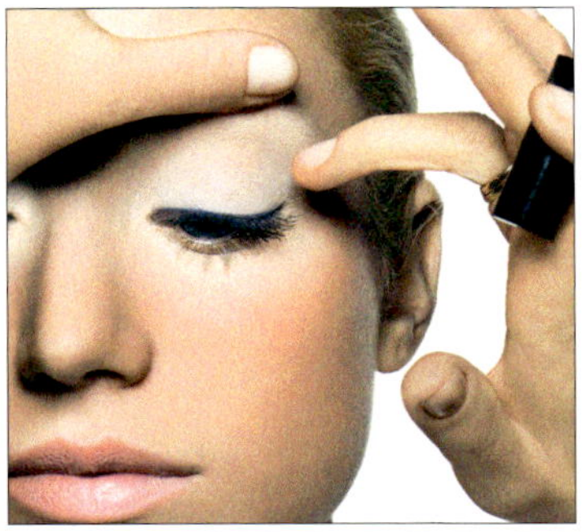

5

If you smudge the mascara, wipe it instantly before it dries.

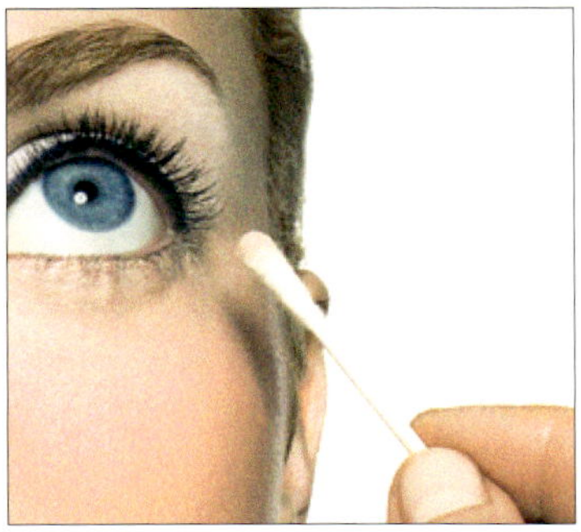

6

If mascara dries on your skin, use a Q-tip to clean it up with a bit of non-oily makeup remover.

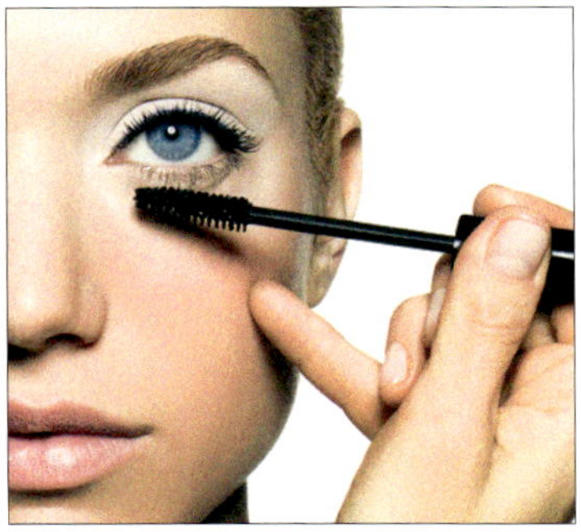

7

Wait a few seconds before beginning the lower lashes. Apply mascara lightly to the lower lashes.

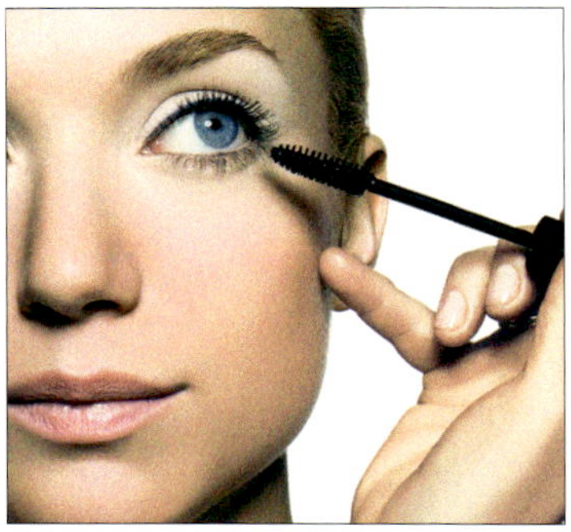

8

Turn the brush at an angle to get all the lashes.

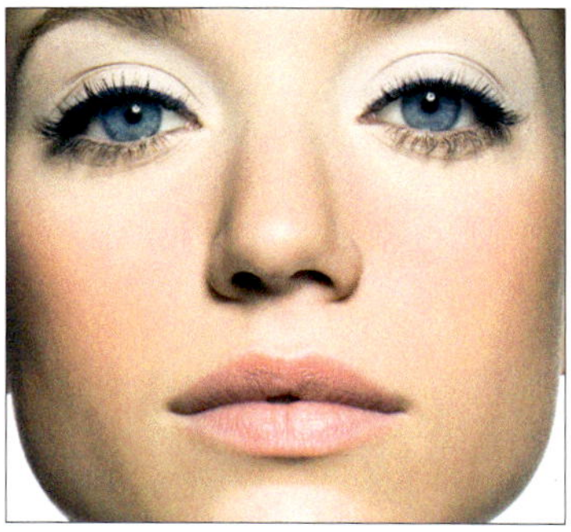

9

The finished product.

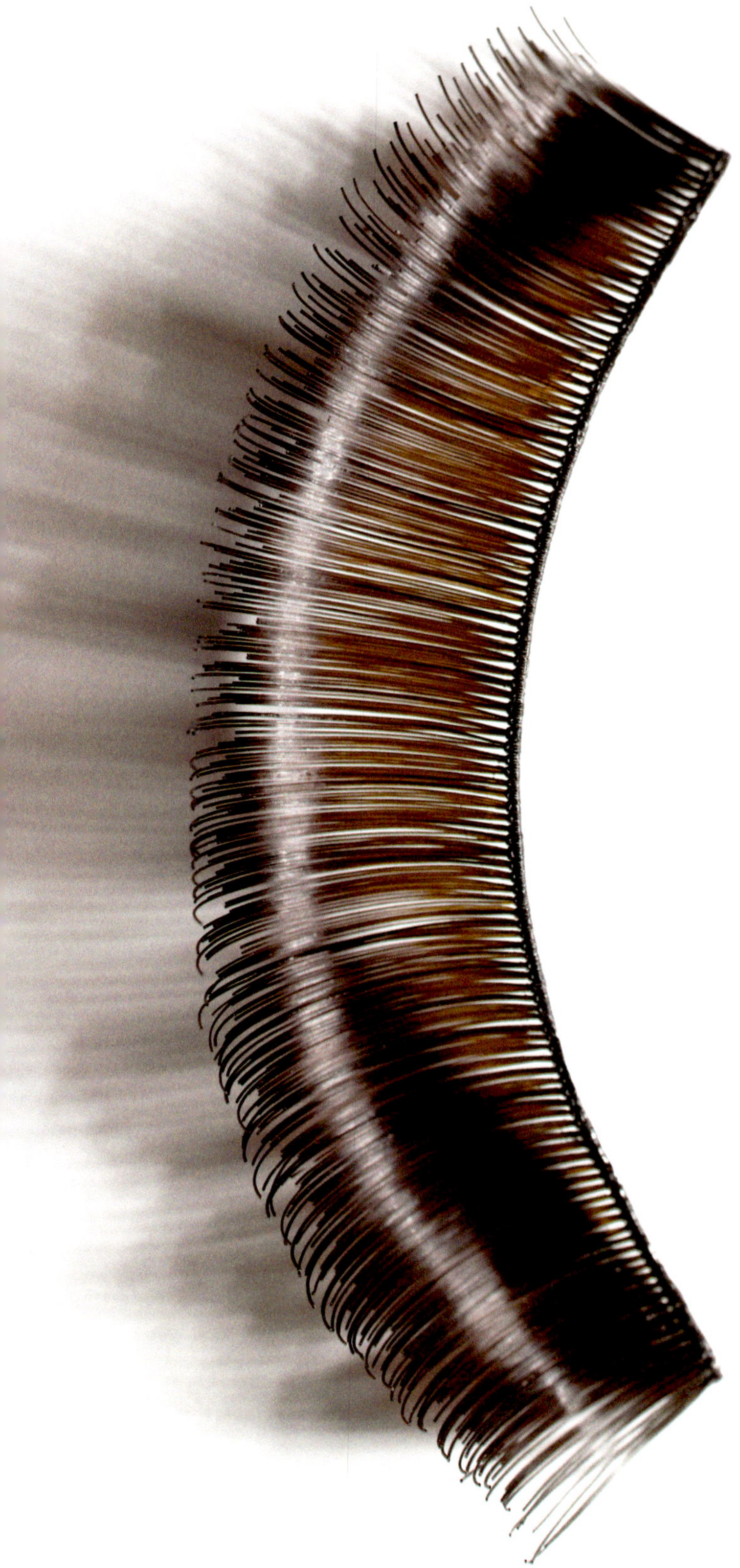

False Eyelashes

False eyelashes are used to create a more dramatic-looking eye and for special effects. Lashes can be applied individually, in a small section, or in a full band. Eyelash glue comes in white, clear, and black. I prefer black as it blends into the lash line.

Eye Makeup Removers

Eye makeup removers are available in liquid, lotion, and cream formulations. Find a product that thoroughly removes your eye makeup without causing any irritation or stinging. Generally, a non-oily product will remove makeup quickly and easily. However, when using waterproof makeup, oil-based removers are the most effective. Place a nickel-size amount of the product on a cotton ball, and gently press through the eye area to dissolve the makeup. If needed, repeat this process until the cotton ball comes away clean.

Troubleshooting: Eyelashes

There are many effective ways to create the illusion of lashes without false eyelashes.

Sparse eyelashes
For those with sparse lashes, try smudging dark shadow at the lash line with a liner brush and then applying two thin coats of mascara.

Pale lashes
Very light colored lashes sometimes don't look natural with black or very dark mascara. Try light brown or henna-colored mascara for a natural look.

No lashes
When lashes have been lost due to alopecia or chemotherapy, a double application of powder shadow in a smoky shade helps create the illusion of lashes. First, use a damp brush and powder shadow to line the lid close to the lash line, and then smudge the dry shadow from the lashes upward.

FALSE EYELASHES APPLICATION

This takes time, patience, and practice. Many women go to a professional to have them applied.

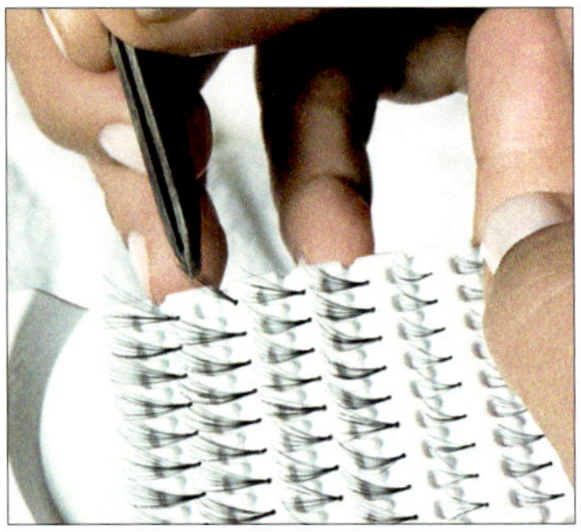

1

Use a lash tweezer to pick up a lash. Begin with small lashes.

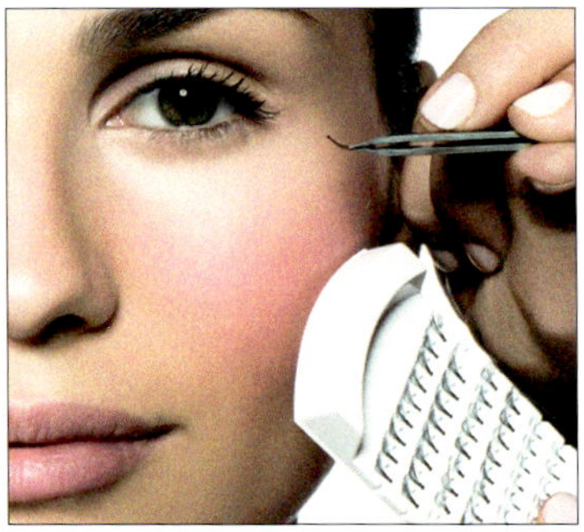

2

After dipping the lash in glue (use dark glue instead of clear) give it a few seconds to air dry partially.

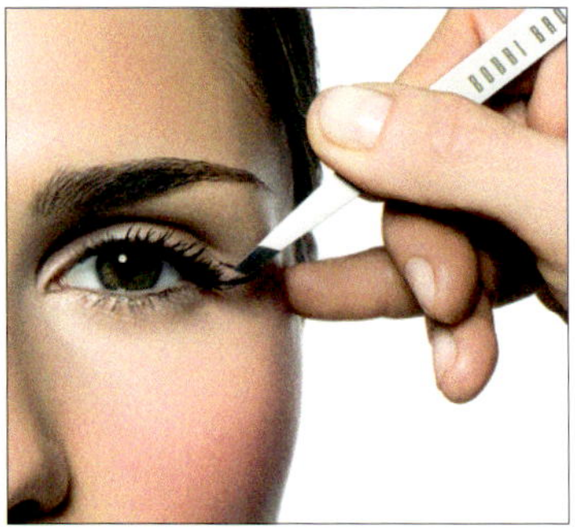

3

Start at the outside of the eye.

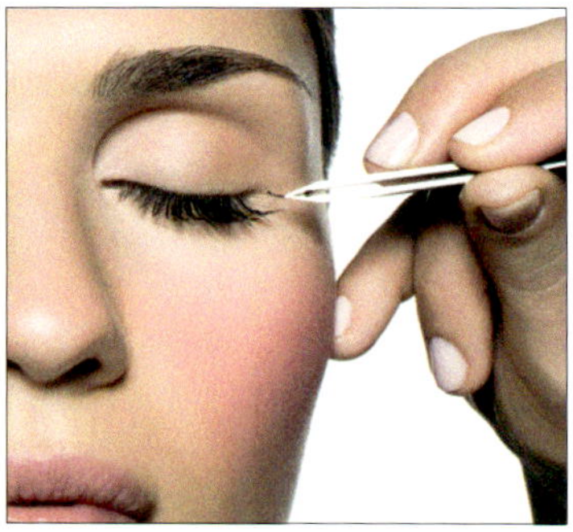

4

Close your eye to continue the application.

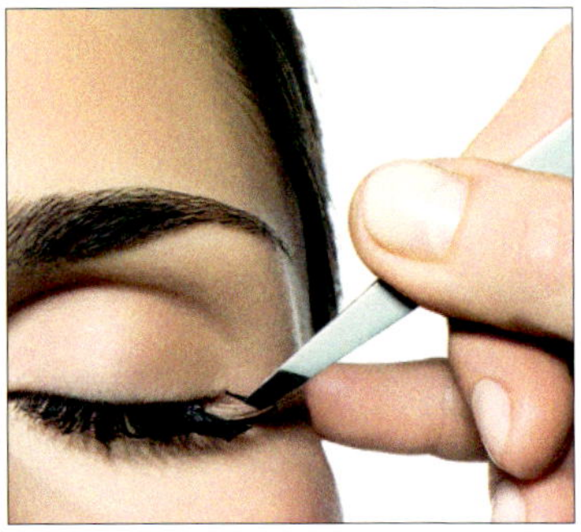

5

Gently build the lashes toward the center, using five to ten lashes.

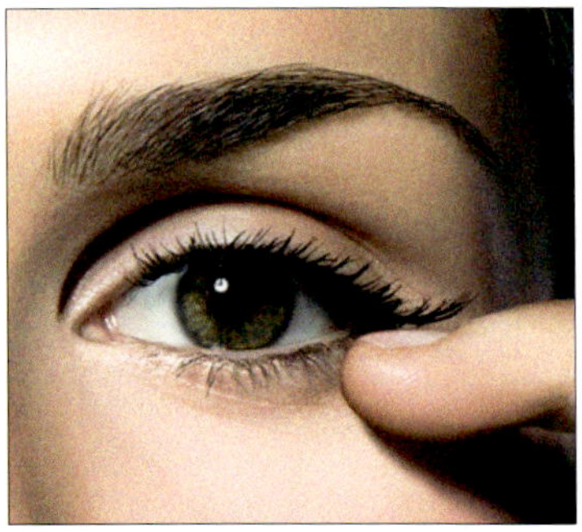

6

Use your finger to hold each lash until it dries.

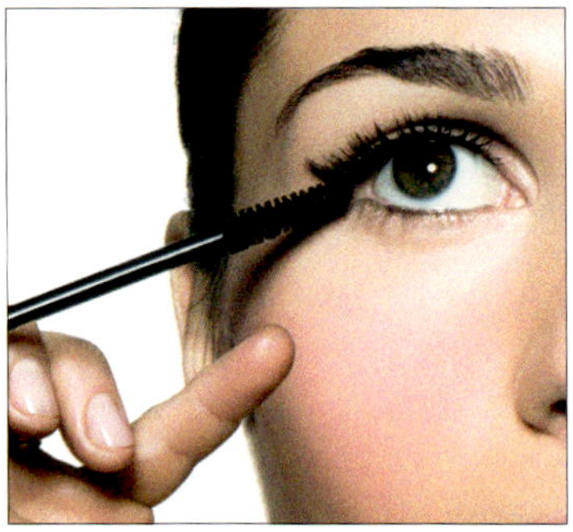

7

After the glue dries, apply mascara.

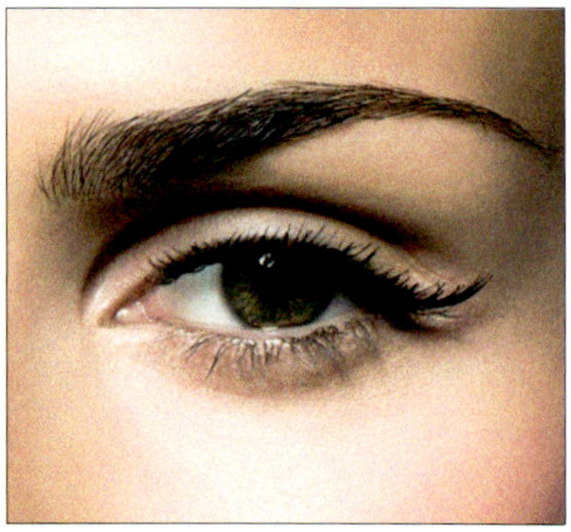

8

The finished product.

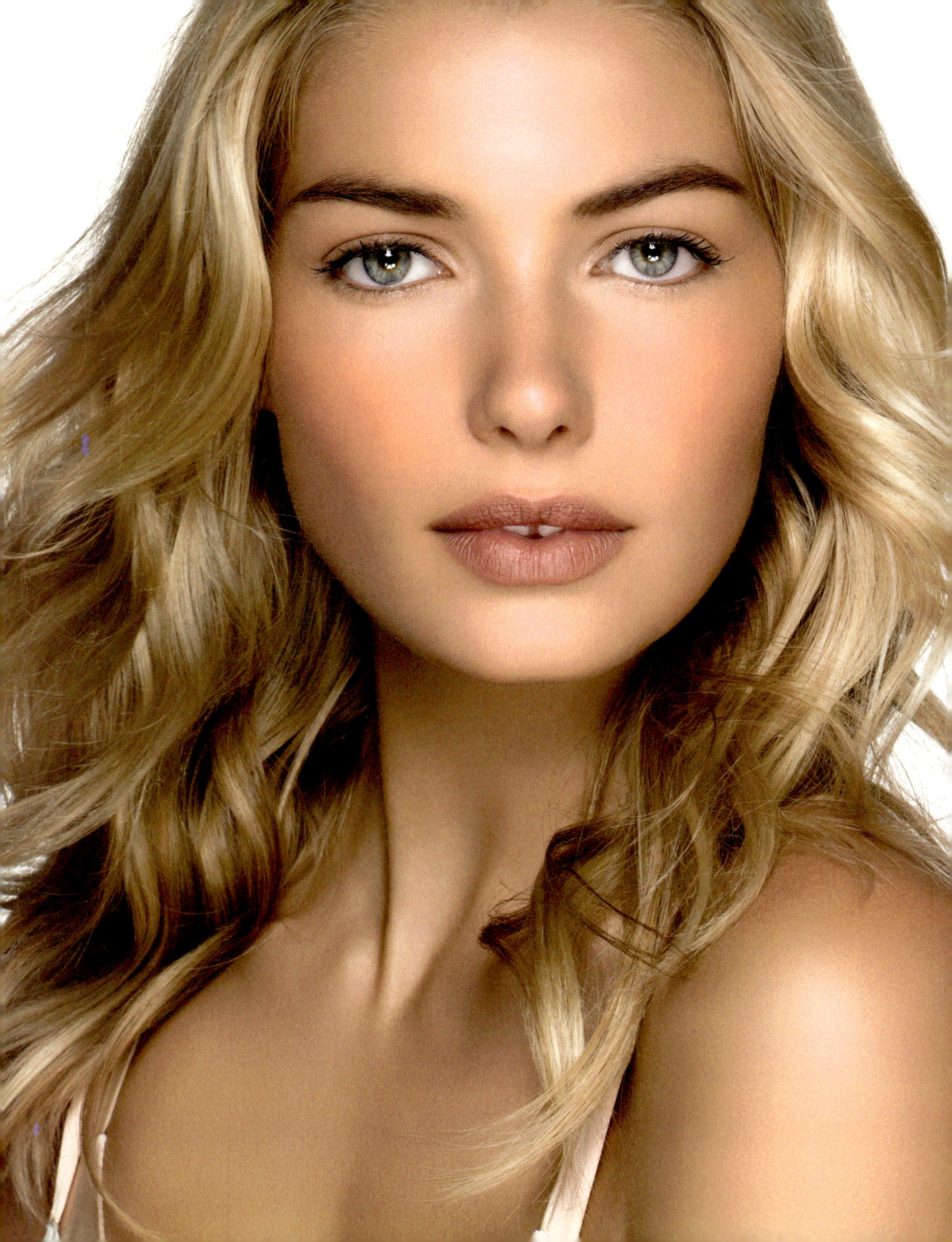

Chapter 7

TEN-STEP GUIDE TO PERFECT MAKEUP

Makeup is simple. When you know how to apply it and have an organized makeup drawer, it should take only five to ten minutes. **Practice is the key.**

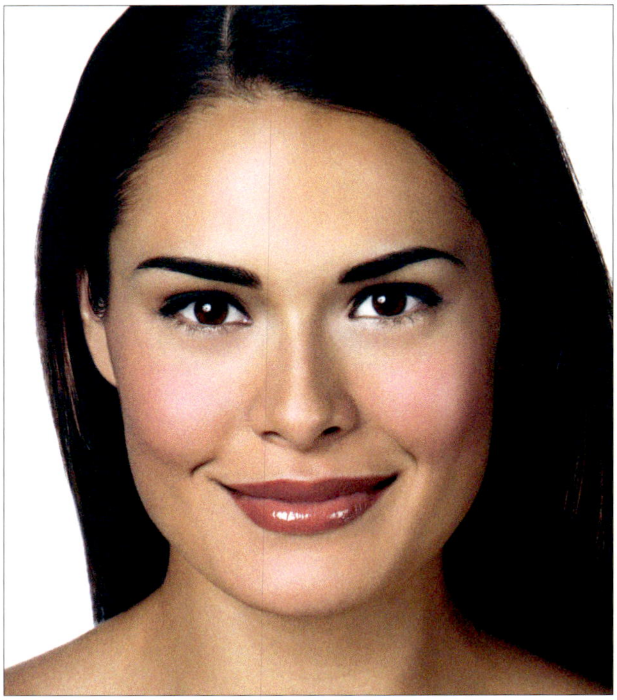

A basic, simple look requires ten steps. Make sure you apply makeup in the correct sequence.

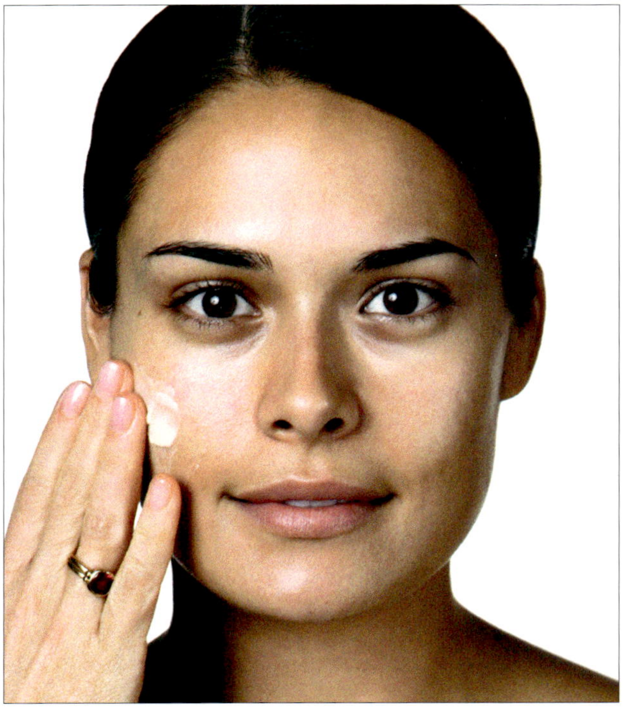

Pre-Makeup

Moisturizer is the key to fresh-looking skin. It creates the perfect base for makeup. For normal skin, use a lightweight moisturizing lotion. For dry skin, use a rich hydrating cream or balm. For oily skin, use an oil-free formula that hydrates and helps control oil production.

Always begin with a lightweight eye cream to ensure that under-eye concealer goes on smoothly and evenly.

When skin looks dull, use an exfoliant to help slough off dead skin cells.

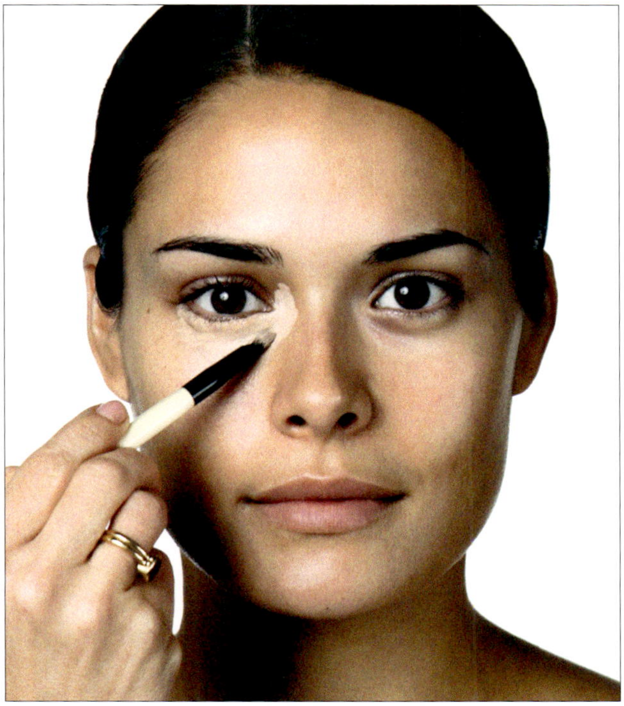

Step 1

Corrector/Concealer

First, neutralize darkness with a pink- or peach-toned corrector. Apply with a brush to the deepest or darkest area to prepare for concealer. (Sometimes you can stop here if the coverage is enough.)

Next, choose yellow-based shades of concealer and layer them over the corrector underneath the eye. Using a concealer brush, apply underneath the eye up to the lash line and on the innermost corner of the eye. Blend by patting with your fingers.

Last, apply pale yellow or white powder with a brush or puff to set the concealer in place. Also apply powder onto the eyelid to take away shine or darkness.

Under-eye concealer should be one to two shades lighter than your skin tone. If the concealer looks ashy, it is too light. If it looks very yellow, it is too dark.

Applying concealer on the spot next to the inner corner of the eye will open up your eyes and give you a fresh, bright-eyed look.

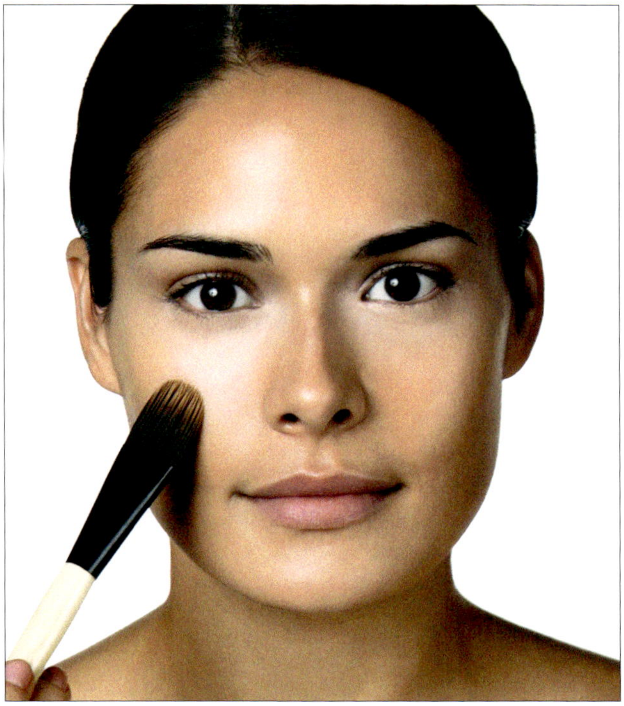

Step 2

Foundation

To find the perfect foundation shade, swatch a few shades on the side of the face and forehead, and check the colors in natural light. The shade that disappears is the right one.

Use a brush, sponge, or fingers to apply foundation where the skin needs to be evened out—around the nose and mouth where there is often redness. For full, all-over coverage, use a brush, sponge, or fingers to apply and blend foundation to the outer edge of the face.

To cover blemishes, spot-apply foundation stick or blemish cover stick in a shade that matches the skin tone exactly. Pat with your finger to blend. Repeat if necessary.

It's a good idea to have two shades of foundation—one for the winter months and a slightly darker one for the summer, when skin color tends to be darker. You can blend the two for spring and fall.

For a sheer, casual alternative to foundation, use tinted moisturizer to even out skin tone.

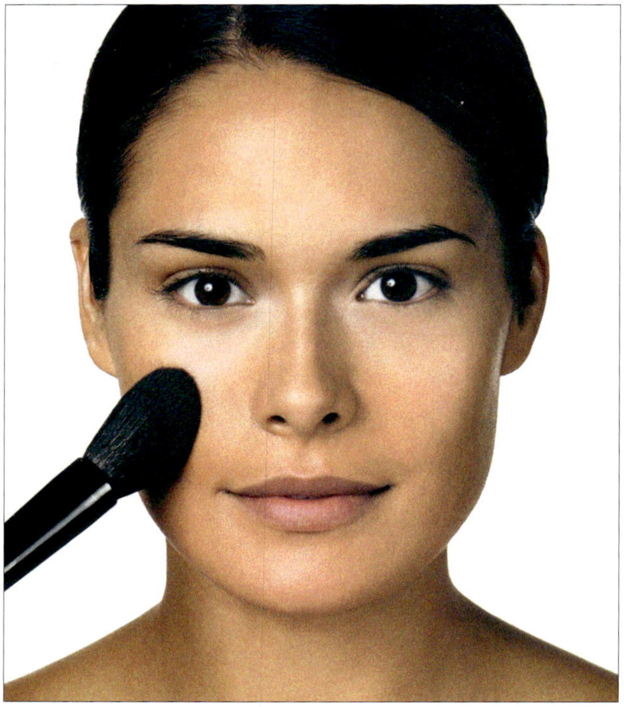

Step 3

Powder

For crease-free, long wear, apply loose powder in a pale yellow tone (or white, if you are very fair) over concealer using an eye blender brush or a mini powder puff.

Apply powder in the correct shade for your skin tone to the rest of the face using a powder puff or powder brush.

If skin feels dry, dust powder only around the nose and forehead.

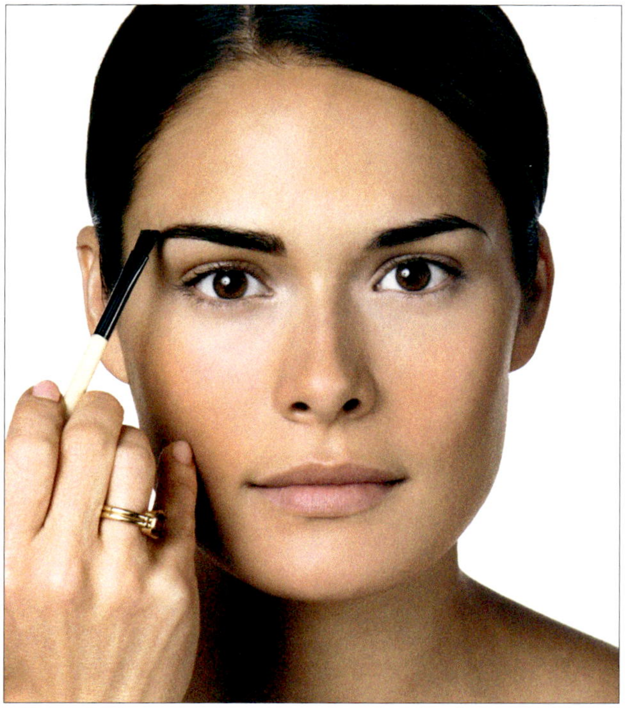

Step 4

Brows

Define brows using shadow or pencil in the color of your eyebrows and hair.

To apply shadow, begin at the inner corner of the brow, and follow its natural shape using light, feathery strokes.

Set unruly brows in place with a brow shaper.

Fill in sparse areas or holes in the brow with an eye pencil. For the most natural look, layer powder shadow on top.

Soften too-harsh brow color by pressing loose powder onto the brows with a powder puff.

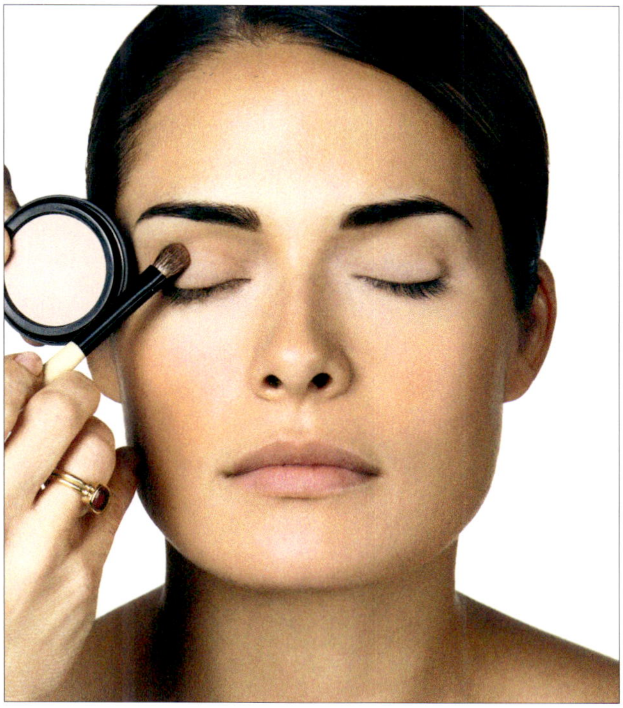

Step 5

Eye Shadow

Sweep a light eye shadow color from the lash line to the brow bone.

Dust a medium eye shadow color on the lower lid, up to the crease.

Apply contour color if needed to fleshy part of lid as a correction and to add depth to eye.

Face powder on bare lids helps create a smoother-looking surface for eye makeup and keeps shadow from creasing.

For a longer-lasting look, use a long-wearing cream shadow.

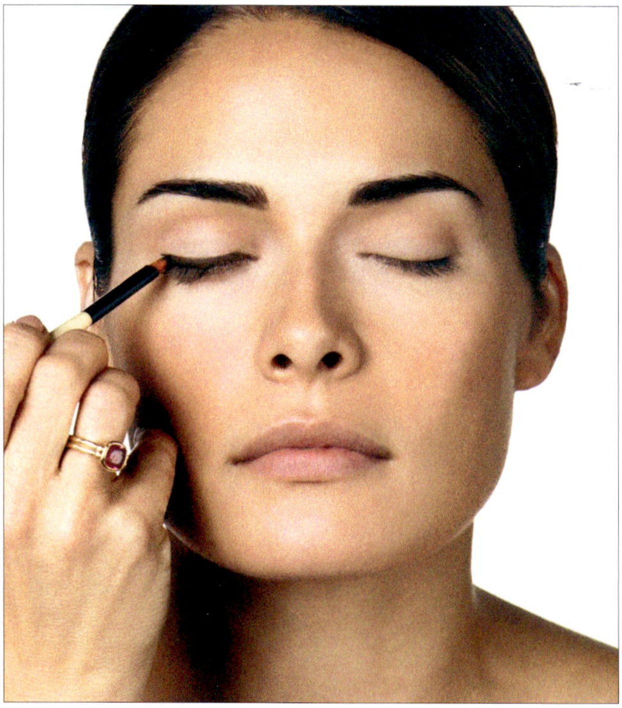

Step 6

Eyeliner

Line the upper lash line with a dark shadow color. Apply damp or dry.

After lining the upper lash line, look straight ahead to see if there are any gaps that need to be filled in. If you also line the lower lash line, make sure the top and bottom lines meet at the outer corner of the eye and that the lower line is softer.

Black eyeliner is the secret to gorgeous, sexy eyes. Layer black liner on top of your normal liner (just on the upper lash line).

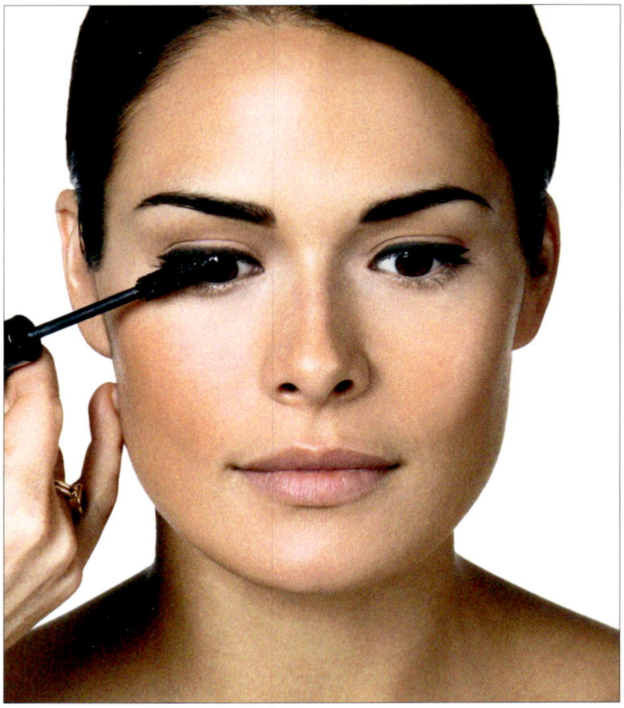

Step 7

Mascara

Choose your mascara formula based on your needs and desired effect. Thickening mascara gives individual lashes a denser look and is ideal if you have a sparse lash line. For lashes that are enhanced but still natural looking, choose defining and lengthening mascaras. Waterproof mascara is a good choice if you want a long-lasting look or if your mascara tends to smudge.

When applying mascara, hold the mascara wand parallel to the floor and brush from the base of the lashes to the tips. Roll the wand as you go to separate the lashes and avoid clumps. Always apply two to three coats.

If you choose to curl the lashes, do so before applying mascara. Curling lashes after applying mascara can break the hairs.

True black mascara makes the most impact. Choose brown for a softer look.

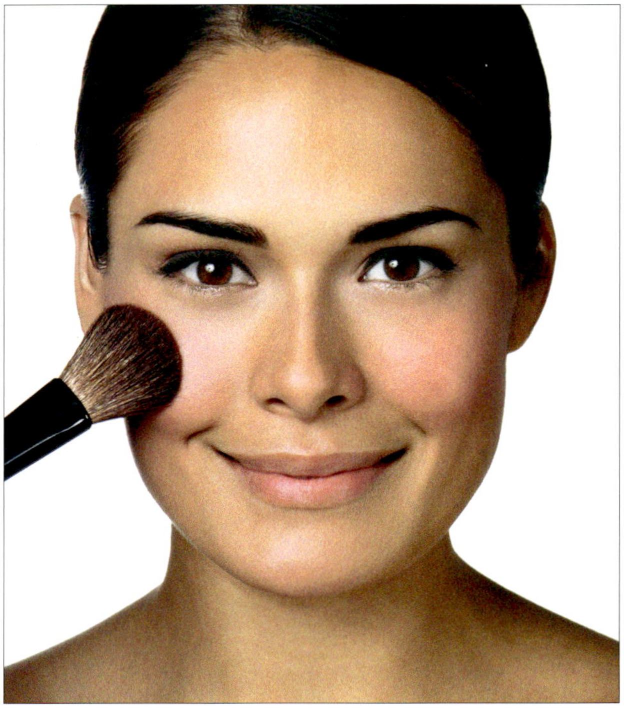

Step 8

Blush

Smile and apply a natural shade of blush on the apples of cheeks. Blend up toward the hairline, then downward to soften the color.

For long-lasting results, layer a pop of brighter blush on top.

For an extra glow, dust a shimmer powder on the cheekbones with a face blender brush, or use a creamy formula applied with your fingers.

Tap or blow off excess powder blush from your blush brush before applying. It is easier to build color in a few light layers than to remove excess color and start over.

Pot rouge or cream blush is a good option for dry skin.

To add a warm tint to skin, use a bronzer on areas where the sun normally hits the face—cheeks, forehead, nose, and chin.

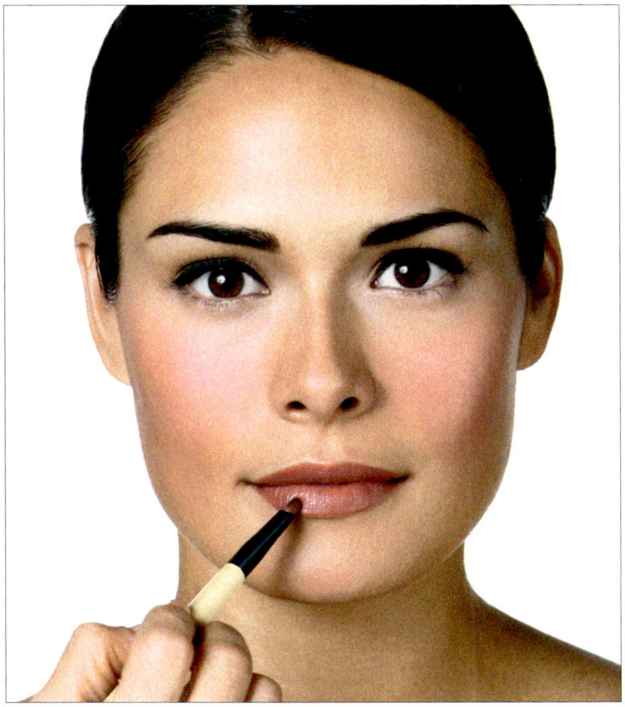

Step 9

Lipstick

Start with clean, smooth lips.

Neutral lipstick shades and sheer formulas can be applied directly from the tube. Use a lip brush to apply darker or brighter colors, which require precise application.

Use the natural color of your lips as a guide when choosing a lipstick shade. The most flattering shade will either match or be slightly darker than your lips.

If you have thin lips, choose light to medium lip color shades, as dark shades have a minimizing effect.

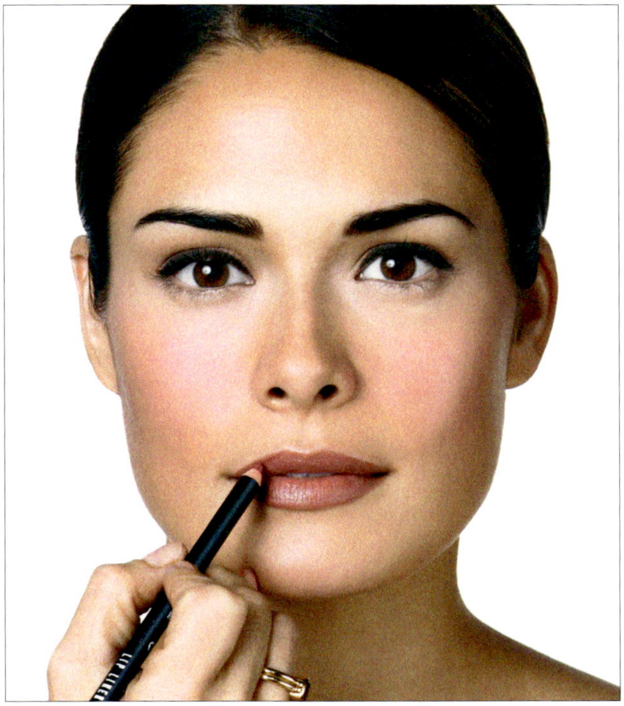

Step 10

Lip Liner

To achieve natural-looking definition and to keep color from feathering, line lips with a lip liner after applying lip color. Use a lip brush to soften and blend any hard edges.

To make your lipstick or gloss longer lasting, line and fill in lips with lip liner before applying color.

FACE CHART

The purpose of a face chart is to have a reference of a makeup lesson. Many women tape them to their mirrors while they try to recreate the look.

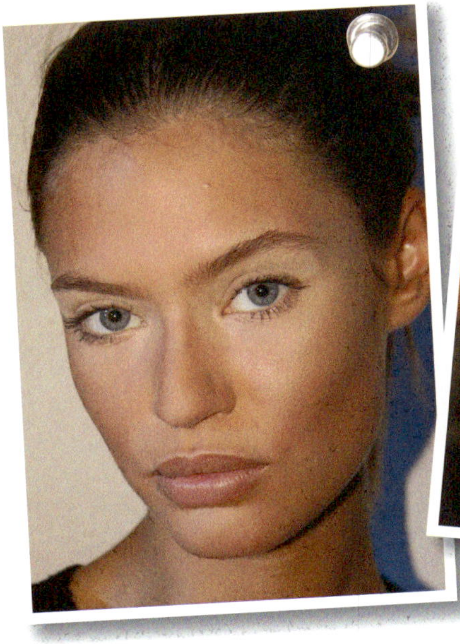

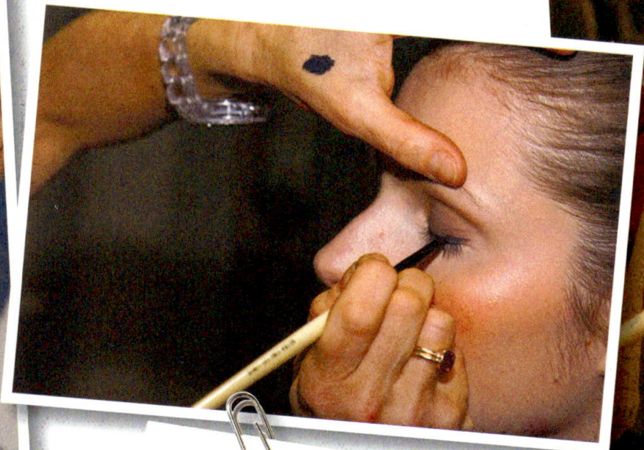

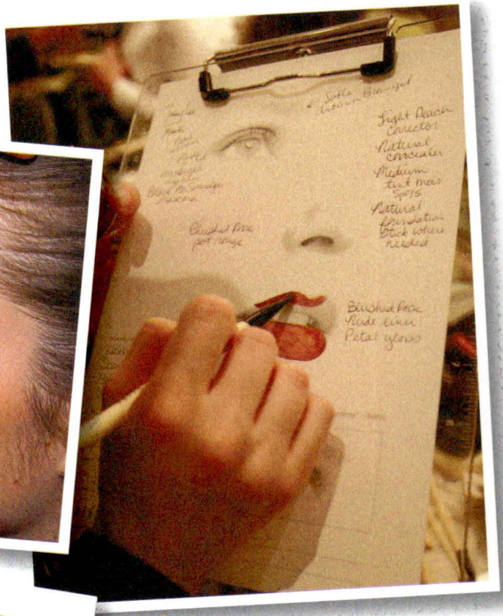

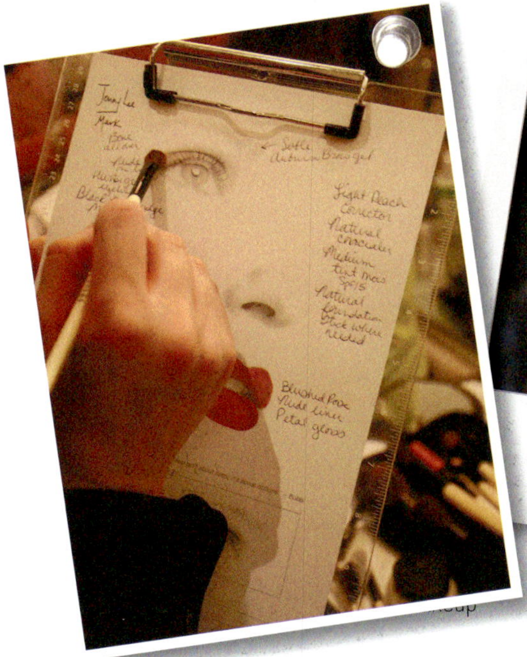

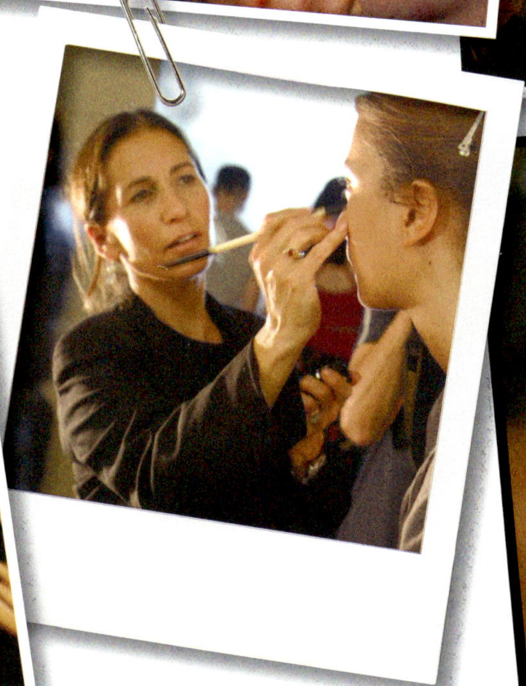

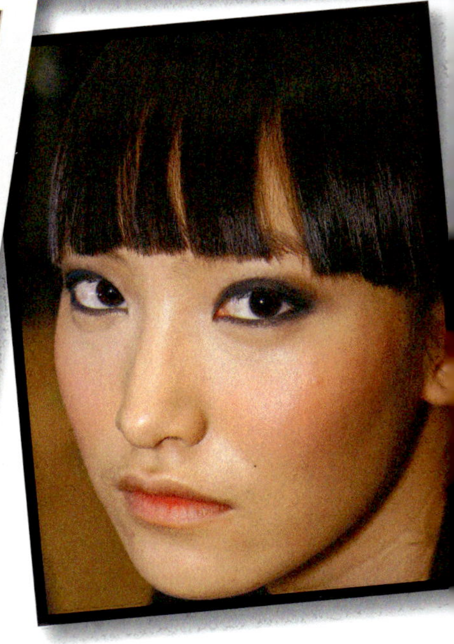

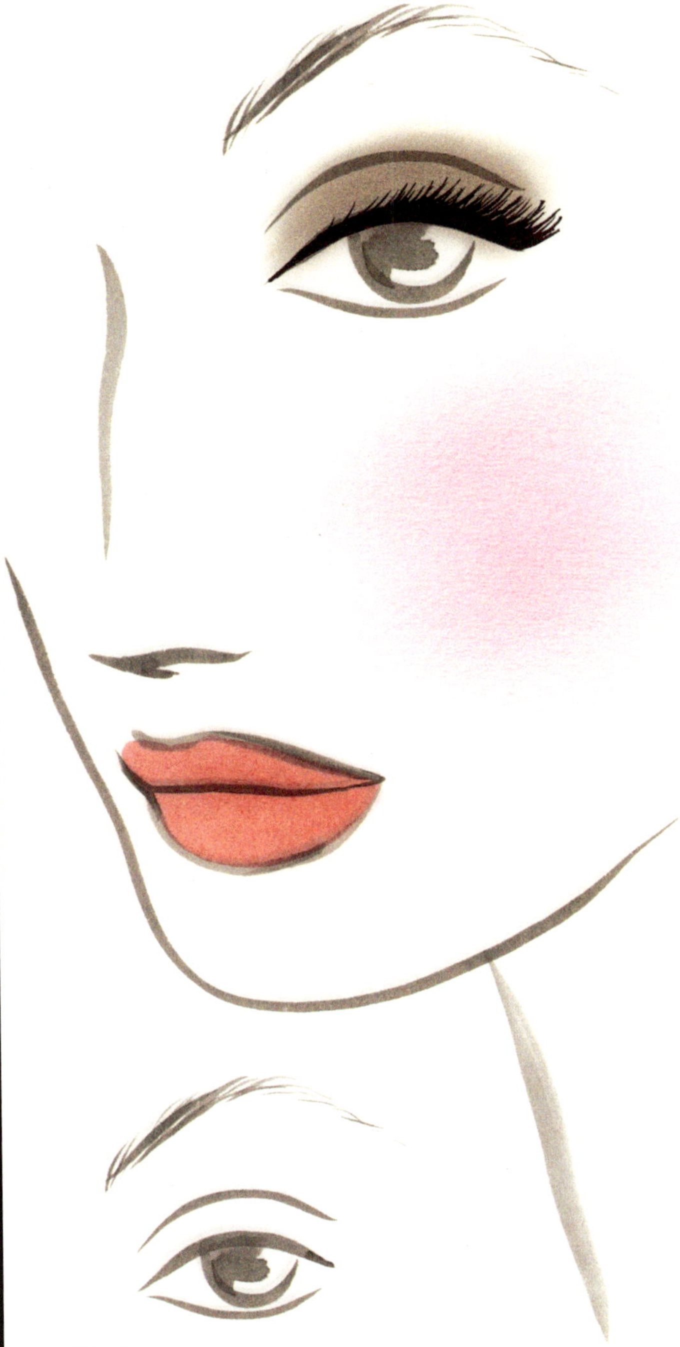

Skincare

Hydrating Eye Cream

Face

Corrector / Concealer

Cheek

Pink Raspberry Pot Rouge

Extra Soothing Balm

Lip

Pink Raspberry Pot Rouge

Eye

Navajo Eye Shadow

Fog Eye Shadow

Black Everything Mascara

Optional Look ______

BOBBI BROWN

www.bobbibrown.com

Makeup Artist ______

Store ______

Telephone ______

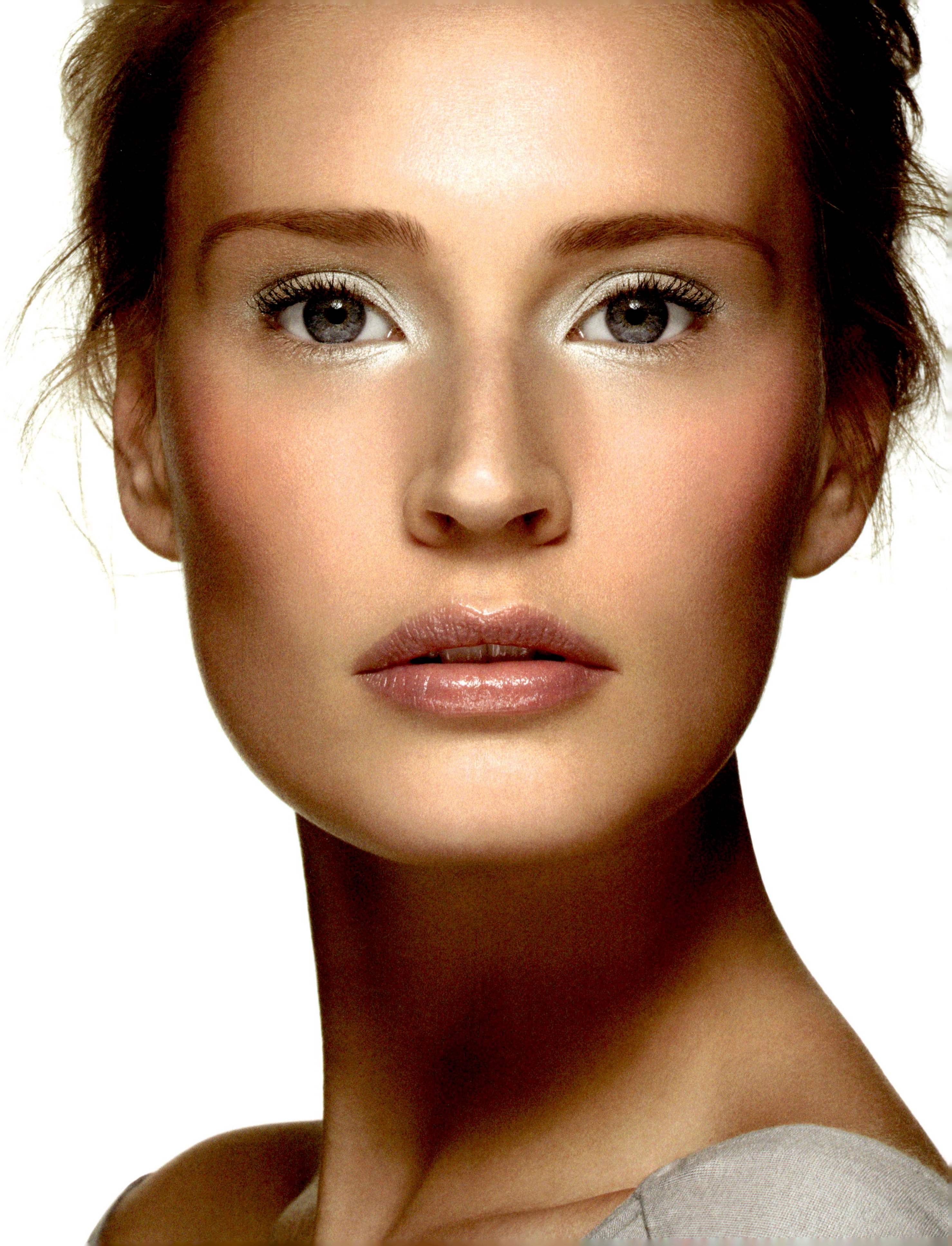

Chapter 8

SPECIAL MAKEUP APPLICATIONS

Once you master the basic techniques of makeup, **it's both fun and easy to take it to the next step for a variety of looks.** Individual beauty is about knowing what to do with your own unique skin tone and features. And it's also about being confident enough to break out of your comfort zone.

DIVERSE BEAUTY

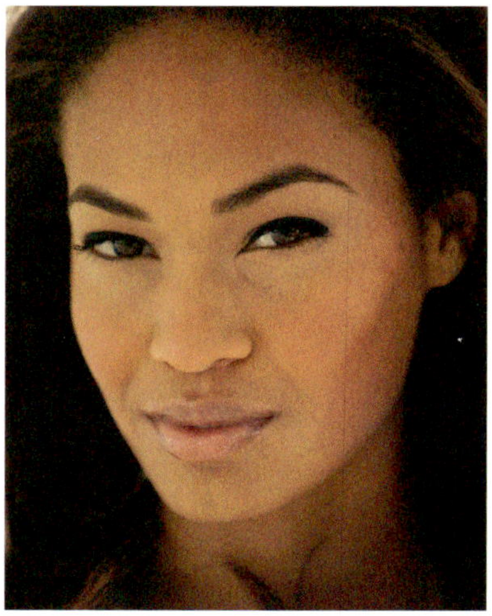

African American Beauty

For dark under-eye circles, use peach corrector and yellow-toned concealer.

Find a foundation that exactly matches skin tone. Skin tone is often uneven, with the forehead and cheeks slightly different shades. Experiment using two different tones of foundation or mixing two shades together. Undertones can be yellow, orange, red, or blue.

Some dark skin looks best with no blush or with a bit of deep bronzer. For medium-toned skin, try bronzing powder or a currant-toned blush. A range of blush tones in plum, rose, or pink look good on lighter skin tones.

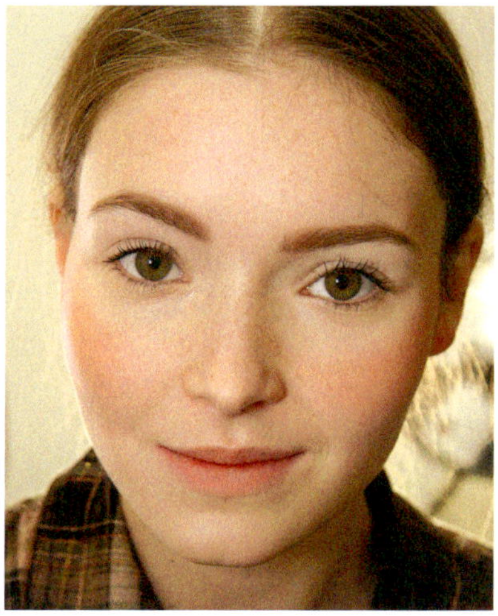

Freckled Beauty

Embrace your freckles.

If you need concealer, look for a yellow-toned product that is just one shade lighter than the skin tone.

Foundation can be used to cover redness around the nose or blemishes. Tinted moisturizer gives some coverage but lets the freckles shine through.

Light tawny, coral, or pink tones of blush work well.

Sometimes foundation has to match the freckles that are a shade or two darker than the skin underneath. Do not look for coverage all over the face, only on the redness.

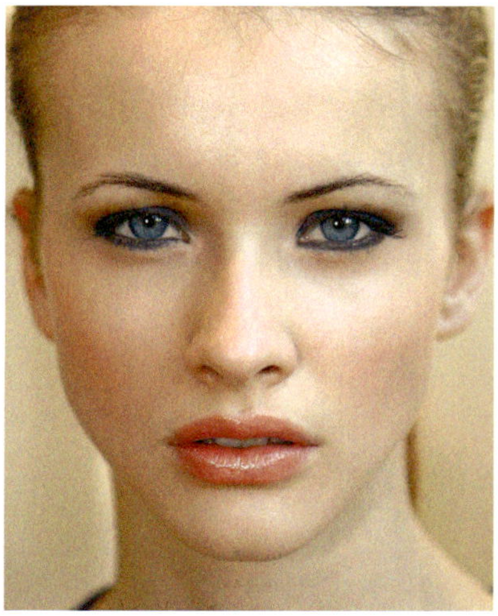

Porcelain Beauty

Sunscreen helps keep skin looking young and beautiful.

Use porcelain-toned foundation to cover redness, dark circles, and blemishes.

Use white face powder.

Avoid using blush with brown undertones. Go for pastels—pale pink is awesome.

Tan bronzer always looks dirty on porcelain skin.

Eye makeup in cool tones works best for porcelain skin tones. Avoid any red-toned products, which can make you look tired.

Pastel lip colors complement very light skin tones.

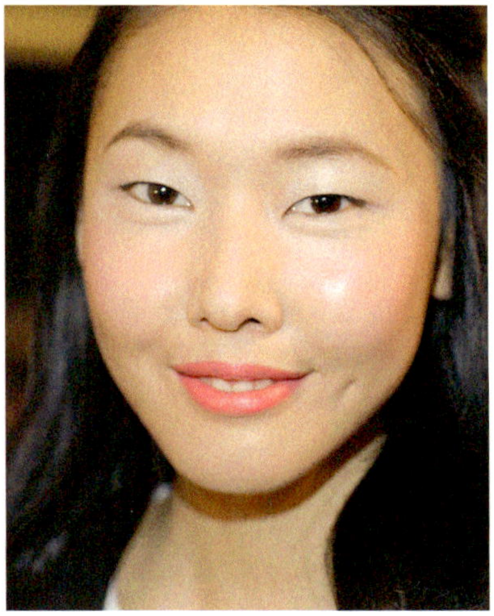

Asian Beauty

Use yellow-toned foundation. Though skin tones vary, all have yellow undertones.

Fill in sparse brows with an eye shadow powder in dark brown. Avoid using black or charcoal, even if the hair is black, because it will look too heavy.

Accentuate eyes with liner on the top only or the top and bottom. Use a stronger line on the top. Make sure it shows when the eyes are open.

Layer shadows to define the eyes. Don't make the mistake of using a very dark shadow to draw in a crease.

A pop of bright coral or pink blush on the apples of the cheeks look fresh and pretty.

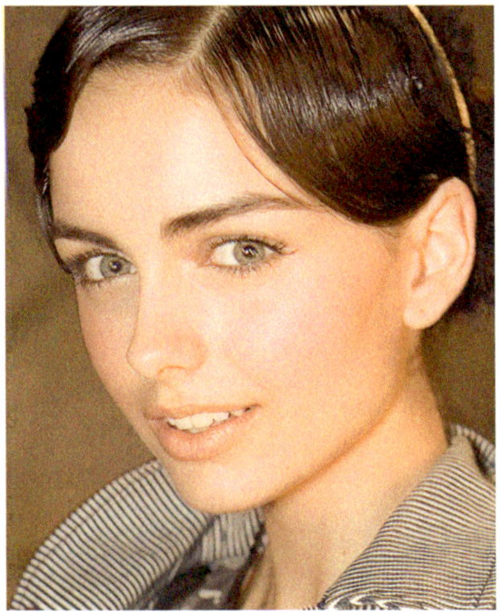

Middle Eastern Beauty

Use a corrector to brighten very dark under-eye circles.

Sometimes you have to layer a few correctors (pink over peach), and then add concealer.

Find a yellow-toned foundation that exactly matches the skin. The right foundation often has a bit of orange as well.

Line the eyes with black liner or a charcoal shadow. Never go lighter than mahogany.

Use blush in deep rose and pink shades. Don't be afraid to find your pop of color.

Deep lip colors look wonderful on those with darker lip tones.

Avoid colors that turn ashy.

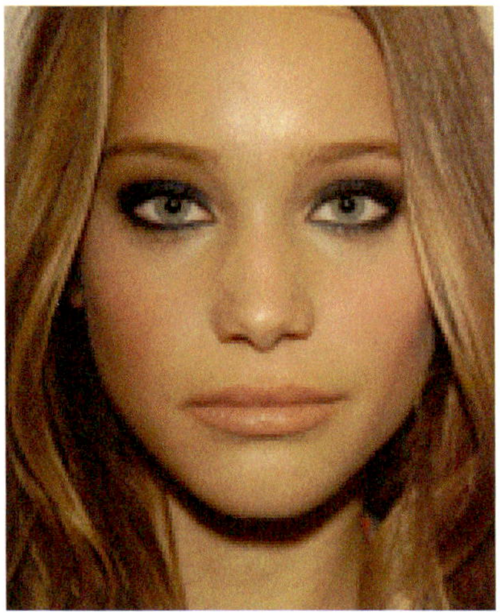

Latin Beauty

Skin tones vary from very fair to dark.

Use foundation with a yellow undertone that exactly matches skin.

Neutral eye shadows look best for every day. Try shades of navy, silver, chocolate, or gold for evenings or special occasions.

Accentuate natural lip color with lipstick. Choose brighter or deeper tones for evening.

Bronzers are great to add warmth and ensure foundation blends into the skin. Always finish with a pop of color.

BRIDAL MAKEUP

Bridal makeup should be special. On her wedding day, every bride should look like herself at her most beautiful. It is not a time to try a look that is very trendy or radically different from her usual style. Wedding makeup must be long lasting, look amazing in photographs, and be timeless. Every bride should love how she looks in the pictures ten years from now.

Makeup Rules

If possible, do a consultation and run-through of the makeup before the wedding day. Reserve an appointment for about four to six weeks prior to the wedding day to design and practice the look. The wedding day is also special for family and friends, so consider booking makeup appointments for the whole bridal party.

Bridal makeup needs to have enough color to compensate for the whiteness of the dress. Remember, there's a big difference between everyday clothes and a wedding dress, so there should be a difference in the makeup, too. Start by making sure the skin looks even and smooth, and then add color to give cheeks and lips a glow. Finish with eyes that are defined but not overdone. To avoid feeling rushed, allow forty-five minutes to an hour for makeup application on the wedding day.

Natural light is best for makeup application. If possible, set up your makeup station near a window, or use a superbright lamp.

Use a moisturizer that will prepare the skin for makeup. Avoid sunblocks and sunscreens that can give a "flash off" to makeup. They reflect too much light under flash photography, resulting in an overexposed shot.

Emphasize the eyes by brightening any darkness under them with corrector and concealer.

Flash photography emphasizes pink tones, so be sure to even out the skin with a yellow-toned foundation. Start around the nose and mouth, where there's redness, and then blend out to the rest of the face.

Blend well, especially at the corners of the eyes, since cameras pick up visible makeup lines.

Set concealer and foundation with a sheer loose powder. Powder applied with a powder puff assures amazing wearability and reduces unwanted shine—a must-have look for pictures.

If the wedding gown has an open neckline, warm up the neck and chest with a dusting of bronzing powder. It will ensure that the face and body have a balanced tone.

For a pretty flush that lasts, use two shades of blush. Start with a neutral shade, and apply it on the apples of the cheeks, blending up into the hairline, then downward to soften. Finish with a pop of brighter blush just on the apples of the cheeks. Balm or shimmer can be layered for a highlighting effect.

Neutral, brown, and pale lip colors look washed out in photographs, so choose a lipstick that's one or two shades brighter than what you normally wear. For those

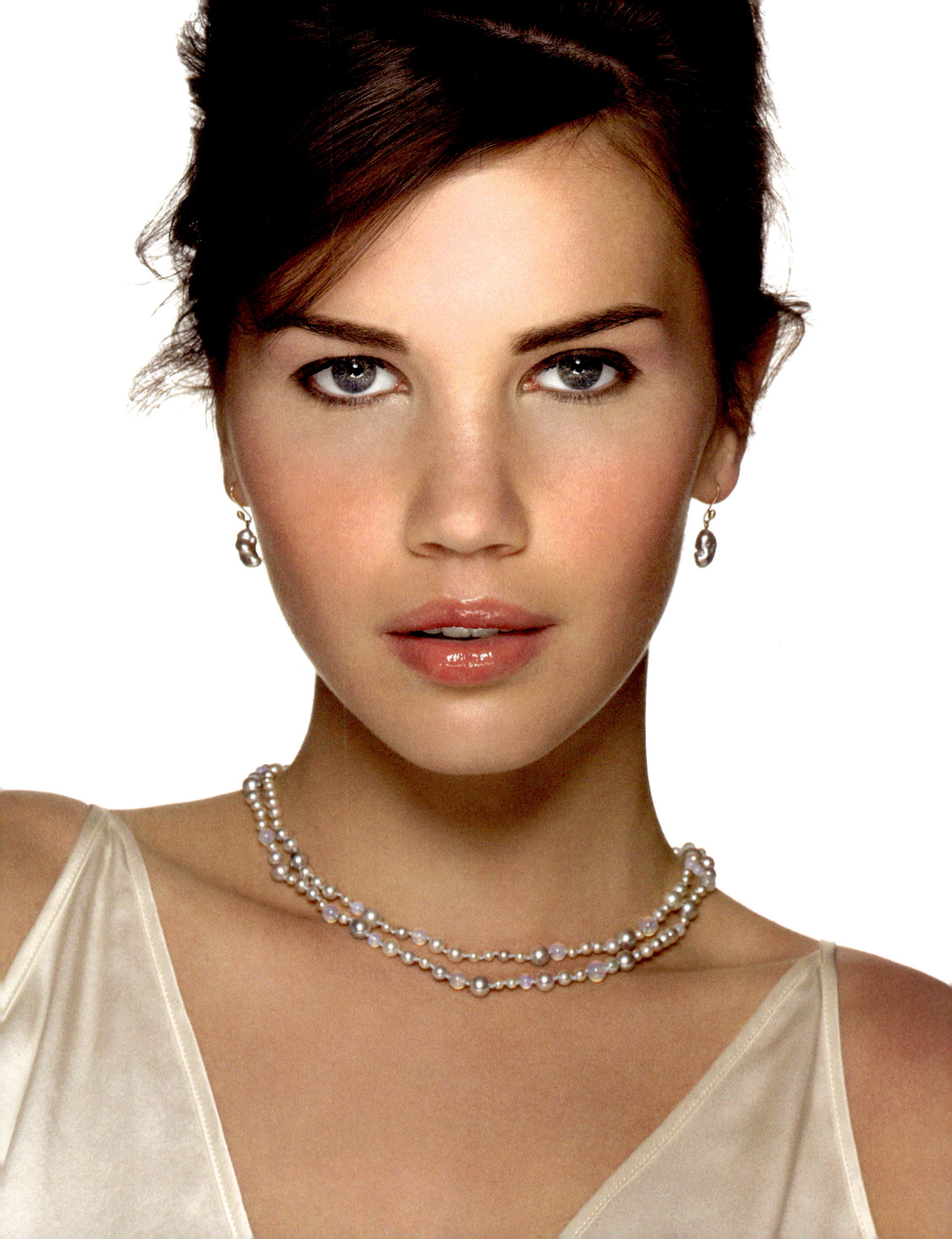

who normally wear a neutral hue, it should be worn as a base, with a pink or rose color on top. For those who normally wear dark lipstick, use that as the base, and apply a brighter pink on top to give the color a lift. Pinks, roses, and plums are great choices for brides.

To make lip color last longer, line and fill in lips with lip pencil before applying the lipstick.

Define brows with a soft matte shadow that matches the hair color.

Use a flat white shadow as a highlighter on the brow bone for those with light skin. A vanilla shade better suits deeper complexions. Use matte eye shadows, as they won't reflect light or look too shiny in photographs.

Define the eyes with a crease color, but avoid using a color that's too dense or dark, as it can detract from the eyes themselves.

Use a water-resistant liner that can withstand tears. If you prefer to line with shadow, make it last longer by applying it with a slightly damp eyeliner brush.

Use an eyelash curler before applying the first coat of mascara.

Choose mascara that's waterproof. It lasts longer and withstands tears.

After applying all the eye makeup, finish with a highlighter shade on the brow bone to make the eyes pop. Rub your finger in a light matte shade, and pat lightly on the outer corner of the brow bone.

Wedding Day Essentials

Pack a small bag with makeup essentials. Keep it simple by filling a face palette with corrector, concealer, foundation stick, pot rouge, lip color, and a soothing balm. Add a lip liner, lip gloss, tissues, Q-tips, and mints.

Include a sewing kit with pre-threaded needles and a pair of tiny fold-up scissors to fix a dropped hem or popped button.

Add prewrapped wipes to remove makeup or food stains.

Bring static spray and lint remover to get rid of static cling and lint on clothing.

Bring a small bottle of perfume in your bag.

Pre-Wedding Wellness Tips

Beauty starts on the inside.
Following these tips will help any bride prepare for her wedding day.

Eat smart.
Choose whole grains, fresh greens and fruits, and clean proteins, such as chicken, fish, and beans.

Hydrate.
Drink lots of water daily to hydrate the skin and flush out toxins.

Move your body.
Exercise at least three times a week to strengthen your body and calm your mind.

Take relaxing baths.
Add soothing Epsom salts or skin-softening powdered milk to your bathwater.

Be present.
Slow down and appreciate what's around you rather than rushing to get from start to finish.

Bridal Dos & Don'ts

Do complete a makeup trial.

Do get as much sleep as possible on the night before the big day.

Do drink plenty of water before your wedding day, and properly prepare skin with moisturizer and eye cream.

Do make sure foundation is right for the skin tone. Your color may have changed since the makeup trial.

Do buy a new mascara for your wedding day, but test it a few days before.

Don't go to a tanning bed right before your wedding. If you want more color, use a self-tanner. Test the product weeks before the date. Apply it several days before the wedding in case you need to make corrections.

Don't apply too much eye makeup. You want the eyes to stand out, not the eye makeup.

Don't use concealer on the eyelid. It causes eye makeup to crease.

Don't use a concealer under the eyes that is too light for the skin tone. It will make you look like a deer caught in headlights.

Don't experiment with eye makeup you haven't tried before.

Don't wear frosted, shiny, or sparkly shadow, as it will reflect camera flashes.

Don't apply shimmer all over the face. One or two accents are enough.

Don't tweeze or wax brows on the wedding day.

Don't wear false eyelashes if they are not 100 percent comfortable and you are not 200 percent confident that they will stay on!

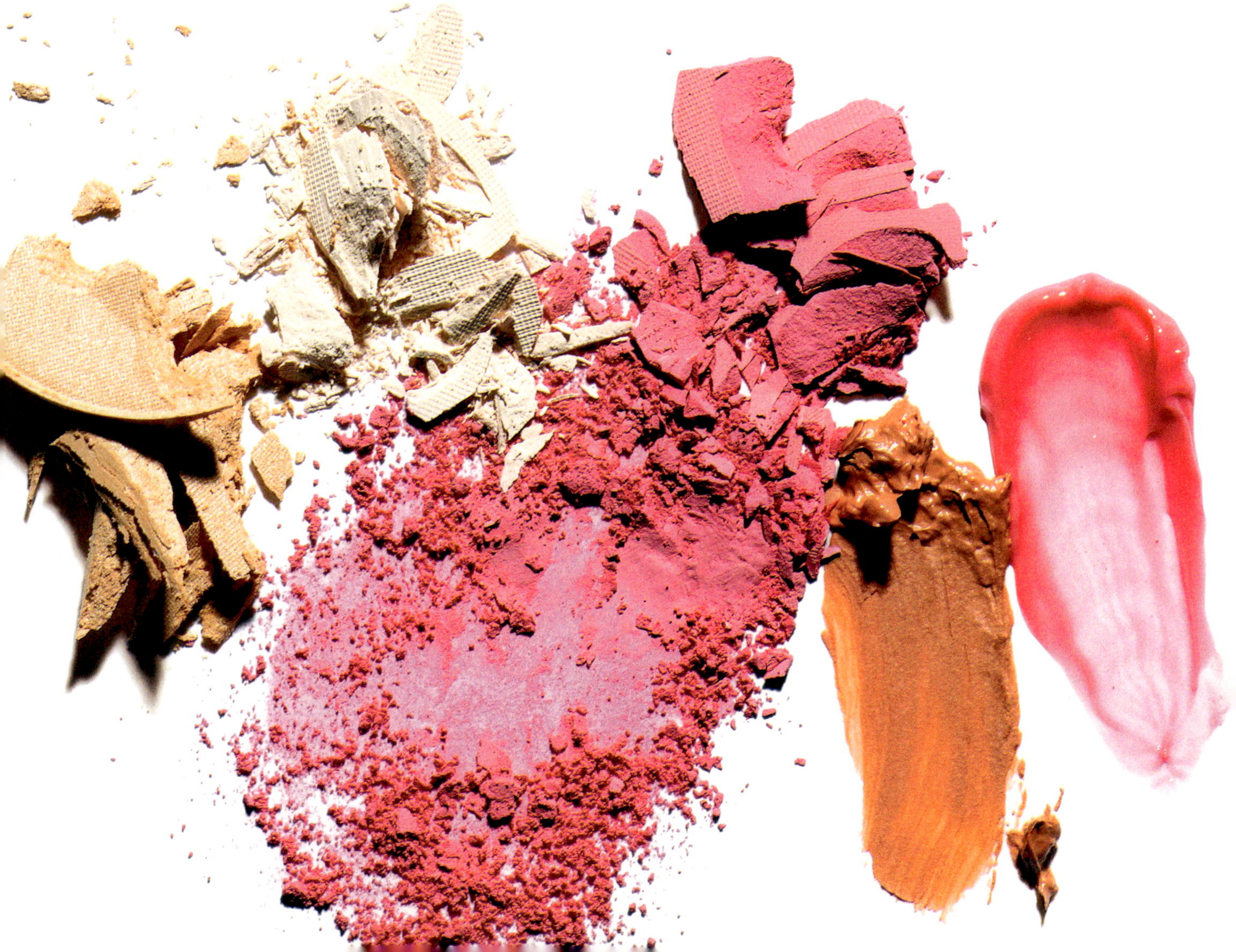

SPECIAL-OCCASION MAKEUP

Few women have the time or energy to clean their faces at the end of the workday and redo their makeup for a night out. Instead, they want a few quick tricks to make a simple transition from office to evening. Since lighting is often softer at night and the occasions are dressier, the idea is to make the face look a bit more dramatic than during the day.

Transforming a Day Face into an Evening Face

Start with a touch of eye cream to smooth out existing concealer. Reapply as needed.

Apply foundation as needed to cover any blemishes and even out skin tone, especially around the nose.

Use a blush that is slightly brighter than the one used for a daytime look. Use it alone or as a pop of color just on the apple of the cheeks.

If skin is showing on the neck and chest, make it glow with a light sweep of bronzing powder.

Use shimmer on lips, eyes, or cheeks to make the face look dressed up. Warning: Too much shimmer will look overdone, so don't use it on all three areas at the same time.

Switch to a darker shade of lipstick. Red or burgundy will add drama to your look. Or try a sheer shade paired with a more dramatic eye.

Add drama to eyes by sweeping on a darker shadow as a liner and applying plenty of black mascara. A smoky eye is always sexy for night looks. Applying white as a highlighter under the brow bone is also a great evening look.

Spritz on a warm, sensual fragrance, and put on a great pair of earrings.

Try red lips with pink cheeks and minimal eye makeup.

Pair shimmery bronzer with smoky brown eyes, bronze cheeks, and copper lips. Add shimmer to either lips or eyes, not both.

Have fun with a bright pink or orange mouth, pale pink or apricot blush, and soft eye makeup with several coats of black mascara or false eyelashes.

For very special occasions, don't be afraid to go all out. Cool colors such as white, platinum, gunmetal, and slate work on the eyes with black liner and individual false eyelashes. Using pale pink with a hint of shimmer on the cheeks and soft beige or sandy pink gloss on the lips will look great.

Use an oil-control lotion on oily areas of the face to keep it shine-free.

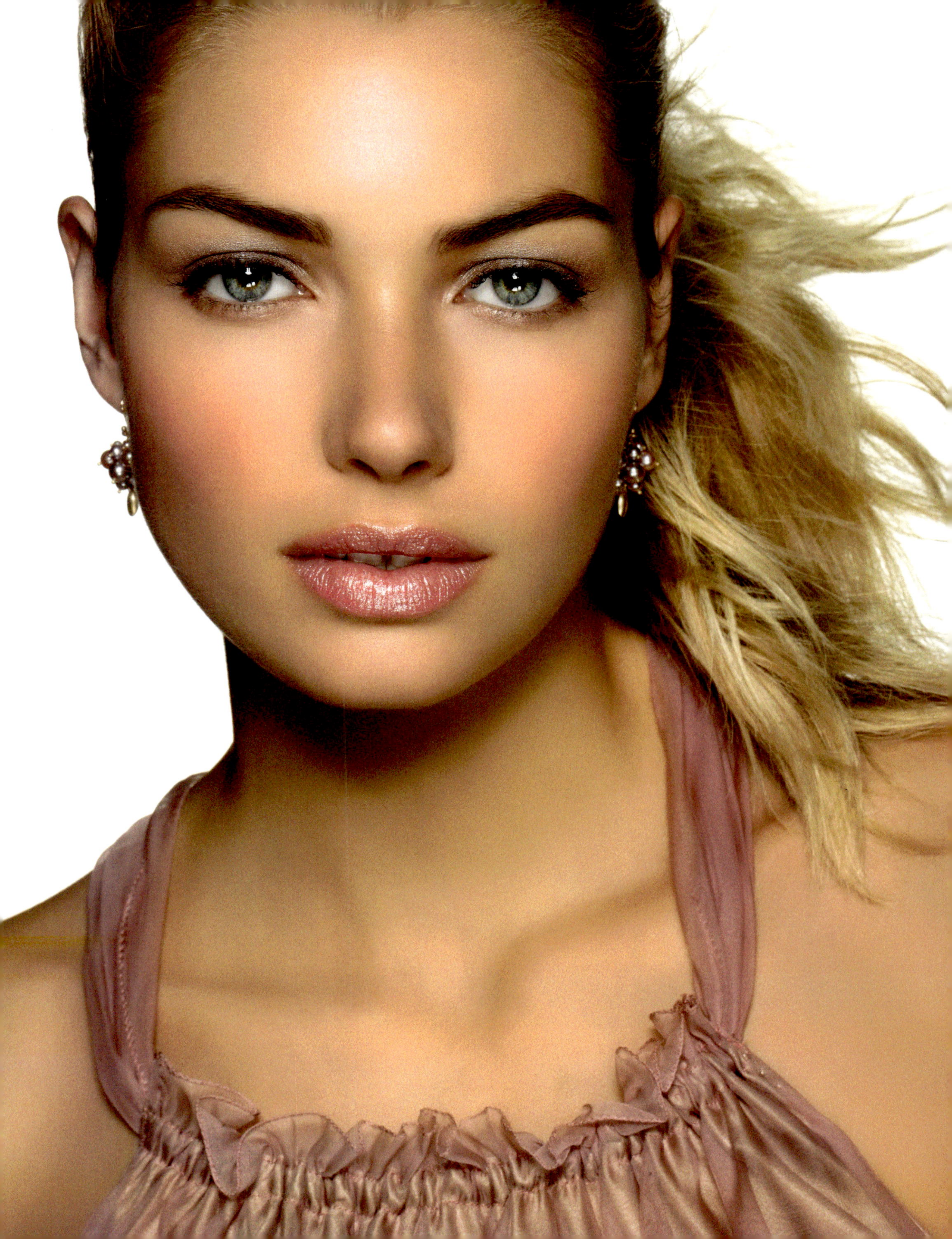

MAKEUP FOR TEENS

Most young women are obsessed with makeup, but they don't often have the knowledge, skills, or confidence to make it work. The teen years are the time to try trendy colors and textures, but a fresh young face should never be smothered in makeup.

Skip an all-over foundation application. Cover blemishes with a blemish stick. Then, apply a stick foundation to those areas that need color correction.

Do not use makeup to look older. The results look harsh and awkward.

Keep colors light and sheer. Avoid heavy, smoky eye shadow and too-bold shades for lips and cheeks.

If the skin is oily, keep blotting papers handy for touch-ups throughout the day.

To avoid drawing attention to braces, skip bright lip colors. Instead, use a moisturizing tinted lip balm or sheer gloss.

Use a clear brow gel to keep brows in place.

Master covering a pimple.

How to Cover a Blemish

1. Choose a stick foundation or concealer stick the exact shade matching your skin tone.
2. With a concealer brush, dab the product on the spot only. Wipe it away from the surrounding areas. Layer a second coat on if needed.
3. Dust a bit of skin-tone-correct powder directly on top of the spot.

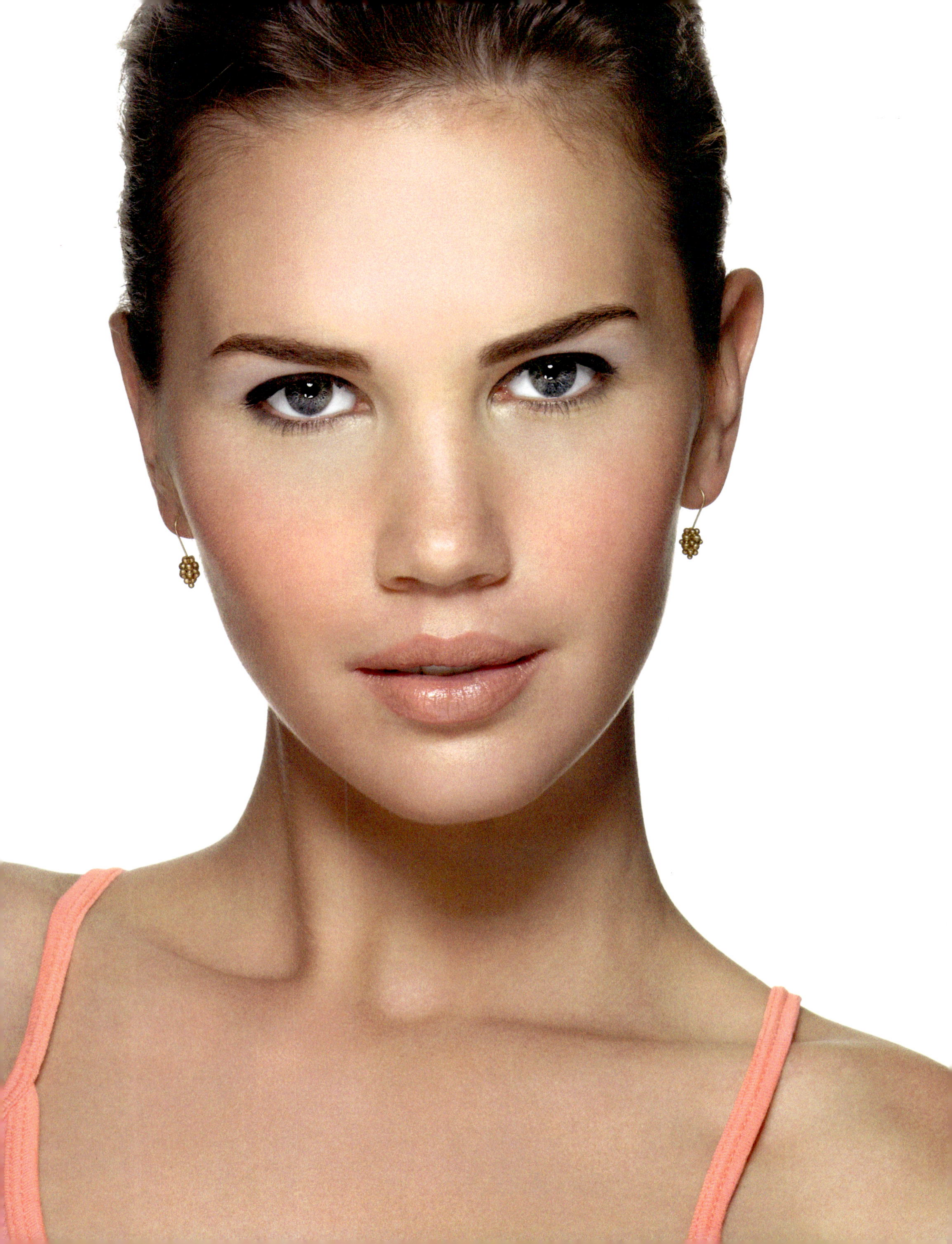

AGELESS BEAUTY

Beauty is about looking and feeling great. That means beauty depends in part on taking care of the body: drinking lots of water, eating healthy foods, using sunscreen, and getting plenty of exercise.

Good beauty routines begin with good skincare. Pamper the skin, and experiment with rich, hydrating moisturizers.

Under-eye darkness often deepens with age. Use a rich under-eye cream overnight and a lighter cream for day to hydrate and smooth the area. Use a pink or peach-toned corrector followed by a yellow-toned concealer and foundation. Lighten the upper lid with a light eye shadow.

Using moisturizers can reduce the appearance of wrinkles. Tinted balms and moisture-rich foundations help soften lines and wrinkles and don't settle into them. Match the foundation exactly to the skin tone.

Skin loses elasticity over time. Using a cream with retinoids that stimulates collagen production helps to give skin a firmer look.

Yellow-toned foundation or tinted moisturizer will tone down ruddy skin and rosacea. Bronzer helps counteract redness as well. Strong facial scrubs often aggravate ruddiness. Rosacea can be treated topically; ask your doctor.

Brown spots can be removed with laser resurfacing performed by a dermatologist or covered with the lightest pink or peach corrector and yellow-toned foundation that is set with powder.

Color will make you look pretty and fresher. Experiment.

Eye contour gives droopy eyelids a lift—the contour shadow needs to look blended and natural.

Sometimes adding a gel bronzer gives a nice boost (aka a fake tan) for a healthy look.

Smooth skin is prettier than too-tight skin.

Eyeliner is great for bringing the eyes out and making them look awake.

Crepey eyes: Make sure you moisturize at night, and stick to formulas that are not too dry.

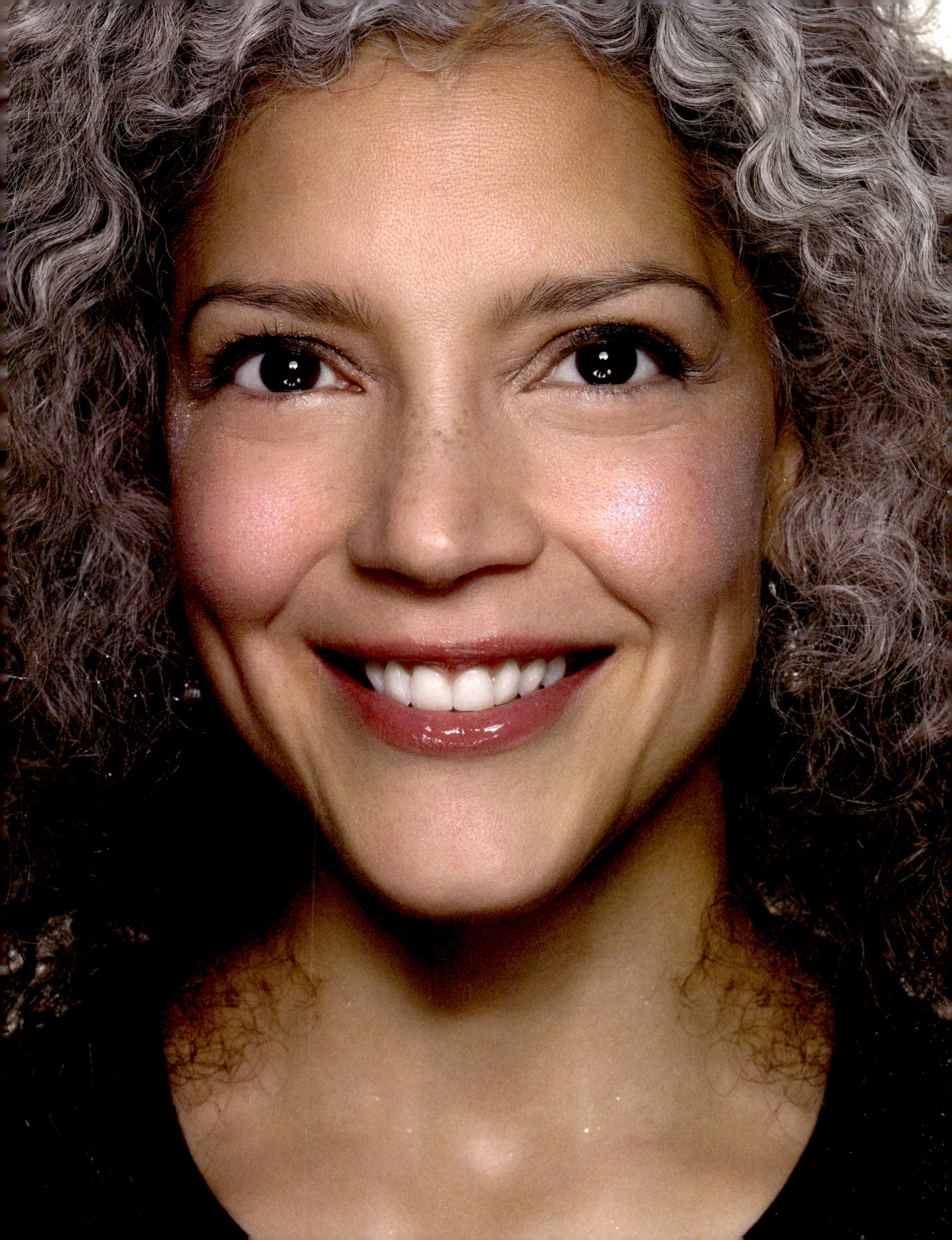

MAKEUP DURING PREGNANCY

For many women, pregnancy is a time when their bodies do not feel like their own. Hormones and physical changes caused by pregnancy create some special needs. Skin often changes during pregnancy, dark patches appear on the skin (sometimes called the "mask of pregnancy"), and some women become extremely sensitive to fragrances.

Adjust any skincare regimen for pregnancy-related changes, either by adding more moisture to combat dryness or switching to oil-free formulas if skin has become oilier.

Use sunscreen! Pregnancy hormones often leave the skin sensitive and more vulnerable to the sun. The vigilant use of sunscreen will help minimize the appearance of hyperpigmentation.

To cover hyperpigmentation, apply a corrective concealer to the area using a concealer brush. Apply foundation over the entire face, using a light touch to avoid wiping away the concealer. Use the fingers to press additional foundation into areas where needed, and then set it with powder.

For those days when there is no natural glow, fake it with a pretty shade of blush, or use a light touch of bronzer over the face.

For added glow, pat face balm over makeup or on a bare face.

Learn the quick on-the-go makeup routine and promise yourself you will do it (most days) and prepare a palette that is customized for you. Make sure you choose colors that don't need to be blended.

Minimum steps are concealer and blush.

BAD-DAY BEAUTY

Everyone, even the most gorgeous model, has the occasional bad day. These are the days when eyes look puffy, skin appears sallow, breakouts seem overly obvious, and nothing seems to help. There are many solutions to improve these situations.

Add moisture. When skin is dehydrated, it looks older and less alive. Drink plenty of water. Use a rich moisturizer to help temporarily plump up skin, making it look softer and younger.

Skip the full makeup application. Avoid the urge to apply makeup in an attempt to banish the bad-day issues. Use just a bit of concealer, a tinted moisturizer, and a pinky blush.

Curl lashes to open up eyes and make them look more awake. Do not follow with lots of eye makeup. Dark liner and shadows can make tired eyes look even more tired. Stick to light shades on the lids, and use mascara just on the top lashes.

Fake a tan. To enliven sallow-looking skin, apply a light coat of self-tanner, bronzing powder, or gel. Follow with a pinky blush.

Don't compensate for paleness with too much color. A sheer pink blush will warm up the skin without looking fake. A bit of moisturizer patted onto the skin over blush will make the skin look great.

Add sheer, glossy lip color to perk up a tired-looking mouth. The best shades match your natural lip color or add just a hint of rose or pink.

Dark eyeglass frames really come in handy on some days.

Cover bruises with a blemish stick or foundation stick.

Cover discolored scars with a blemish stick, and then apply foundation over the area to blend in with skin tone.

Ease a sunburn with a cool shower and cold compresses. Any redness still remaining can be helped with a light application of foundation or tinted moisturizer. Avoid red-colored lips. Instead, try a bronze or brown-based lip color.

Bobbi's Best Friends

Black eyeliner

Bright pink blush

Cheek glow (balms)

Bright pink scarf

Ray-Bans

PASTEL
A L'ÉCU
SENNELIER
AP

PART II: ARTISTRY

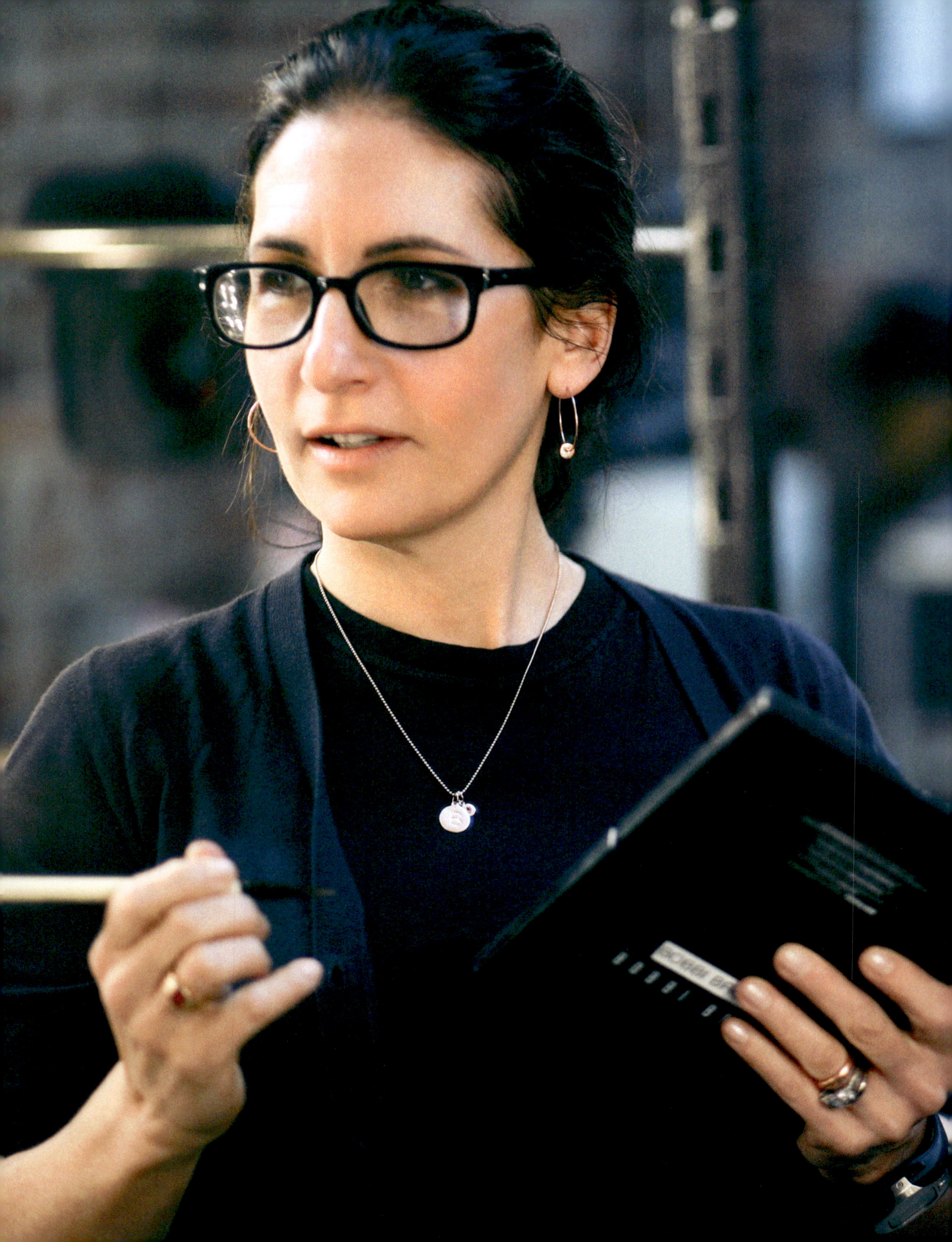

Chapter 9

ARTISTRY

What it takes to be a professional:
this chapter is all about learning to see, formulating your style, listening, collaborating, and finding inspiration.

ARTISTRY

Professional makeup artistry is a field for those who love makeup. ***Makeup artists must be obsessed with both the art and business of it, and they cannot be afraid of hard work.*** Makeup artists must learn to see in order to evaluate their choices and techniques. They must be open to learning and growing in their craft. Successful professionals in the field of makeup should be excellent teachers and communicators.

THE IMPORTANCE OF SEEING

The most important quality of a good makeup artist is the ability to observe. You can learn a lot about makeup and style just by observing. Look at the faces and styles of women on the street, actresses, and friends. Study women in magazines, old photos, paintings, and movies. Chances are you will begin to see some patterns emerge as to what you like. They will help you formulate your own signature style as a makeup artist. I studied photographs to discover the many ways light creates color on the skin. I love good light and brightness under the eyes, with a smooth complexion.

While your style is evolving, you can expect some trial and error. Hair color, cuts, bright lipstick, beige lipstick? Go for it. Try new things until you arrive at a look you love. You'll know you have found the right look when you feel comfortable and confident in yourself and your appearance. It's an evolution, and it's up to you to find the way.

THE IMPORTANCE OF LISTENING

Just as you have to train your eye in order to become a successful makeup artist, you also have to train your ear. Effective listening is an essential skill for all makeup artists. While it is important to have a vision and to develop your own style, a makeup artist cannot be a dictator. Your job is to take other people's ideas and visions into consideration and to collaborate with them. If the project is a photo shoot, the photographer, editor, and stylist all have input. Even though the model has no say, I believe she should feel good about the way she looks. For fashion shows, the designer usually has a vision, and it becomes your job to realize it. In theater, makeup artists collaborate with the costume designer and sometimes the wig designer to realize the director's vision.

When the subject is an actress, you have to please her and usually others, including her agent, stylist, and photographer, which is not always easy. One time I was doing Tina Turner's makeup and she requested a sexy look, which I had to balance with the photographer and stylist's request that she have a more natural, no-makeup look. And then there was the actress who insisted on black-winged eye-liner that just wasn't pretty. Or the singer

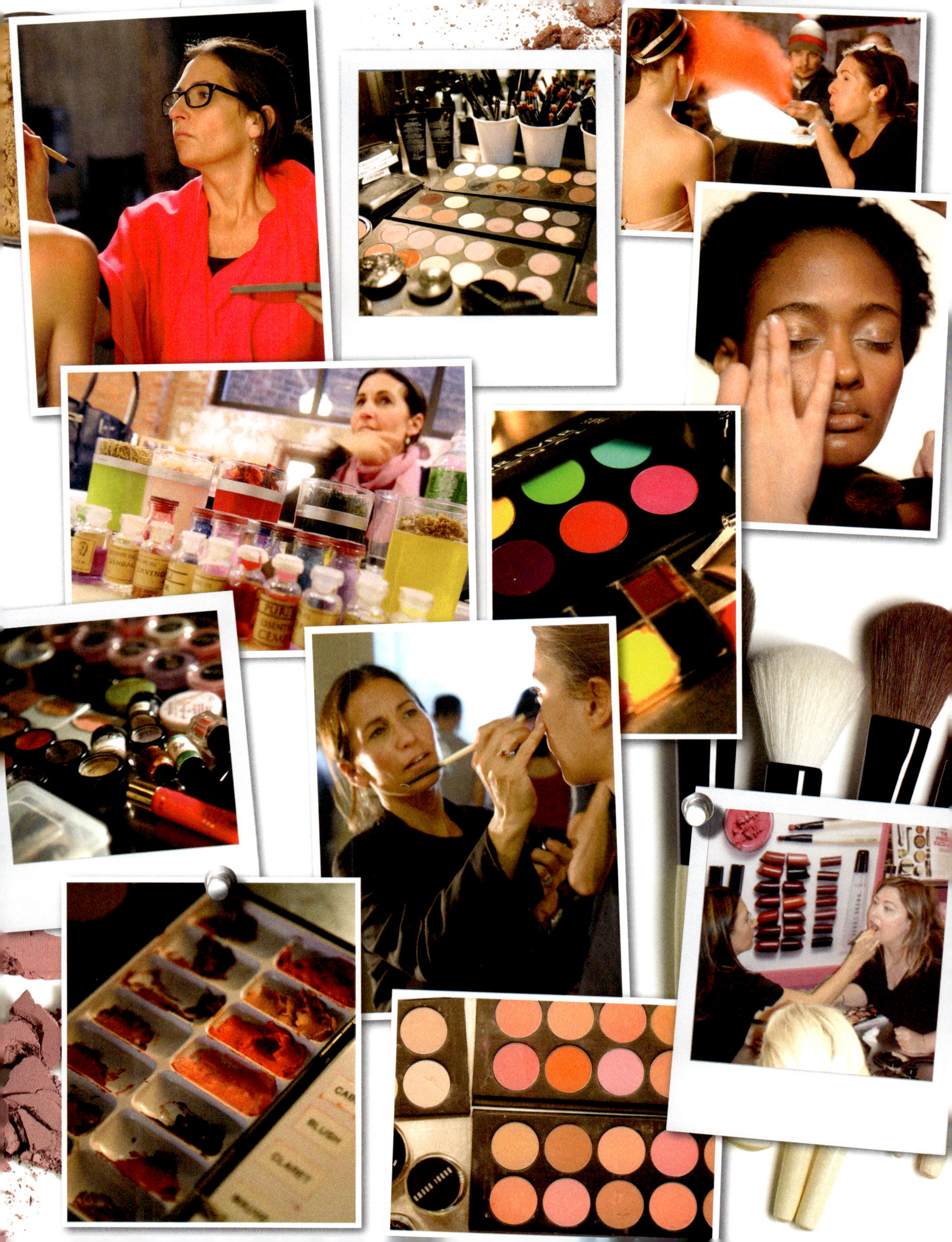

who wanted her foundation five shades lighter than her beautiful ebony skin. Just remember that in the end it is a collaboration, and if you listen well, everyone can be happy.

When your job is to make up a woman, it is important to pay careful attention to what she wants. Begin with a discussion of the woman's lifestyle and skin type. Ask about her makeup preferences, including the type of coverage and finish she likes in foundation. Before you begin any makeup application, it is important to know how much time she wants to spend on makeup on a regular basis. You want to address any concerns she has and know what is comfortable. Find out what kind of foundation she usually wears and her favorite lip color. Listen for real meaning. Sometimes what she says is not actually what she wants. One woman's idea of natural is another's evening look. Continue to ask questions at every step. Have the client watch the application in a hand mirror. Let her assess the progress at each stage, and listen to her likes and dislikes. She might find a concealer too light or dislike a darker brow. Adjust accordingly. Listening will help prevent unnecessary work (like starting over), keep the client happy, and eventually produce results that you both can love.

INSPIRATION AND CREATIVITY

One of the best ways to train your eye and encourage your creativity is to keep a scrapbook. Think of it as a visual journal for thoughts, images, and completed work. Tear any inspirational images from magazines. These could be faces, colors, or design concepts you find appealing. Sometimes even stationery, logos, or labels can inspire. Carry a digital camera to record inspirational visuals you encounter in daily life, such as colors and textures found on buildings or in nature.

The way you organize the scrapbook is up to you. Options include slipping images into plastic sleeves in a binder, taping them into a bound notebook, or tacking them onto a large bulletin board. Some artists prefer creating virtual scrapbooks, using a Web site to organize and store images and ideas. Other artists prefer to organize scrapbooks by topic rather than chronologically. They keep binders on various topics, such as bridal looks, natural looks, celebrities, color, or objects that inspire them.

As a makeup artist, you will go through dozens of scrapbooks during your career, but be sure to hold on to them. It will be helpful to reference your previous work and inspirations when preparing for a shoot or fashion show. The scrapbook becomes a historical record of your career, and reviewing old ones can be an important source of inspiration. I used to staple Polaroids into my day planner, and I still love looking back, remembering each shoot. I still have the red leather notebook I kept when starting my lipstick line. In it are the names of the women who inspired the colors and all the notes from meetings in which I discussed the line. It is a history that can reinspire me.

FINDING INSPIRATION

There are inspirations and ideas everywhere you look. I get inspiration from faces—women, men, children. I love to see how light affects different skin tones. I look at fashion magazines old and new—from the 30s and 40s up to the present. I especially love images from the 70s and 80s, possibly because that's when I became involved in the beauty industry. I shop at art supply stores, gourmet food stores, and vintage stores, looking for inspiration. I get ideas while I am exercising and listening to the music I love.

Be observant. Watch your client's reactions, and be open to change.

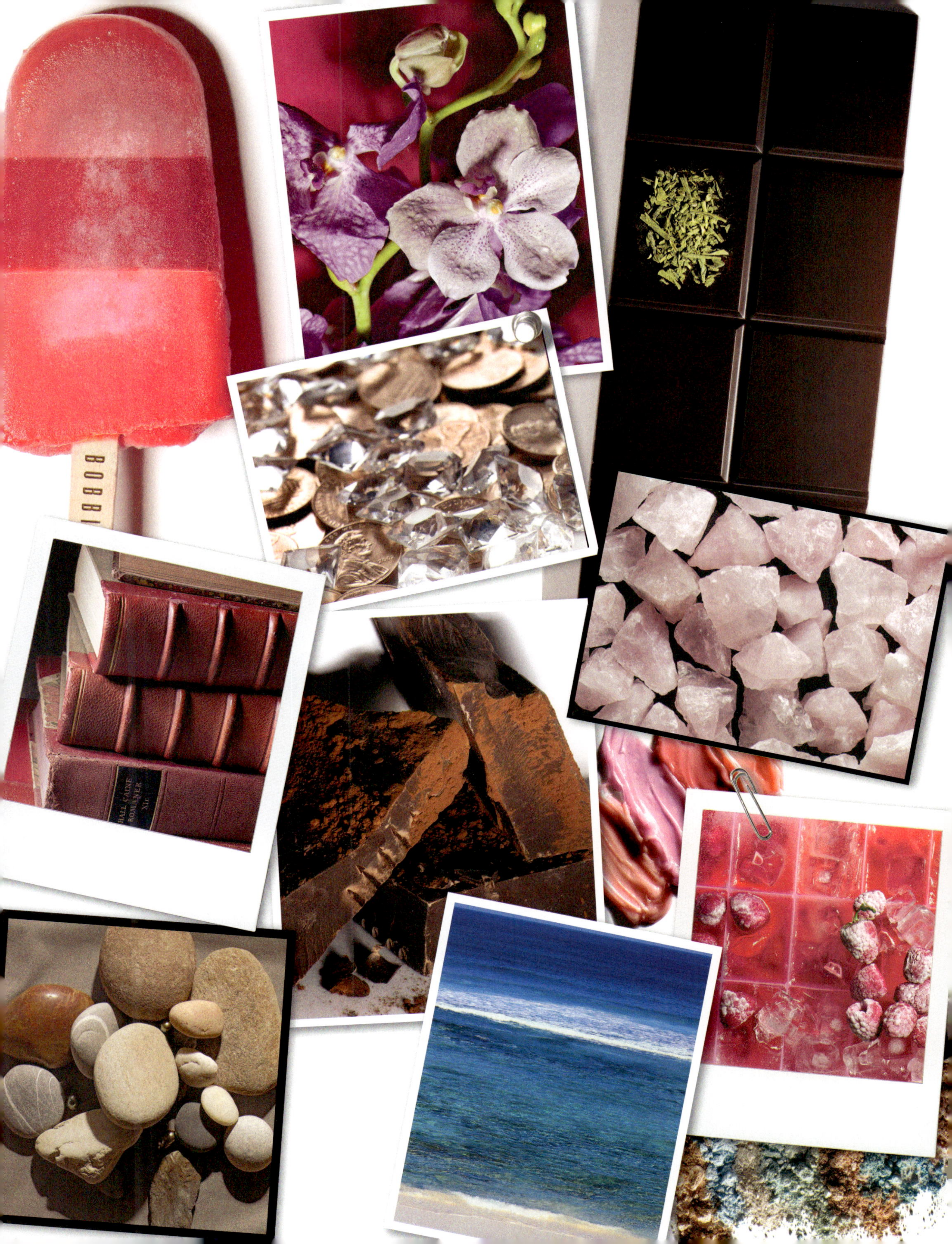
BOBBI

BREAKING into the BUSINESS

New artists have so much to learn about products and techniques and need to become comfortable with the basics. Beginning artists tend to do everything by the book. They often apply all the layers and don't see that a woman might not need some of the elements. ***More advanced artists are confident in their product knowledge and have had time to practice their technique, so they know what works and what is not needed for different clients.*** They have the ability to handle any situation that comes up. They are not afraid to reevaluate in the middle of an application. A strong knowledge base allows artists to make great choices, see when an application doesn't work, and know when to stop.

I was once hired by a big celebrity to do her makeup for the opening of a restaurant. She appeared with the biggest scratch on the side of her face. I didn't panic, but I had to try dozens of products to get the very pink scratch to blend in with her natural skin color. I was ready to handle the challenge with confidence in my ability.

It is important to stay open and eager. I received both good and bad advice when I started out. I was the pioneer of the natural, bronzy look, but I faced lots of criticism for it. I was told that I would have to change my makeup style—that nobody liked the healthy look. A hairdresser once told me that I needed to get a better hairstyle myself if I wanted to be successful.

One of the best ways to get started is to apply makeup on anyone and everyone who will let you. Practice on your friends and family until you get to the point where you feel completely comfortable working on people's faces. Practice all different types of makeup applications—natural, theatrical, bold fashion looks, bridal looks, men. Hands-on experience is invaluable.

Early in your career, experience is more important than pay. If you have the opportunity to apprentice with established makeup artists—even if it means just observing while you spend time cleaning brushes—do it. It can be a valuable learning experience. You never know whom you'll meet. Today's assistant can be the beauty editor of a major magazine in a few years.

Confident, successful artists are those who continue to train. Even top artists go back to the basics from time to time. Skills can always be improved. I learn from my artists, assistants, photographers, models, and friends. Never take a suggestion personally—it is always an opportunity. Things are always changing in the beauty industry, so you need to be open, aware, and looking for ways to improve.

Success is achieving the goals you set for yourself. Artists need to continually redefine their goals. Everyone might want to work in the fashion industry, but there are successful makeup artists working in film, television, and theater. There are those who have used their training and experience in makeup artistry to move into careers in education, marketing, merchandising, and other aspects of design.

By maintaining a clear picture of reality while seeking, creating, and fully exploiting every opportunity, artists can secure success one step at a time.

Artists are often eager to grow and move up in the industry. Patience is so important, and time is needed to perfect skills. Be happy at whatever level you are working, even if it is just observing. Look for a mentor. Work to completely understand the basics so that you can begin to make your own interpretations. Ask for help and guidance. It will be perceived as strength, not weakness.

Desire is perhaps the strongest determinant of success. When I hire a new artist, I look for someone who really wants to be doing the work. It is apparent in every aspect of the person. I want to work with people who are as passionate about beauty as I am. I look for applicants with great attitudes who are eager to work hard and to learn as much as they can. Some of the artists who assist me at fashion shows have worked for me for five to ten years. Yet they still watch carefully as I do the first model. Others seem uninterested. Guess which ones have the most talent?

ADVICE FOR BREAKING INTO THE BUSINESS

It helps to have a positive, professional attitude.

Always arrive on time. If you plan to arrive a bit early, then inconvenient delays will not be a problem.

Be who you are. Your appearance is an essential part of your presentation. Your personal style and makeup are reflections of your own tastes, and, like it or not, people will judge you by it.

Practice confidence. Hold your head up, make eye contact, have a firm handshake, smile, and take a genuine interest in what others have to say.

Don't be afraid to ask questions. Ask photographers, stylists, and models for their opinions.

Be nice to everyone. Even when my skills were just okay, I was invited back because I was pleasant.

Never stop learning. When I think about my own skills, I know I'm not done learning. I love watching other people do makeup. A good artist is secure enough to be open to new ideas and learning new techniques.

It's not about you. Great makeup artists focus on the client and don't ever let their own egos get in the way. It doesn't matter if the client is a celebrity, a supermodel, or a regular woman. It is about her, not about you!

Love what you do. Great makeup artists never lose their passion for makeup.

CAREER OPTIONS

Makeup artists have the opportunity to work in so many different areas. Career options vary from long-term jobs in television, with regular pay and benefits, to freelance jobs working on short-term runway, print, or film projects in a variety of locations and with a wide range of styles.

Department Store Counter

Artists generally work for a specific makeup line, teaching customers to choose and apply their own makeup. This job involves sales, and the compensation is often commission-based.

Bridal

Working with brides is both rewarding and very demanding. You need to do consultations and a run-through in addition to the makeup on the day of the wedding. The job usually involves traveling to the bride's location. Sometimes it will include doing makeup for the rest of the bridal party as well.

Beauty Salon

Makeup artists working in salons often find themselves in a teaching role. They do makeovers, help clients practice techniques, and are often called to do makeup for special events and weddings. Fashion and media work is sometimes booked through salons.

Television

Working on a set involves creating character looks and might include anything from doing basic makeup to designing looks for elaborate characters, aging the actors, creating the appearance of illness, replicating injuries, and much more. Artists sometimes work for years on one television show. Careers generally begin with assistant positions in the industry. Artists develop books of their work and a résumé. After gaining experience, artists are allowed to join a union, which provides opportunities, some job security, medical benefits, and a pension. Most television shows require makeup artists to have union membership.

Film

Shooting a film can take just days or several months, sometimes in multiple locations. The film industry is hard to break into, but not impossible. Any large-budget film requires makeup artists to have union membership. Which union you should join will depend on the area of the country in which you are working.

Television Commercials

Artists who work in this field are usually experienced in another aspect of the industry and have built a strong reputation either in print advertising or music videos.

Early in my career, I used to watch famous models correct the makeup I had done on their faces. The result was good—they always looked better, and I learned so much by watching them.

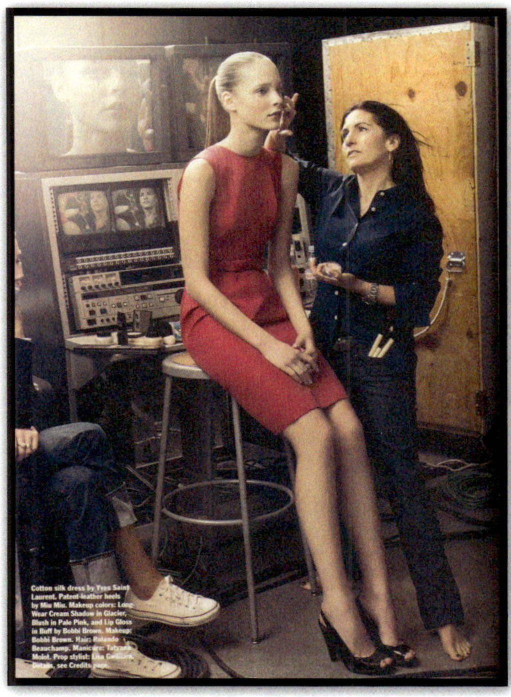

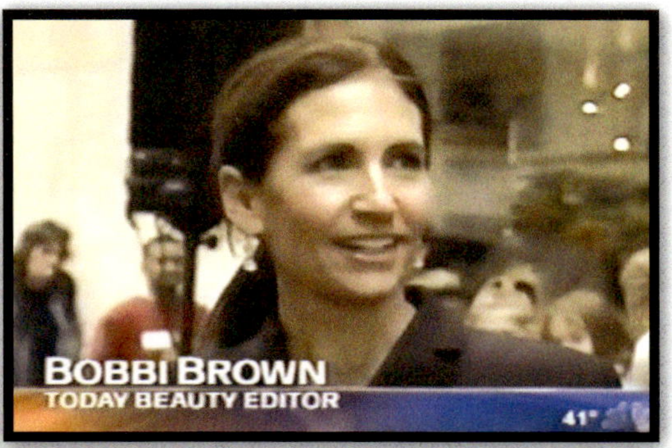

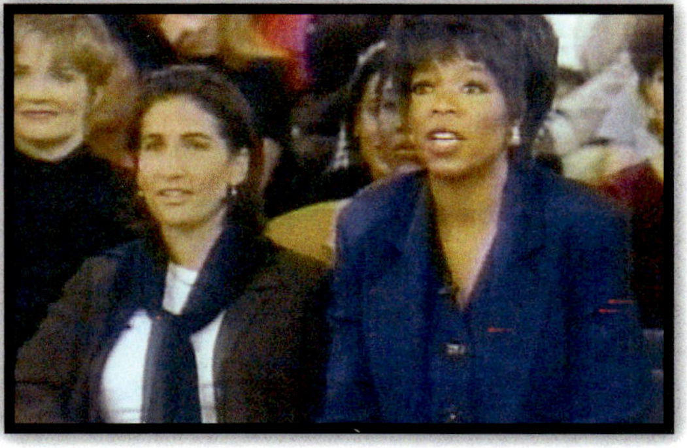

Print

Makeup artists who work in the editorial or print advertising field work with models, photographers, stylists, and editors. Collaboration is everything. Shoots take place in studios and also on location—sometimes very exotic ones. Work is obtained by sending a portfolio, or book showing your past work, to agencies that provide representation and to clients. The better the book, the higher the demand and pay rate. Print jobs include work for magazines, advertisers, catalog companies, corporate in-house publications, movie posters, and album covers.

Video

Music videos are often filmed very quickly and require flexibility, spontaneity, and simple artistry. While many videos are low-budget freelance projects, they provide opportunities for young artists to build their portfolios. Makeup artists are often hired for music videos because their print work, doing magazine and album covers, has attracted a music artist's attention. Educational and industrial video shoots also hire makeup artists and stylists.

Live Performance

This field includes work for theater, dance, and musical theater, as well as for live concerts and road tours. The artist works under time pressure and needs to maintain continuity. An artist sometimes stays with a production for months or even years.

Fashion Show

Applying makeup for the runway is both adrenaline boosting and exhausting. It involves collaboration with a designer and models. Work begins with a pretest to discuss and try out the look. On the day of the show, another pretest is completed with the actual runway lighting for final designer notes and approval. Then the work becomes incredibly hectic and fast-paced as all of the models are made-up. Makeup artists obtain work in this area by sending out their book and through reputation and connections.

Remember when I said to be nice to everyone? Often assistants become editors-in-chief.

the BUSINESS of MAKEUP ARTISTRY

While makeup artists are first and foremost artists, they also need to be businesspeople. ***Makeup artists need to be talented, confident, and charismatic, as well as effective entrepreneurs who are able to effectively market their talents.*** To begin, you will need to find ways to gain experience, develop effective work habits, create a business system, and build a portfolio and résumé. Eventually, you will want to secure agency representation.

Your success is completely up to you. This means you need to attract and keep clients, develop and maintain several portfolios and a résumé, handle the business effectively, and stay current.

DEVELOPING A PORTFOLIO

A portfolio is a book in which you keep photographs of all your work as a makeup artist. The book can be low-cost plastic or high-end leather with your name engraved on it.

The first step in finding work is developing a great portfolio you can show to potential employers. Having professional photographs taken of your work can be prohibitively expensive and is probably not worth the investment when you are first starting out. Instead, try to find an aspiring photographer who might also like to have photos for his or her own book, and help each other out. Call every modeling agency and ask if you can do makeup for testing. Testing is when a model, photographer, hairdresser, and makeup artist all do a shoot for free to show others their work. The payment is a photo for your portfolio. It's also an excellent way to learn how to build rapport with a team at a photo shoot—an important lesson, because the same team will often work together repeatedly on jobs.

After the test, getting pictures from the photographer can sometimes be a challenge. It is up to you to confirm when the pictures will be ready to view. Set a date to pick out your own shots, and crop them if needed. Since most photographs are now digital, you can collect and store them on your computer. Prints can be made in a lab or with your own printer.

Your book should include at least fifteen amazing test shots before you show it around. Whenever possible, use professional models and photographers. Amateur work is quickly evident. Once you begin to find paid work, you will be able to include tear sheets (published work) from magazines, book covers, television commercials, and other jobs. You can begin looking for agency representation when you have at least ten to fifteen tear sheets that show a variety of work. Building a portfolio takes time. It will take at least six to nine months of consistent work to develop a book that you can show to clients. Once you have the book together, you need to show it to everyone—photographers, other artists, producers, and art directors. Get their advice, and listen to it. Thank them for their time and help.

PUTTING TOGETHER A PORTFOLIO

Presentation counts for a lot in this business, so your portfolio needs to make a brilliant first impression.

It is a representation of you as an artist.
The book needs to be neat, well organized, and an accurate reflection of your aesthetic and personal style.

Portfolio books themselves are available in a variety of sizes.
The two most popular sizes are 9" x 12" and 11" x 14". Art supply stores are a good source for portfolio books. Look for one that has plastic or acetate pages into which you can slip your photos. You will also want at least one pocket (on the inside back cover) to hold a résumé, promotional cards, and business cards. Include several of each so that whoever is looking at your book can take and keep a copy of your résumé and card. Some agencies prefer receiving portfolios on a CD rather than in book form, so always have several electronic copies available.

Keep one portfolio with all of your original photographs in it.
High-quality color copies are used in books intended for mailing. Tear sheets should be originals, so if a magazine prints your work, buy lots of copies of it. Have at least two books ready to be sent out at any time. Consider having four or even five copies. It is also not a bad idea to carry a reduced version with you in case an opportunity to show it presents itself.

From my portfolio:

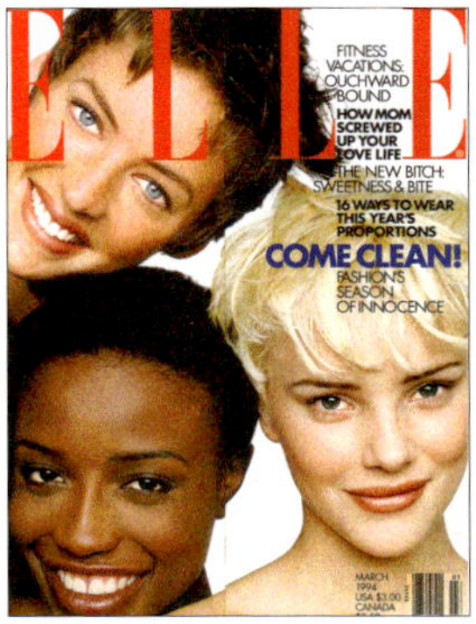

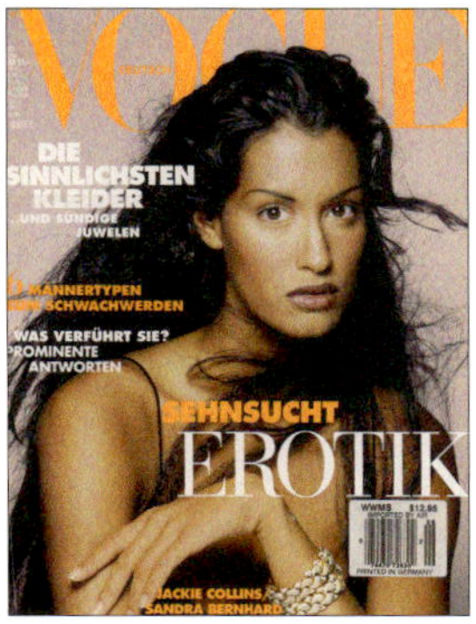

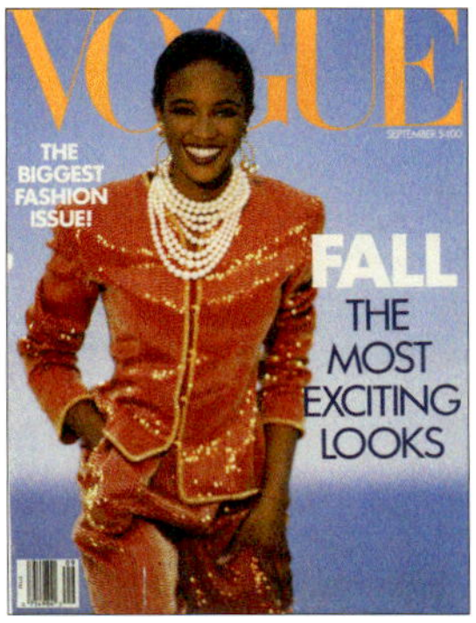

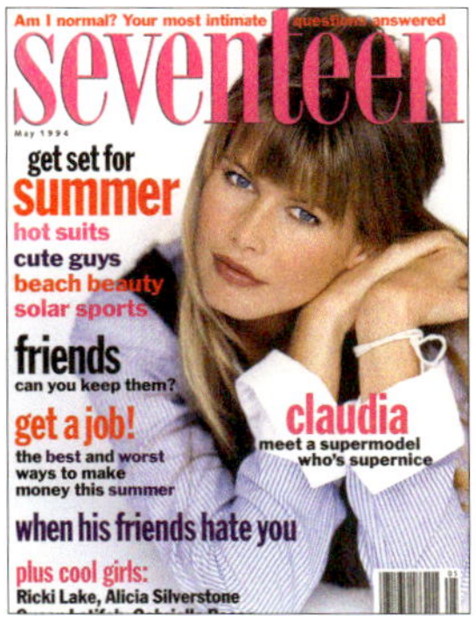

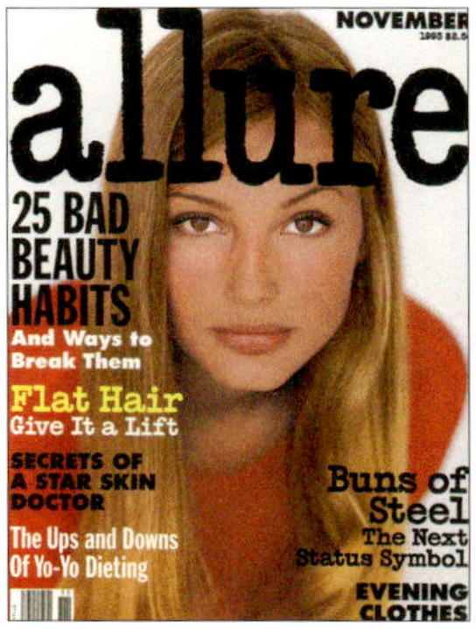

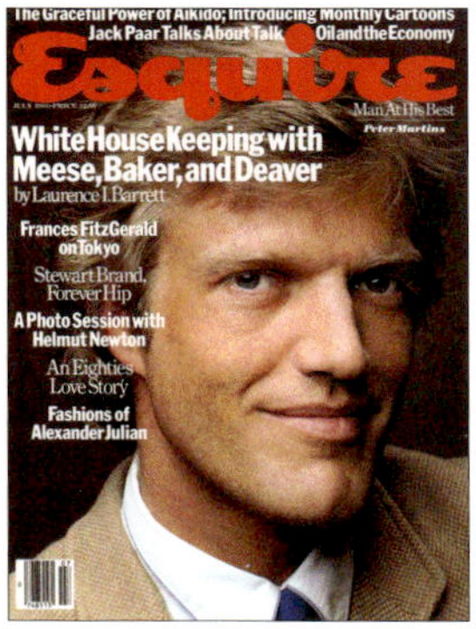

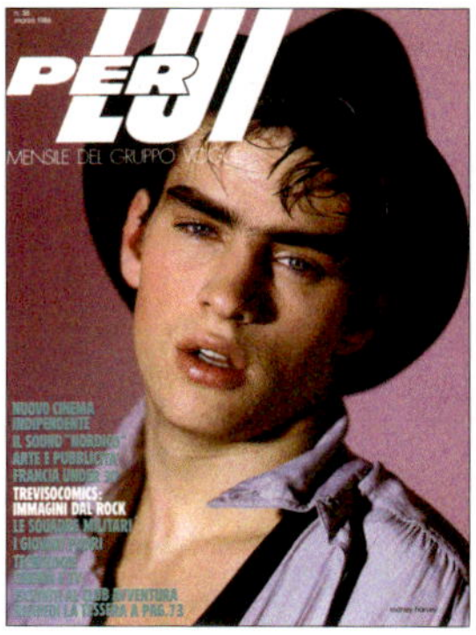

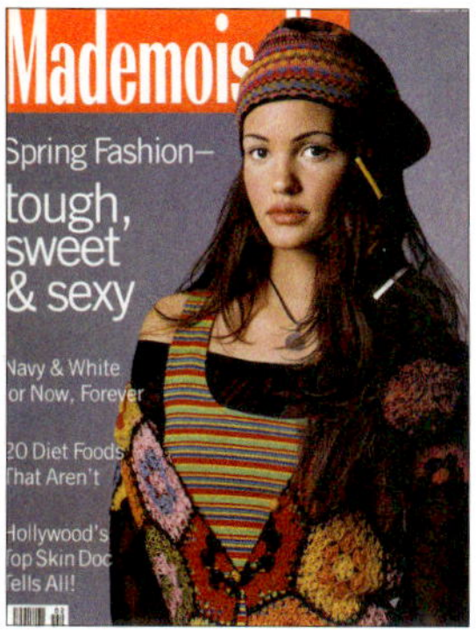

Promotional Cards

A promotional card is an essential addition to your promotional arsenal. These cards are postcard-size and have one to three photos of your work, as well as your name and contact information. Also referred to as a comp card, a promo, or a leave-behind, these cards show your artistry and style. Both print and electronic versions of the cards are necessary for self-promotion. Promo cards have four-color photographs on one side, and your contact information in black and white on the other. As photographers own the rights to their photographs, you must obtain their written permission to use any photos and credit the photographers on the card. You can send out the cards in the mail and have several in your portfolio for the editor, photographer, or agent to keep on file. That way, art directors and fashion editors always have a sample of your work on hand. Also keep the card as a PDF file on your computer, or better yet on a flash drive. This will allow you to e-mail a copy almost instantly, wherever you are, to potential employers. Carry several with you in your bag for those unexpected opportunities.

Web Sites

New artists are using the Web to promote their services. Make sure you hire a reputable Web designer to help you design and launch your site, or lease space on an existing site that will help you build your own. Some makeup agencies offer such space to their artists. Remember that the quality and style of the site, not just the content, directly reflect who you are as an artist.

On the Web site, include your promotional card and a PDF version of your résumé. Include current portfolio content. Determine how large you want the site to be and how often you will want to update it. Consider how you want people to contact you and whether you want to include links on the site. Build a site that is globally accessible.

Successfully managing your site means that it is always current and can be easily accessed. If your Web server does not automatically list you with search engines, try using Addme.com. This is a free Web site–submission engine that will add your site to the top thirty most popular search engines.

Reels

If your primary goal is to work in television, music videos, or movies, you will also want to put together a reel. A reel is a compilation of your styling work for film, television, and video on a master tape (actually a DVD), edited to several minutes that includes the best footage. Choose music for your reel that creates the perfect mood. The reel will need to be professionally edited to include transitions and titles. Make copies of the reel, and create case labels with your name, address, and phone number for identification. Most producers do not return reels, but making copies is inexpensive, and reels are great promotional tools.

Résumés

Résumés let the decision makers know the full range of your credits. A résumé needs to be complete, accurate, and professional. Pick a font that is easy to read, and print the résumé on good-quality stock. Write a clear, concise cover letter to include with the résumé when mailing your résumé or portfolio. While a cover letter and résumé are important tools in your self-promotion efforts, it is the portfolio or reel that will get you the job. In film and television, a listing of your experience in résumé form is the first thing that producers look at. They might interview and see the portfolios of only a few artists. In print work, a look at your portfolio usually precedes an interview.

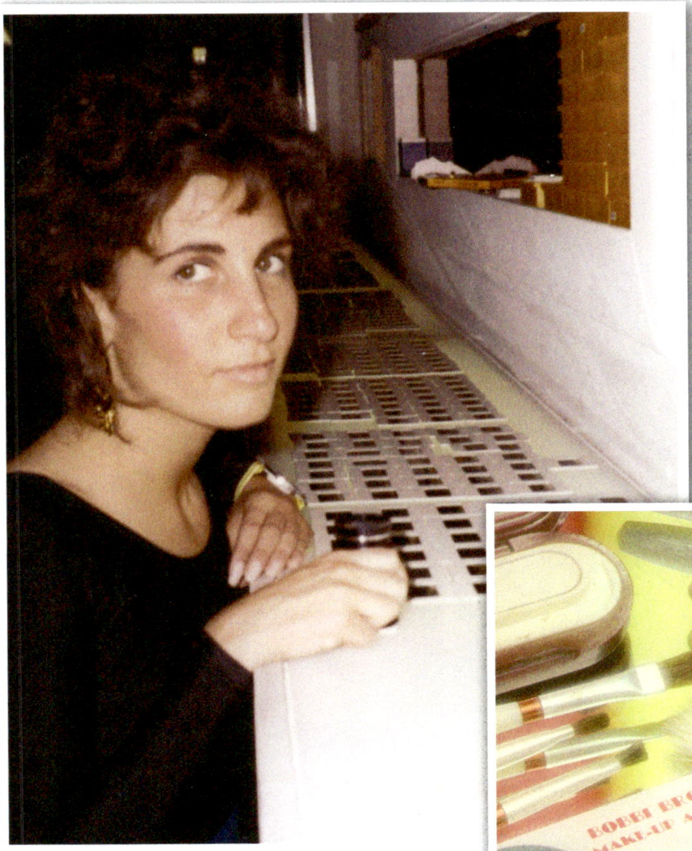

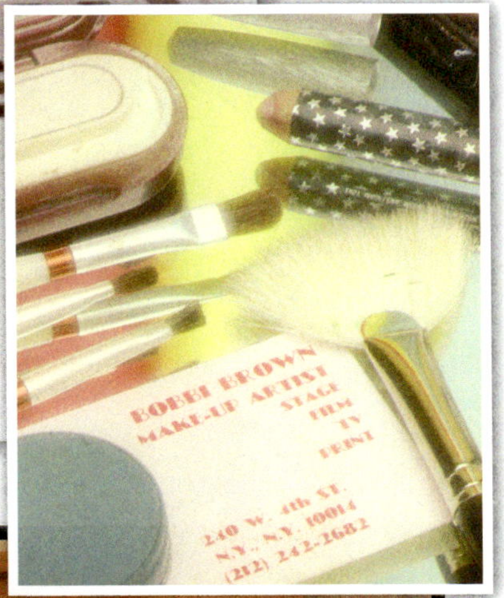

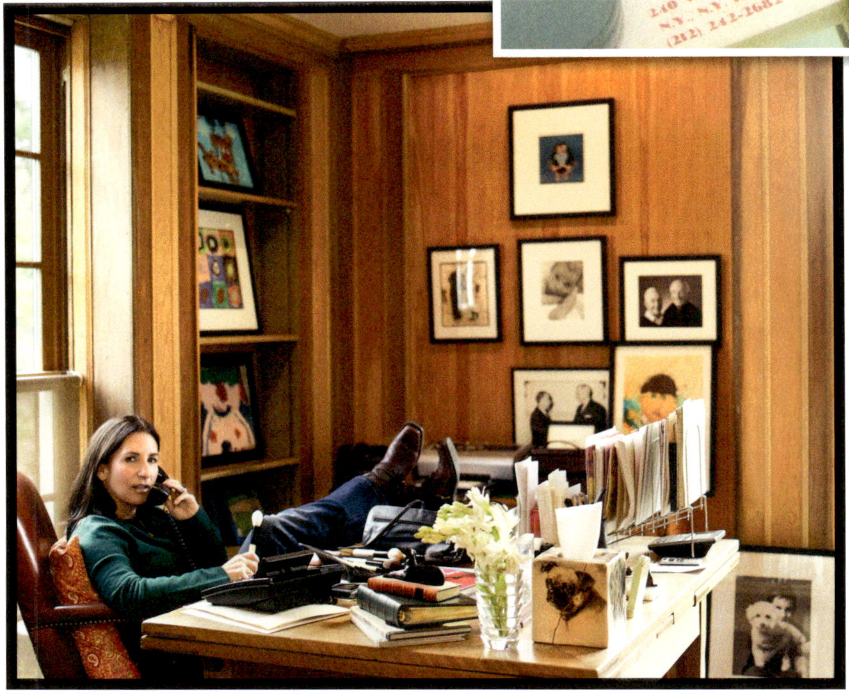

BOOKING WORK

Once your promotional tools are completed and your portfolio looks great, you need a plan. ***Determine what your career goals are. Do you want to work in retail, with private clients, or for commercial clients in print or in film and television?*** You might end up with a combination of work, but maintaining a focus is important. It will determine whether you spend more time developing your book or your reel. In either case, you will need to identify a group of potential clients and contact them. Follow these guidelines:

SHOW YOUR WORK
Develop a mailing list, and send out your portfolio and/or résumé. Sending promotional cards and your résumé is a quick way to remind possible employers of your work.

FOLLOW UP
Call within a week of leaving or mailing your materials.

THANK POTENTIAL CLIENTS
by sending a card thanking them for their time and advice. Ask them if there are any available opportunities.

Fashion stylists or editors are often the key to being hired on a high profile shoot. The bigger the stylist, the better the artist has to be.

Commit your goals to paper. Learn as much as you can about photographers who work in the industry, as they often decide which stylists to hire. To get print work, start bringing your portfolio to magazine editors, photographers, and other potential employers. The only way to do this is to have an appointment, so be prepared to spend lots of time on the phone. You can look on the mastheads of magazines to find the fashion and beauty editors and art directors to call. Find out the drop-off days specified by the agencies. These are the specific days and times set up for portfolio reviews. A publication called *The Black Book* lists everyone in the print world and is an invaluable resource for contact information (see Resource Guide).

Don't be afraid to explore several avenues of employment at once. Saturate the market with your card, sending it to not only magazine editors, photographers, and agents but also to local stores and salons. Contact department stores about doing fashion shows or other promotional events. Volunteer to do the makeup for fund-raising fashion shows or productions at local theaters. To help break into the more prestigious and higher paying areas of makeup artistry, do whatever you can to meet the top players in the field. Call or send a friendly personal note along with your promotional card. It will help if you keep up to date on the industry—read all the fashion and entertainment magazines to keep track of the top photographers, models, designers, and makeup

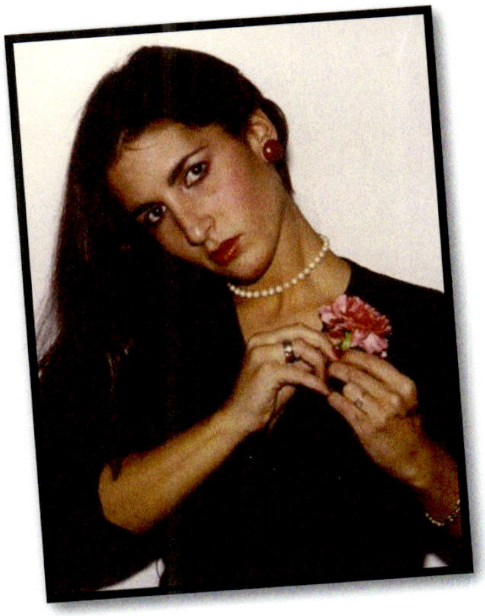

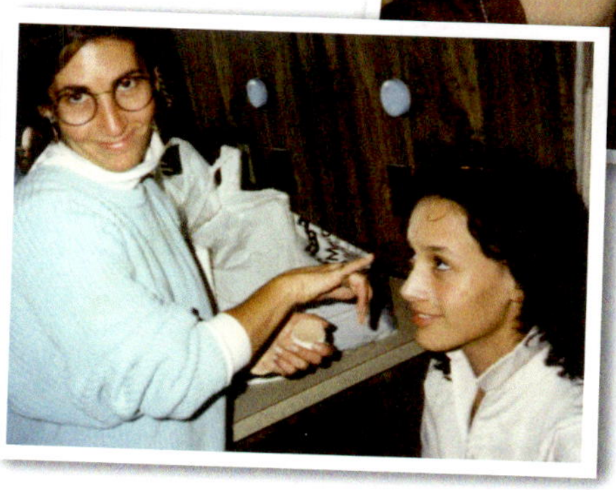

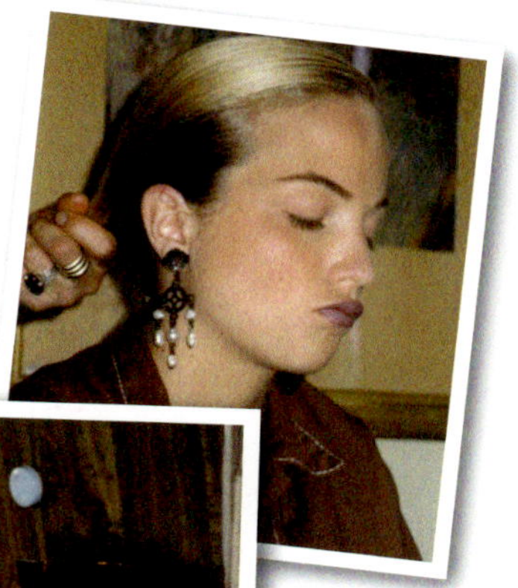

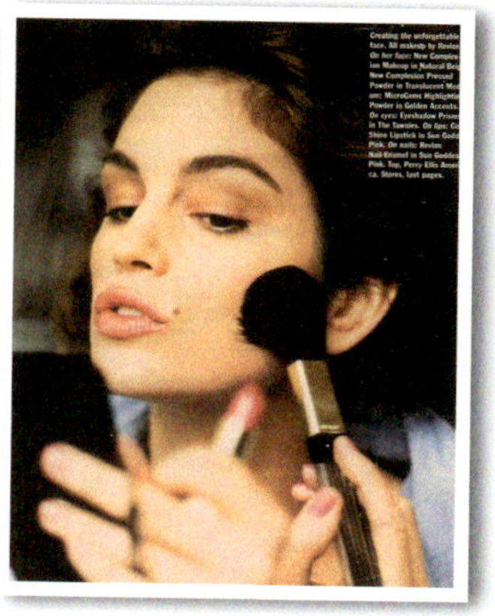

artists. Know who does which advertising campaigns, study photographers' and makeup artists' styles, and be able to recognize their work.

Remember that in the fashion industry—like any other business—people hire people. So always be nice, smile, and say thank you. Potential clients will remember you for it next time, when you come back with more experience and more photographs in your portfolio. Also, when you're just starting out, don't think too much about what you'll get out of a makeup job. Take all the jobs you can, because you never know what you might learn or what contacts you might make.

It's also worth noting that when you are getting started and looking for freelance work, there are going to be dry spells. It's important to be frugal with your money, to learn how to budget when you do get paying freelance work, and to have another source of income to fall back on (waiting tables, working retail, dog walking, etc.). And when you do have downtime between assignments, use it constructively—make calls, send out your résumé and promotional card, and do more test shoots to build your portfolio.

MANAGING YOUR BUSINESS

It is never too early to begin to develop a business plan and system. On a computer, in a planner, or directly in your current scrapbook, create a simple log of all your contacts and work completed. The log should include the date, name, company (when relevant), contact number, topic, result, and follow-up. Print your digital photographs from shoots, labeled with the date and persons involved, to include in the scrapbook or log. Networking is such a huge part of being a freelance makeup artist that it is important to keep a detailed record of all your contacts and previous work.

You will need to negotiate the terms and fees for each job, prepare confirmations to make sure that the terms and conditions are met, generate invoices, keep accurate financial records, and collect all payments. Terms might include payments for travel and per diems, materials costs, and assistant rates. You need to know the scope of the project before these terms can be set. Ask questions and take notes, only making your decision when you have all the information you need. Then send confirmation, also called a deal memo. It is a document that includes the job description, day rate, overtime rate, the flat dollar amount if overtime is not included, length of project in days, the number of assistants and pay rate, a materials budget, and for stylists, clauses regarding reimbursement for clothing damage. Create job folders for each job, with copies of receipts, any advance checks, signed vouchers, and invoices. Prepare a professional invoice form, and send it to the client at the end of the shoot. Send a credit sheet, indicating the job you worked on and how you want your credit to read, to the appropriate person. Templates of business forms used in the industry can be found at makeuphairandstyling.com.

Remember that many expenses are tax deductible. Keep a categorized record of automobile, travel, and entertainment expenses, plus records of money spent on office supplies and office equipment. Record the purpose of the expense on each receipt, and file it by category, with a copy in the job folder.

Maintaining and updating your portfolio and résumé is essential. Stay current. Know what is going on in entertainment, fashion, and beauty. Look at magazines, fashion shows, and music videos. Always dress appropriately, be prepared and on time, be decisive and efficient. If you can't say something nice about someone, don't say anything at all. Networking is a major part of the job, so make contacts, listen with interest, be positive, make phone calls, send thank-you cards, and keep your promises.

AGENCIES

Agencies provide a wide range of services, including finding work for their talent, doing promotional work, negotiating and collecting fees, and offering career management. In exchange for those services, the artist pays the agency 20 percent of his or her fee.

When starting out as a freelance makeup artist, you will undoubtedly experience frustration. You need a good portfolio to get an agent, but without an agent, it may be hard to get the jobs you need to produce a good book. Having agency representation does help you secure the best assignments. Begin with research. Take the time to learn something about different agencies. What is their philosophy? What type of work do they do? How many artists do they represent? Who are these artists? Why is a certain one the right agency for you? Interview several agencies that seem to be a good match. Ask what you can expect from them. How do they promote their talent? Bring a résumé that lists all the photographers, editors, art directors, stylists, models, etc., who have worked with you. Include all your work done for magazines, catalogs, ads, or videos. Don't be discouraged if the agency doesn't sign you on the spot. It pays to be persistent; after making the initial contact with an agency, keep in touch. Follow up by sending additional tear sheets from new assignments, and try to make another appointment a few months later. It's also helpful to ask for constructive criticism. Find out what the agent likes or doesn't like about your book or promotional card, and take the advice to heart.

One of the best ways to get a foot in the door at an agency is to be willing to work as an assistant to one of the agency's makeup artists. Before you call, know which artists the agency represents, what projects they might be working on, and which ones you are most interested in and/or most qualified to assist on. The need for extra assistants often arises at the last minute, and whoever is available and interested may get the job.

RATES

Rates vary depending on experience and location. Rates paid in New York and Los Angeles are generally higher than rates in other places. Research the going daily and hourly rates in your area, and always charge competitively.

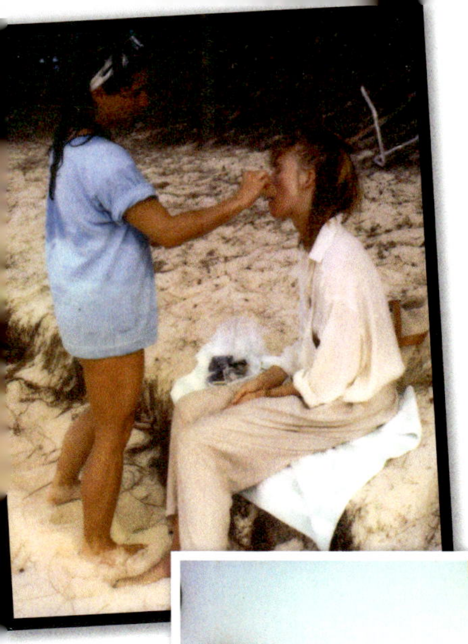
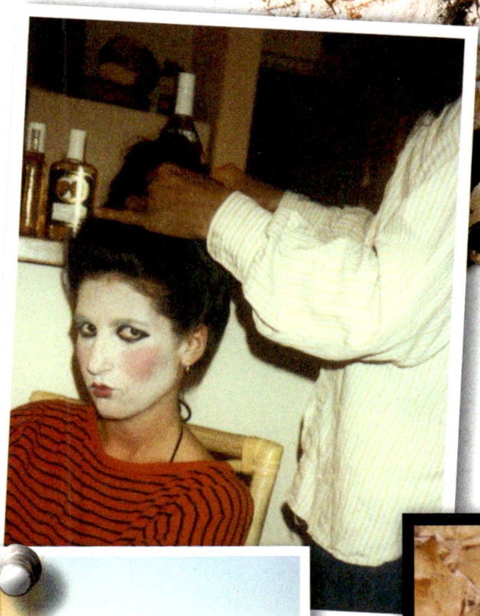
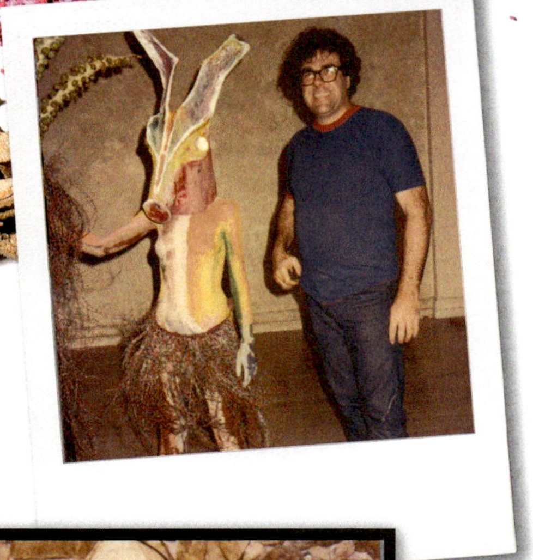
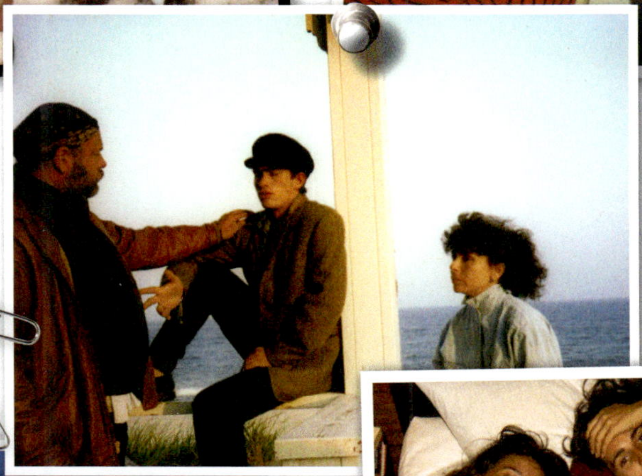
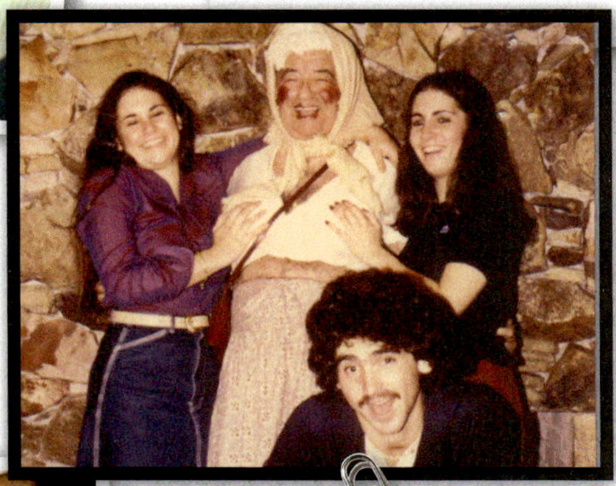
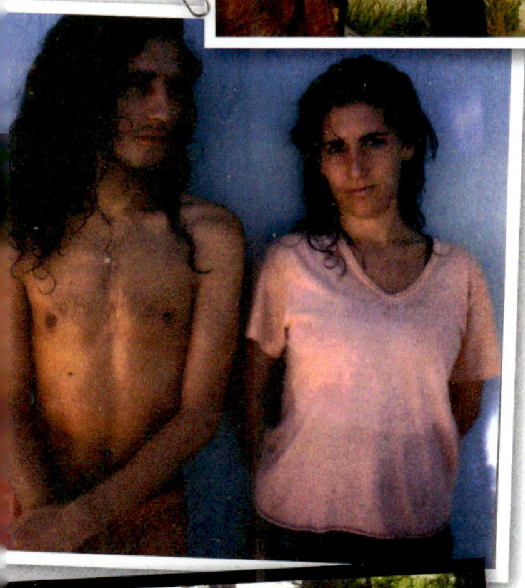
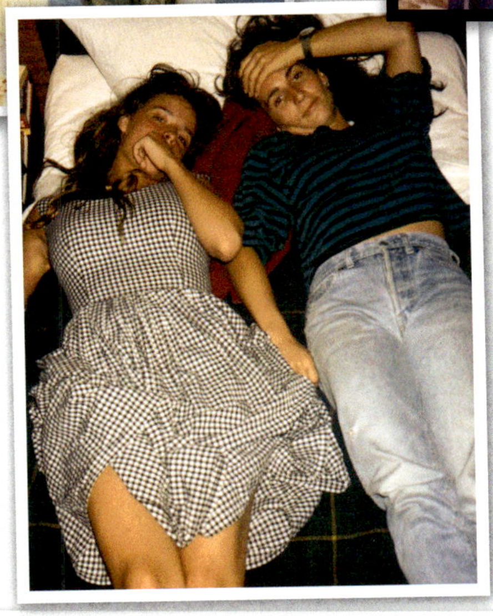
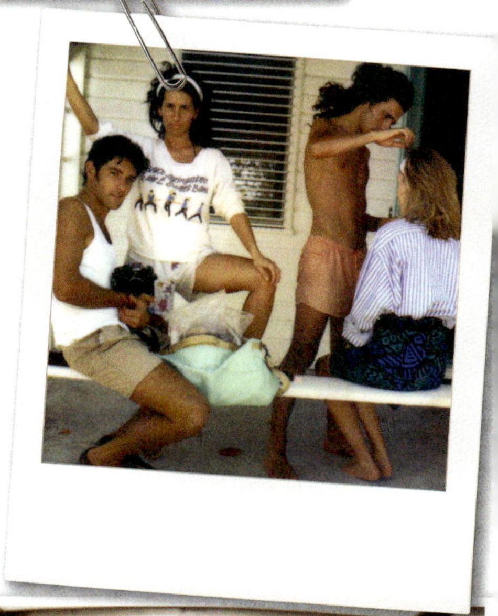
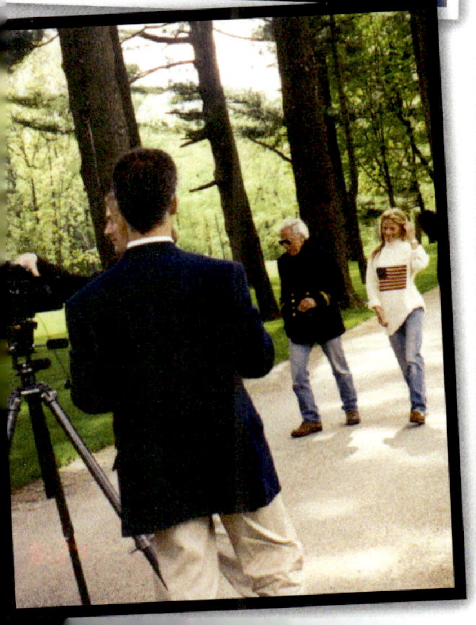
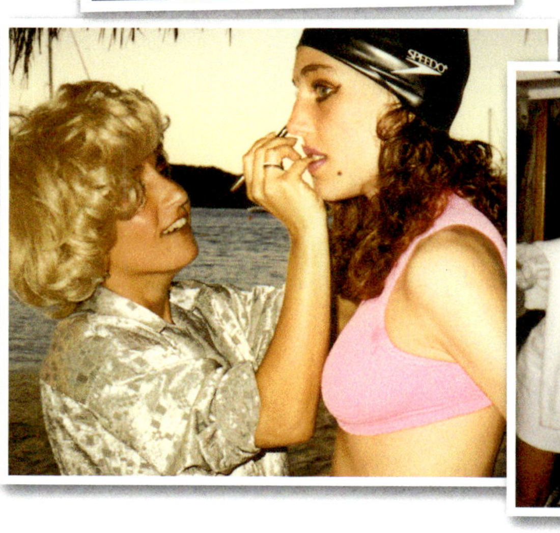
SPEEDO
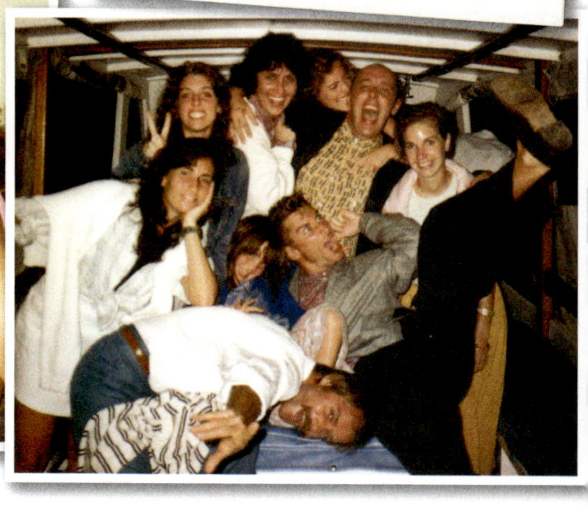

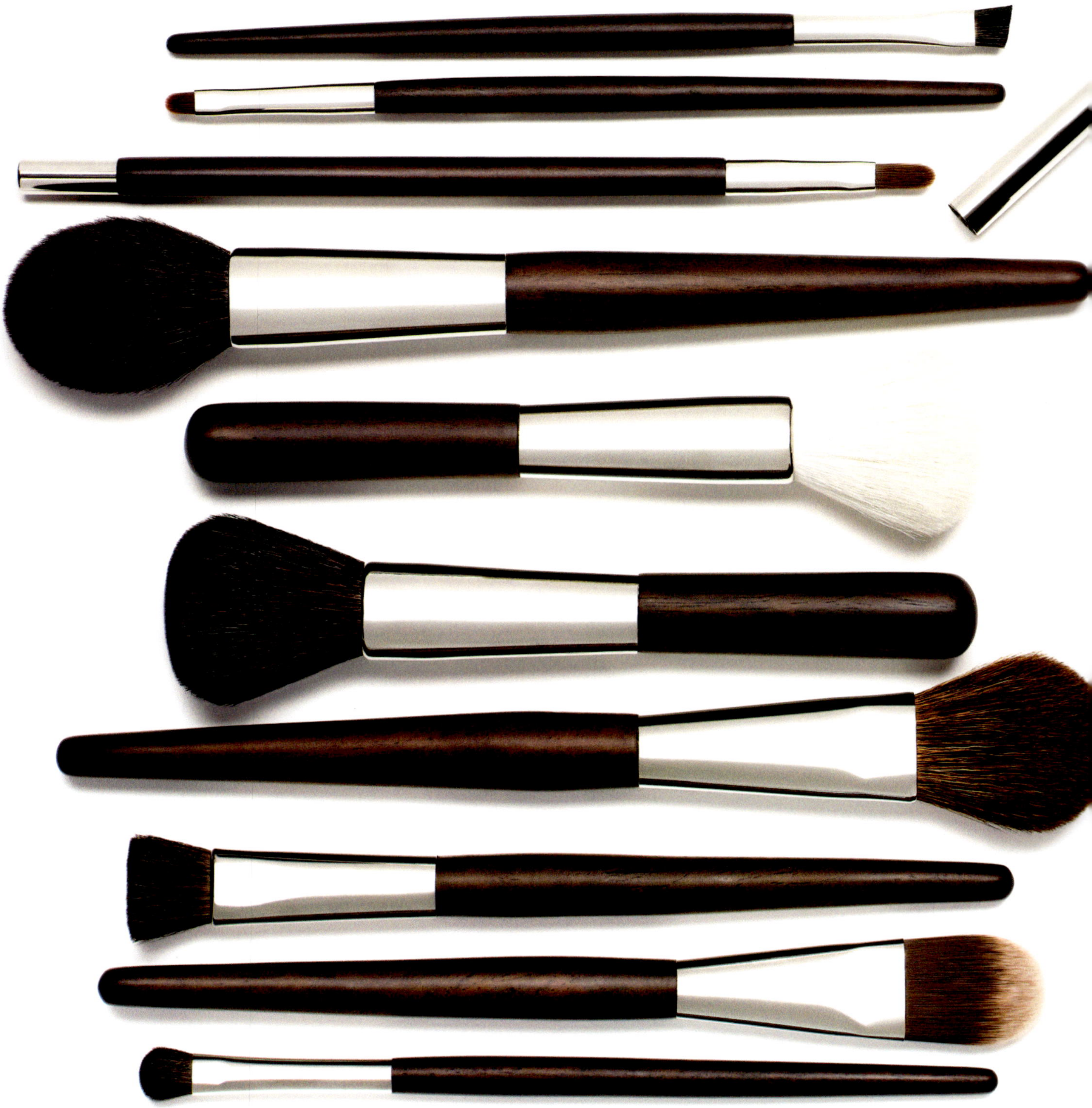

Chapter 10

ESSENTIAL EQUIPMENT for the PROFESSIONAL

DEVELOPING & STOCKING the PROFESSIONAL MAKEUP KIT

A good makeup kit contains all the products and tools you need to do your work. The appearance and organization of your kit are a big part of the first impression you make when you show up for a job. No one wants to work with a makeup artist whose kit is dirty and disorganized.

One of the best ways to carry your supplies is in a small rolling suitcase. (A shoulder bag or backpack will be too heavy and not good for your back.) Organize all your equipment and supplies in containers. Zip-top plastic bags, palettes, vitamin boxes, brush rolls, small makeup bags, and dop kits are all excellent tools for keeping everything in its place. To make it easy to find what you need, label each container clearly so you know what's inside without having to open it. A helpful trick is to transfer makeup into smaller containers to save space. Create a complete foundation palette by taking slices off your stick foundations. Pour liquids into smaller jars. Create a palette of multiple corrector and concealer shades. Arrange slices of lipsticks as well as balm in a lip palette. The more organized your kit is, the more efficient you'll be as a makeup artist.

After each job, take the time to put everything back in its place. Clean any tools you used, sharpen pencils, spray cream products with alcohol, wipe off powder shadows, and replace products as needed. That way, your kit will always be ready to go, and you won't have to scramble when you get a call to do a job at the last minute.

You never know what you will encounter when arriving on a job, so it makes sense to have all your supplies with you. Since that means toting around hundreds of products, it pays to organize them in categories. A checklist for everything you need to complete a professional kit follows.

THE ESSENTIAL KIT (at right)
These are the basic supplies that you should always have with you.

Skincare

Foundation palette

Lip and cheek palette

Eye shadows

Full brush kit

Lip liners

Lip glosses

Bronzer

Gel eyeliner

Mascara

Eyelash curler

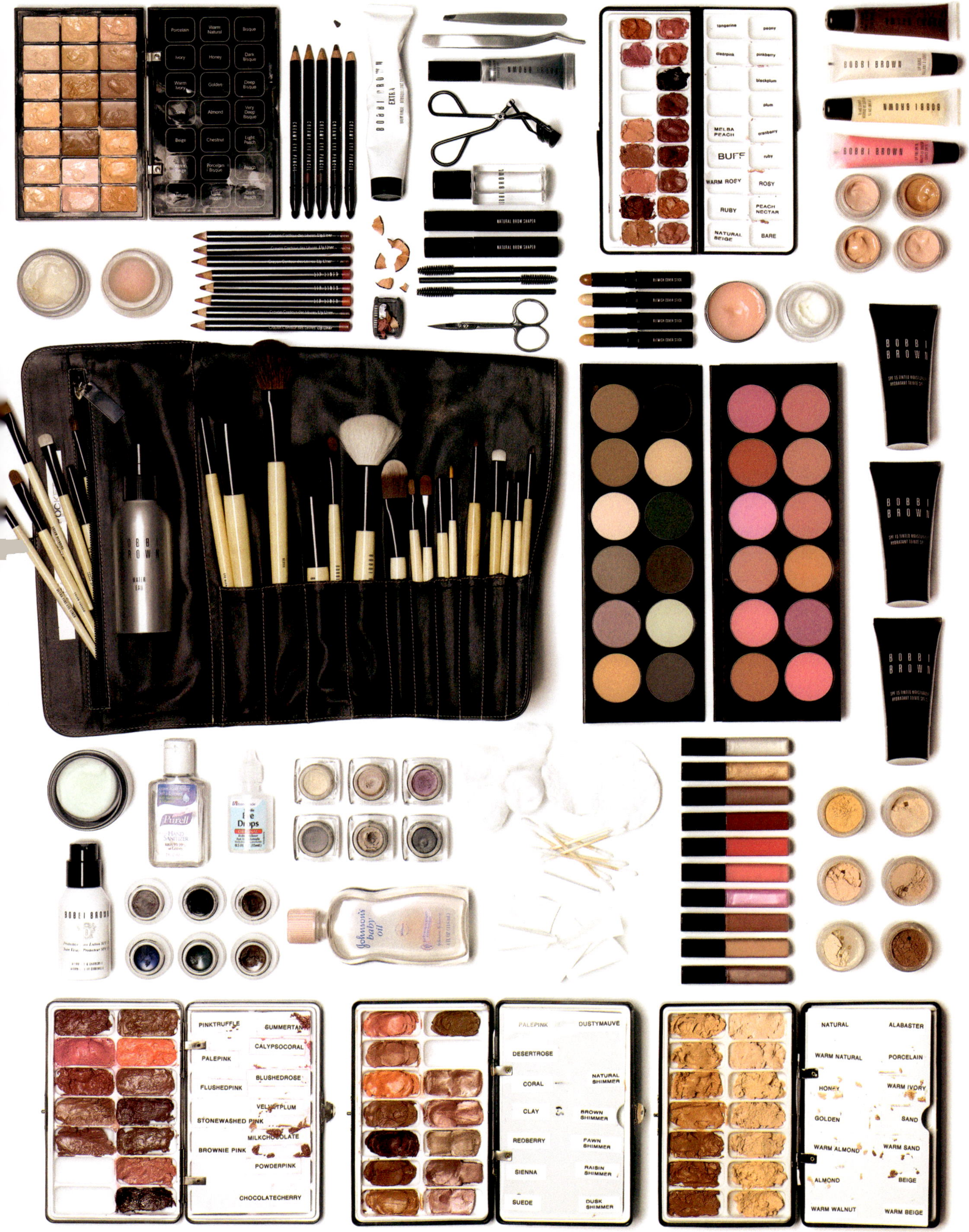

Porcelain
Warm Natural
Bisque
Ivory
Honey
Dark Bisque
Golden
Deep Bisque
Almond
Very Deep Bisque
Beige
Chestnut
Light Peach
Peach
tangerine
peony
clearpink
pinkberry
blackplum
plum
MELBA PEACH
cranberry
BUFF
ruby
WARM ROSY
ROSY
RUBY
PEACH NECTAR
NATURAL BEIGE
BARE
BOBBI BROWN
PINKTRUFFLE
SUMMERTAN
CALYPSOCORAL
PALEPINK
FLUSHEDPINK
BLUSHEDROSE
VELVETPLUM
STONEWASHED PINK
MILKCHOCOLATE
BROWNIE PINK
POWDERPINK
CHOCOLATECHERRY
PALEPINK
DUSTYMAUVE
DESERTROSE
NATURAL SHIMMER
CORAL
CLAY
BROWN SHIMMER
REDBERRY
FAWN SHIMMER
SIENNA
RAISIN SHIMMER
SUEDE
DUSK SHIMMER
NATURAL
ALABASTER
WARM NATURAL
PORCELAIN
HONEY
WARM IVORY
GOLDEN
SAND
WARM ALMOND
WARM SAND
ALMOND
BEIGE
WARM WALNUT
WARM BEIGE

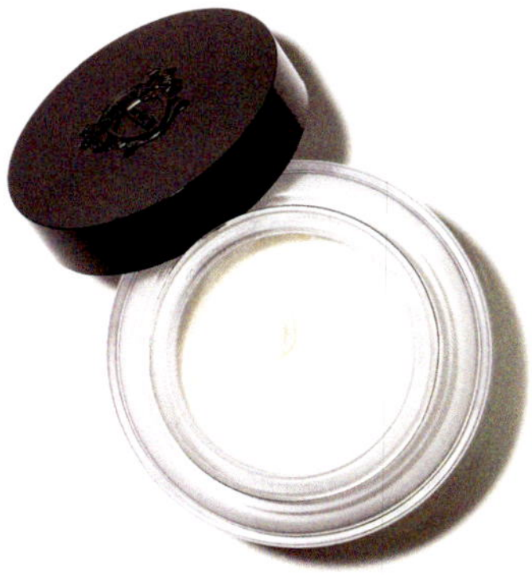

SKINCARE

Transfer moisturizers into smaller plastic jars and bottles, or purchase the smallest size container of each product. Keep all moisturizing products together in a large zip-top plastic bag or makeup bag. Appropriate skincare makes a huge difference in how makeup looks, so be prepared to cleanse and hydrate the face before applying any makeup.

Eye makeup remover, both non-oily and a product for removing waterproof makeup

Eye cream

Face lotion

Rich, moisturizing face cream

Shine-control lotion

Face balm

Lip balm

Body lotion

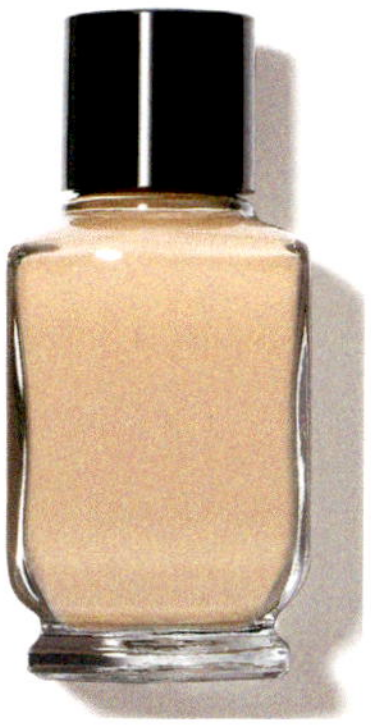

CONCEALER, FOUNDATION, POWDER

You will need a full range of foundation shades in order to properly match any skin tone you encounter. If using stick foundations, slice off sections, and put them into a palette; transfer your moisturizing and oil-free foundations into smaller bottles.

Five shades of corrector

At least ten shades of concealer

At least fifteen shades of foundation in a variety of formulas

Four to five shades of tinted moisturizer

Six shades of loose powder (from white, for use on porcelain skin, to dark brown)

Mix-in pigments—yellow, black, red, blue—are a help to correct wrong color foundation.

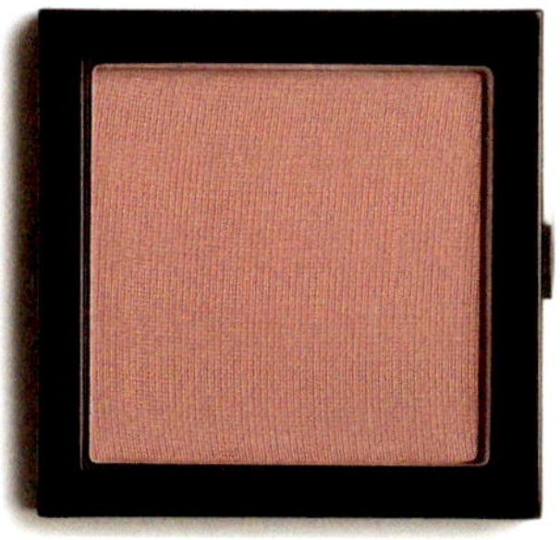

BLUSH

A complete kit includes a full range of blush in both neutrals and brighter shades in powder, cream, gel, and shimmer formulas, and a range of bronzers. Blushes are also used as eye shadow to achieve bright color in magazine work. It's also possible to mix a blush with clear lip balm for an extreme effect.

Six to eight shades of powder blush, from soft neutrals to brights

Five shades of cream blush (can be placed in a palette)

Two to three shades of gel blush

Four shades of bronzing powder

Five shades of shimmer blush or bronzer

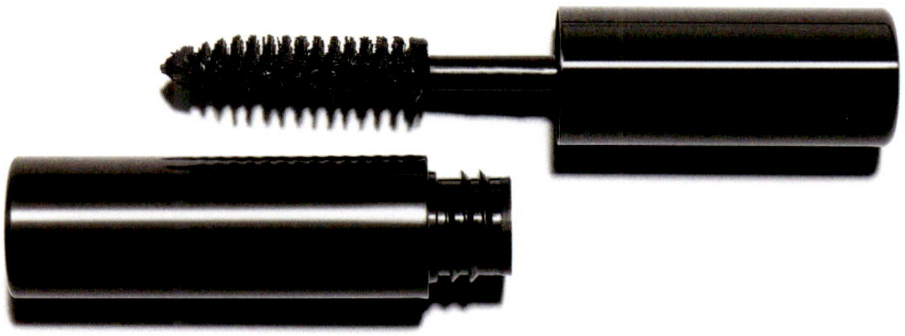

EYES

Include a wide variety of eye shadows in a range of colors and formulas, with pencils, brow pencils, and mascaras. The best way to arrange the shadows is in specially made palettes that have slots for the eye shadow containers. Arrange each palette by shade family, and label the palettes accordingly, so you can see at a glance which one you need. Making separate palettes for brights, shimmers, neutrals, and liners will help keep the kit organized.

Make sure you have all of your makeup tools, and don't forget to include cotton swabs or a non-oily eye makeup remover as well as a waterproof one. It's always better to be overprepared, than underprepared.

Four shades of all-over shadow color, such as white, bone, toast, and banana

A wide range of shadows to use as a lower lid color, include at least twelve choices

Three to six shades of shadow to use as liner, such as black, navy, medium brown, dark brown, dark green, and plum

Twelve shimmery shadows in a range of shades

Six to ten bold shadow and liner colors

Tinted and clear brow gels

Brow pencils in brown, blond, reddish brown, gray, taupe, and ash

Eye pencils in dark gray, brown, black, dark green, plum, and navy

Gel eyeliner in black, dark gray, and dark brown, optional extra colors could include violet and dark green

Black and dark brown mascara in both a thickening and a waterproof formula (colored mascaras are optional)

False eyelashes, both strips and individual

Eyelash glue; precolored glue in black helps fill the lash line

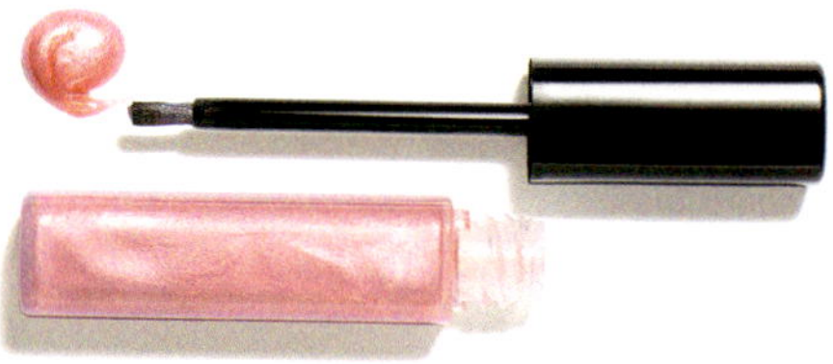

LIPS

It's easy to carry an extensive selection of lipsticks, because slices can be arranged in a palette. Using lipstick is the quickest and easiest way to change both a model's face and the feel of a photograph. In addition to the everyday colors, I like to keep an array of more unusual lip colors as well as other creamy pigments from the color wheel. It's amazing what a black lipstick does.

At least twenty different shades in a wide range of colors. These can be mixed to create dozens more. Essential colors include pale beige, pale pink, light orange, bright pink, bright orange, bright red, deep red, deep wine

At least ten shimmery lipsticks in a wide range of colors

At least ten lip glosses in a wide range of colors

At least ten lip pencils in a wide range of colors

A cream-based color wheel for blending

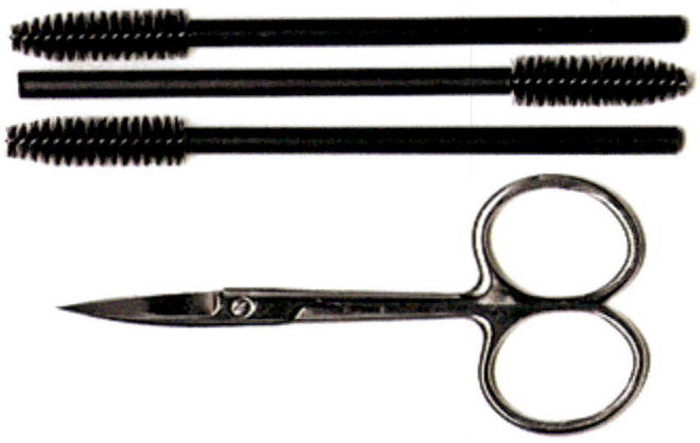

TOOLS

A complete set of brushes stored in a brush roll

Spray-on brush cleaner

Disposable makeup sponges

Cotton swabs

Cotton pads

Tissues

Tweezers

Eyelash curler

Baby scissors (for trimming unruly brows)

Disposable mascara wands

Water spray bottle

Makeup artists keep backups. Keep an extra set of brushes and all the products you can't live without in your home or office so you can access them if anything happens to your kit.

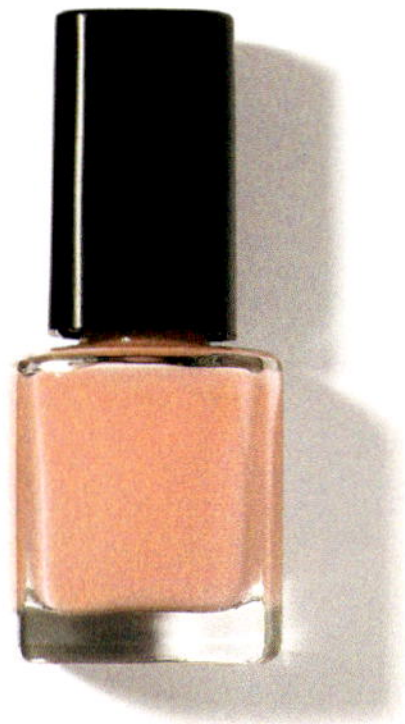

ESSENTIAL EXTRAS

Keep these things in your kit because you just never know when you might need them.

Hand disinfectant

Baby wipes

Mints

Baby oil

Eyedrops

Sheer, red, and chocolate nail polish

Nail polish remover

Extra zip-top plastic bags

Hand mirror

Protein bars, almonds, or other snacks—you will often be working through lunch and other meals

Paperback book for downtime, notebook for writing down inspirations

Business cards, as you never know whom you'll meet

TRICKS FOR PACKING YOUR KIT

Slice any product that comes in a stick (foundation, lipstick, bronzers, blushes), and put the slices into palettes. That way, you can have a whole array of shades in front of you at once.

Use zip-top plastic bags to store things and rubber bands to hold lip glosses and pencils together.

Use a label maker to label every bag, box, and palette neatly.

It's important for makeup artists to have a system. Pack your kit the same way each time, so you can find things in a hurry.

THE FUN KIT (at right)

These are the extra things you won't need very often, so store them all together in a separate plastic bag or makeup kit.

Sparkle and glitter powders

Nail polish in an array of colors

Intense theatrical eye shadow shades and blushes

Lip lacquers and matte stains in bold colors

Self-tanner and/or bronzing gel for the body

Body paints

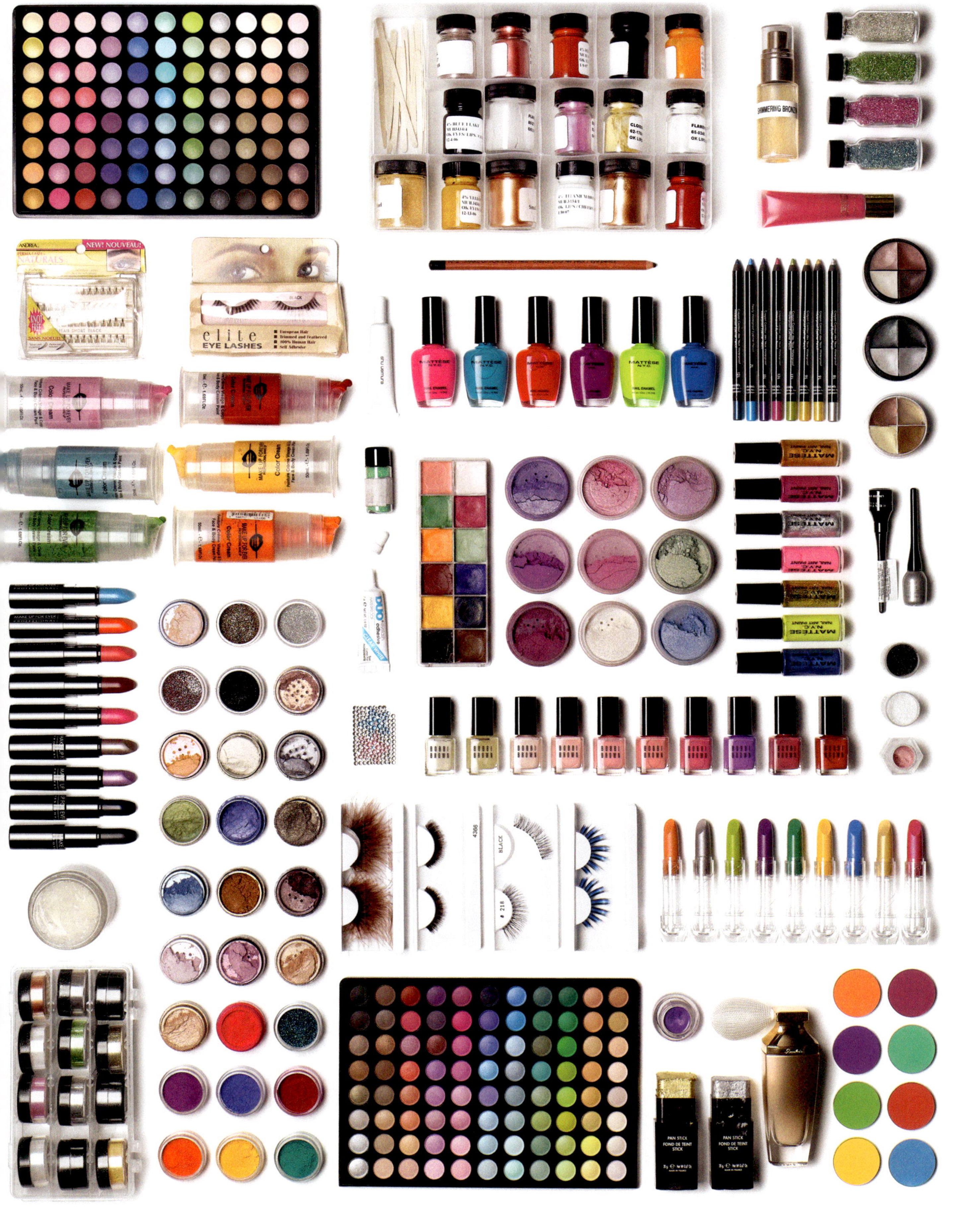
NEW! NOUVEAU!
elite
EYE LASHES
European Hair
Trimmed and Feathered
100% Human Hair
Self Adhesive
SHIMMERING BRONZE
MATTESE
N.Y.C.
Color Cream
BLACK
4366
218
PAN STICK
FOND DE TEINT
STICK

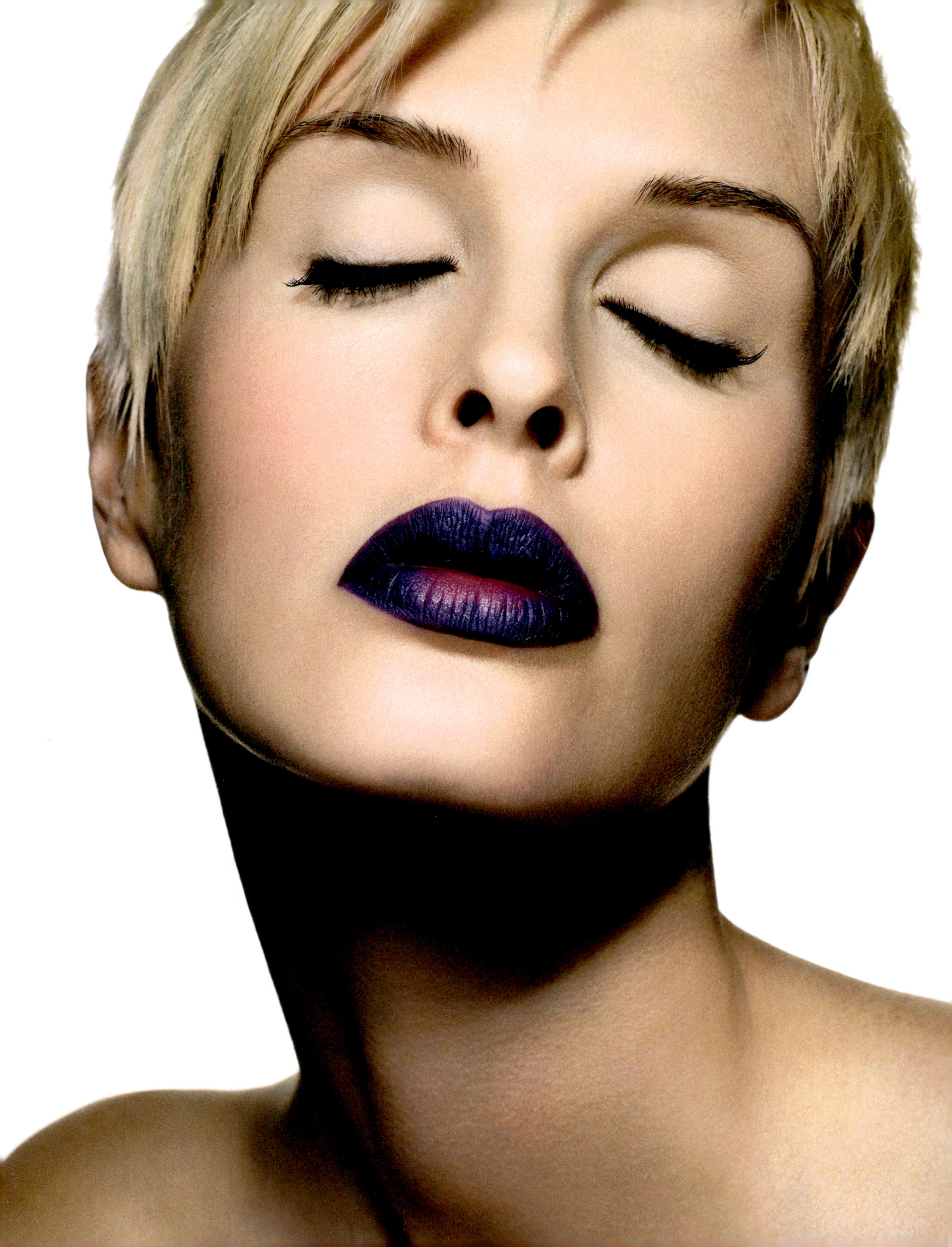

Chapter 11

ADVANCED MAKEUP APPLICATIONS

Every artist needs to learn skills to successfully apply makeup on subjects for photography, fashion shows, film, and television. These opportunities allow an artist to express her or his creativity. **There are no limitations when working in advanced artistry.**

MAKEUP for PHOTOGRAPHY

Applying makeup for photo shoots involves specific techniques that depend on a number of factors: ***Lighting: Indoors or outdoors? Film or digital technology? Color or black-and-white? Style: What image does the photographer want?***

The makeup will differ depending on the purpose of the photograph—whether it is a passport photo, a wedding shot, a model in a natural outdoor setting, a corporate portrait, or a highly stylized fashion or beauty shoot. There is no one rule for how to do makeup that will be photographed. But the lighting in which you do the makeup is very important. I often do makeup with the model facing a window or, better yet, on the photo set with the lighting that will be used in the shoot.

Some guidelines follow that will help you understand the process and develop just the right look each time.

THE ROLE OF A MAKEUP ARTIST AT A PHOTO SHOOT

Making a photograph is a collaborative effort. As the makeup artist, you are part of a team that includes the photographer, the stylist, the hair stylist, the dresser, and the editor (if it is a magazine shoot), publicists and handlers (if the subject is a celebrity), and the subject being shot. Your job is to be true to your own style, yet be open; to understand the requirements of the stylist, editor, and model; and to create a makeup look that works.

The only way to accomplish that is to communicate with everyone on the set and be observant. Don't ever be embarrassed to ask questions or to give your opinion. Throughout the process, ask the photographer, stylist, editor, and subject for feedback. After you have applied the model's foundation, let her look at it in a mirror to see if she thinks it looks right. It is much easier to change things at that stage than to wait until the whole face is done. When analyzing the first shot, get the photographer's opinion on how the makeup is working—or isn't—with his or her lighting. Adjust accordingly. Once the shooting starts, don't think that your job is done. You need to stand by the set with your tools—powder, blush, lipstick, etc. Watch the model through a pair of mini binoculars to keep a close eye on how the makeup is holding up and what might need fixing. And be ready to jump in and try something that just might make the shot great. When a photographer teams up with a makeup artist, magic can happen. They understand each other's style and needs. They can work in sync to get the best results.

I have had a handful of collaborations with different photographers, and my work really grew as a result. I was able to be comfortable with them and try new things, and saw the results the next day. Each photographer moved my work in a different direction and I am grateful to all of them.

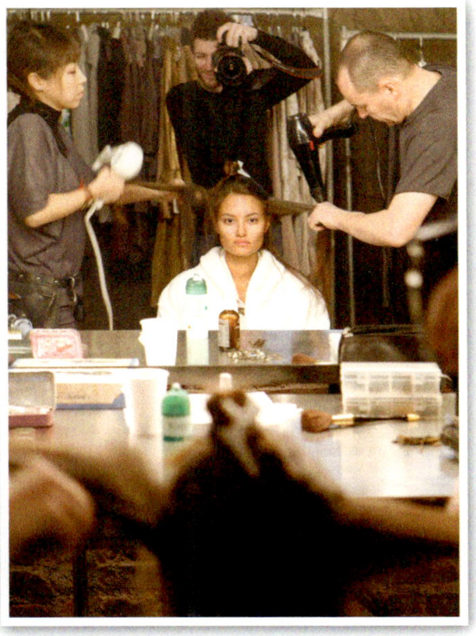
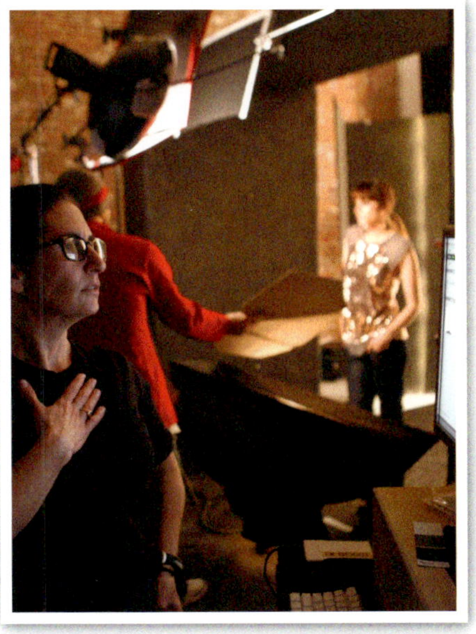
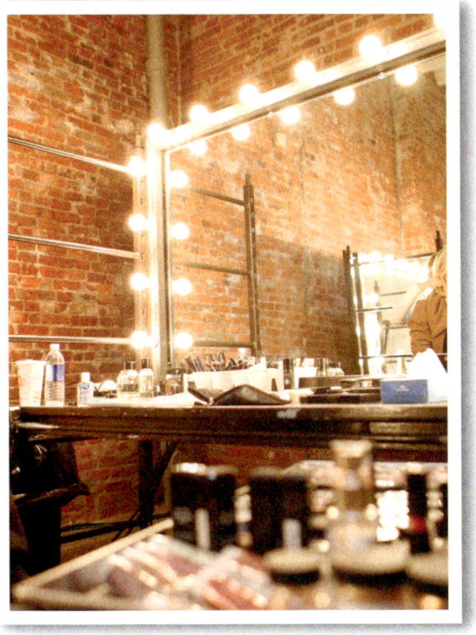
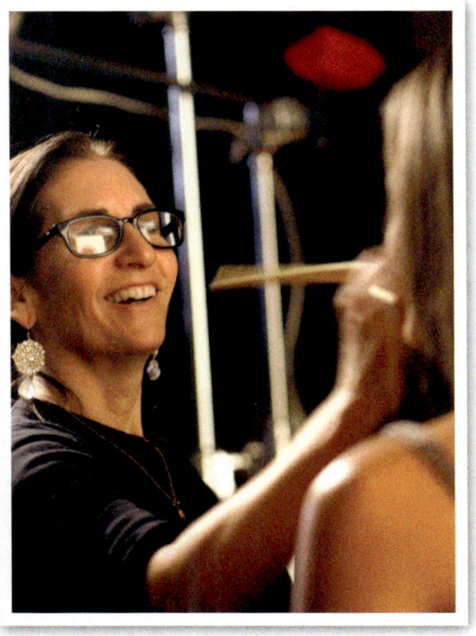
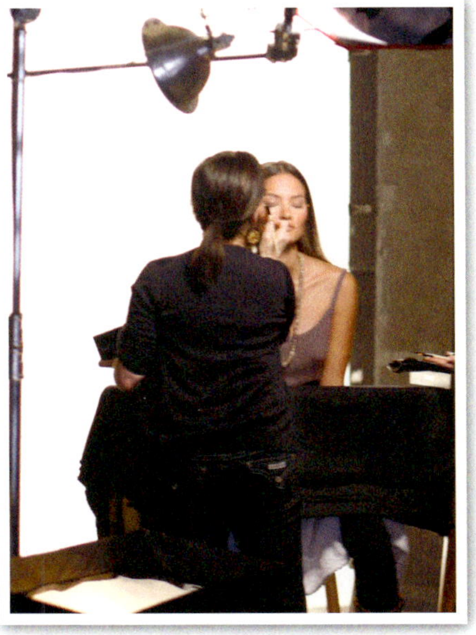
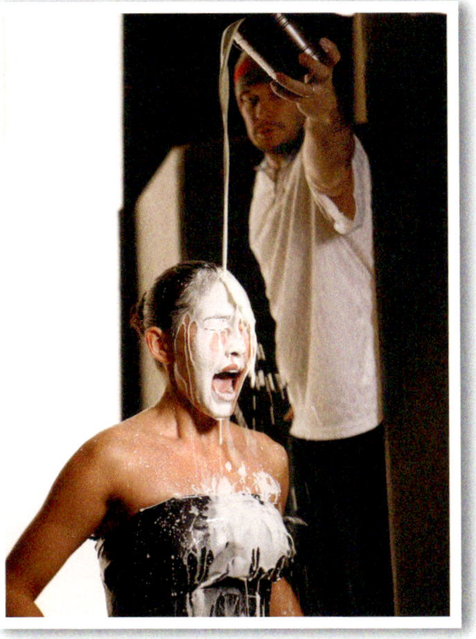
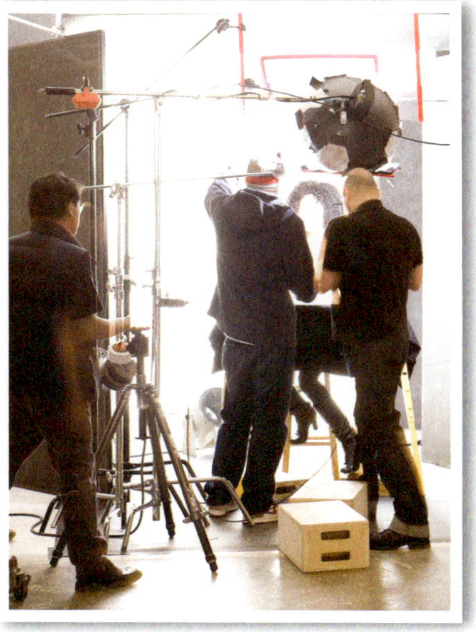
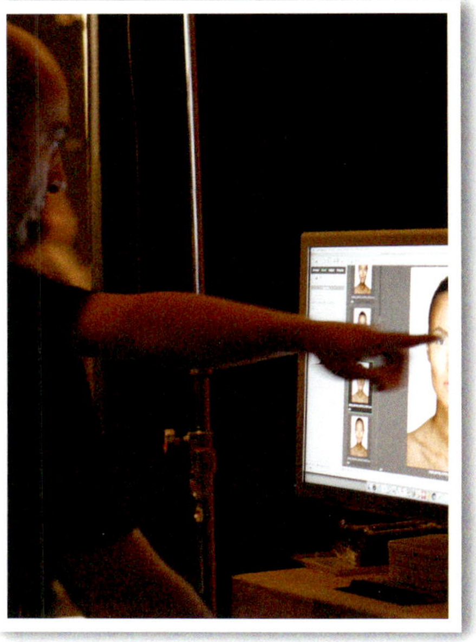
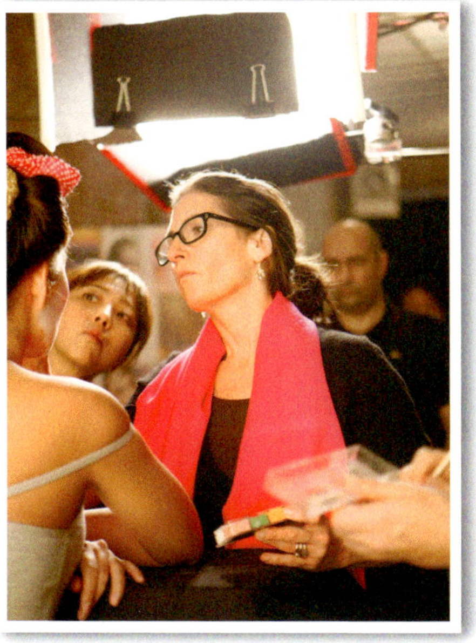

WHAT THE PHOTOGRAPHERS SAY ABOUT MAKEUP ARTISTS

It's important to adapt the makeup to the girl. You can't just decide what makeup you want to do and put it on, like a mask, on the model. It has to be adapted to suit the person you are working on. Working with celebrities can be difficult, because they have a very strong idea of what they want to look like, and it's harder to get them to change their look. You have to really work with them and be gentle.

–Patrick Demarchelier

The lighting that I use is strong, very revealing; therefore, I require perfection from a makeup artist. A makeup artist that I will want to have on my set must have that innate ability to enhance a woman's face and do it quickly. It seems that time is always of the essence, we are always under pressure, and the subject can't see the makeup artist hesitate. She needs to exude complete confidence. This helps put everyone at ease. A great makeup artist needs to inspire the women seated in front of the mirror in my studio. She needs to build up their egos, make them feel truly beautiful, give them the confidence to stand in front of my lens and feel proud about who they are. These elements are the first steps in a great collaboration and capturing an incredible visual. The makeup artist needs to be able to make women not only look beautiful but feel beautiful. That's what makes my photograph. I love shooting women who feel beautiful; you can really feel that in a photograph.

–Walter Chin

When I look at a makeup artist's work, first and foremost, I look for creativity. I look for someone who can think outside the box and who is able to look at a face and see what not to do, how much makeup not to apply. As a portrait and fashion photographer I am always interested in the geography of the face, and people's so-called flaws are often the most interesting things about them. I would never want to hide any of that. A makeup artist should always look for inspiration anywhere and everywhere and not just in their immediate realm. Museums, exhibits, nature, history: it's all there for the taking. Never become complacent; always be excited.

–Henry Leutwyler

I rely on the makeup artist's input from the beginning. I will always trust her opinion of which model we should use. Especially when you're doing close-up beauty shots, the less you have to do, the better it looks. So if we choose the model that already has great skin or long lashes, the less work it takes to nail it. We shoot so much digitally now, and that's really changed the way both the photographer and the makeup artist work. It's so easy to retouch and remove a blemish that usually I tell the makeup artist not to even bother trying to cover it up. But the most important thing for the makeup artist to know is that for beauty shots, you really have to exaggerate the effect you're trying to create. Film has a tendency to neutralize, so the color needs to be much stronger than what it would be in real life. You need to overdo it, and then assess it not by how it looks to your eye, but how it looks on camera.

–Troy Word

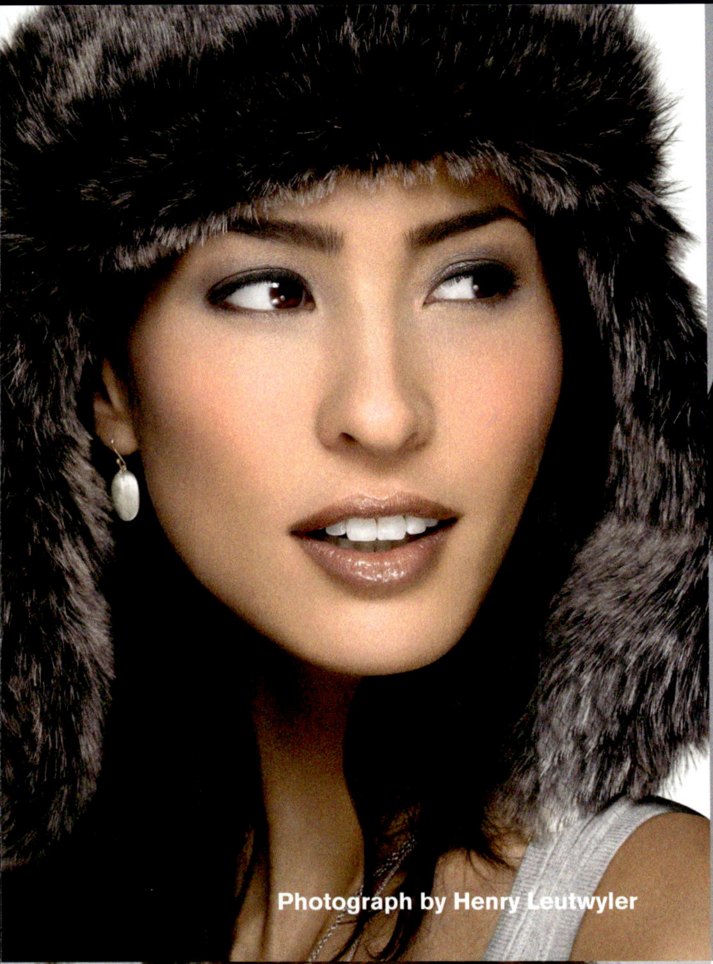

Photograph by Henry Leutwyler

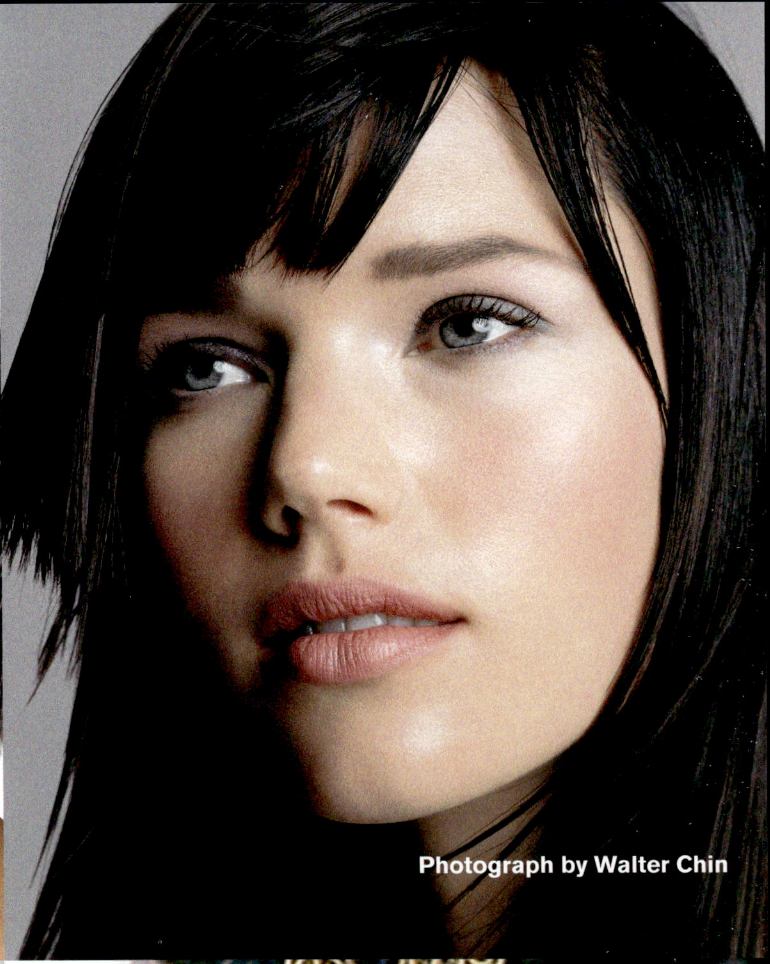

Photograph by Walter Chin

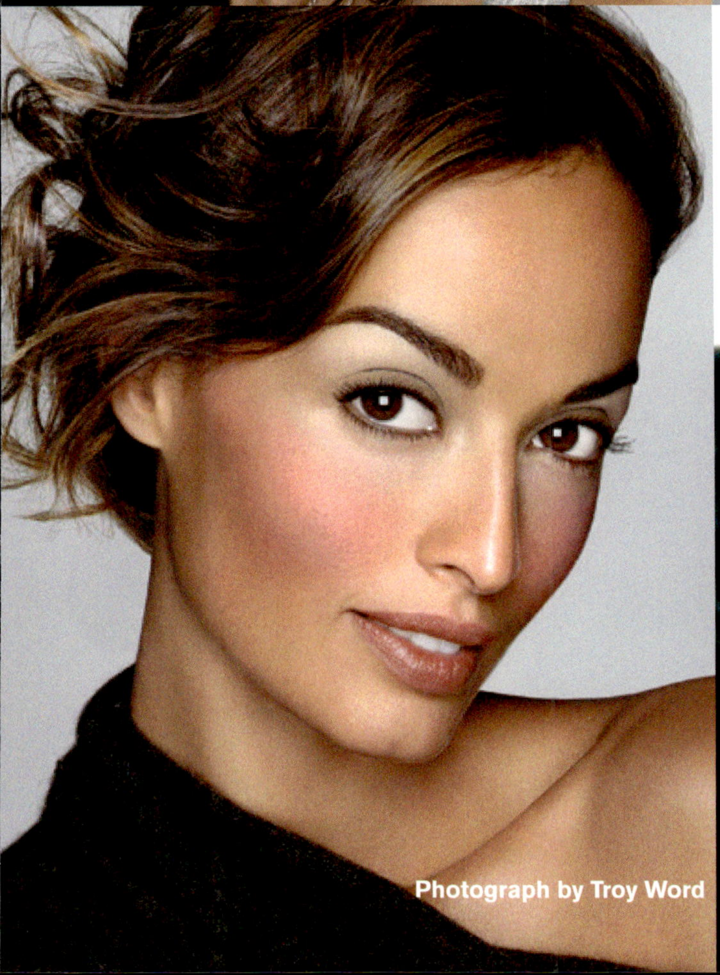

Photograph by Troy Word

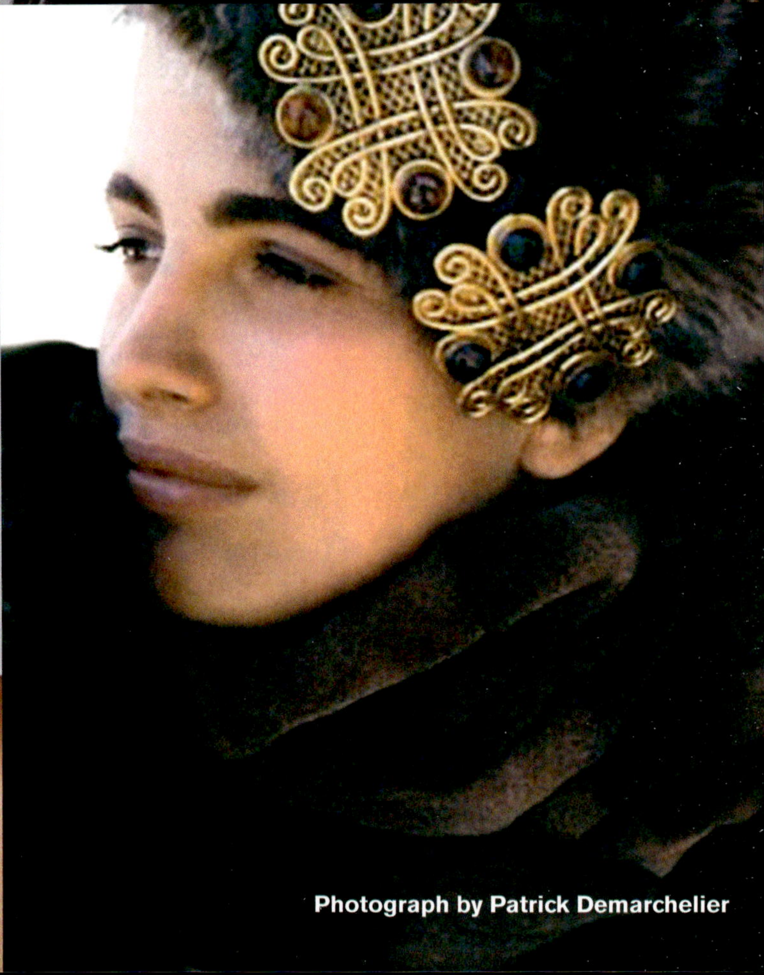

Photograph by Patrick Demarchelier

INDOOR OR OUTDOOR PHOTOGRAPHY

Whether photographs are being taken indoors or out, the most important rule is that foundation must exactly match skin tone, and the face has to match the body. Sometimes that means bringing the foundation lower on the neck or using some bronzing powder on the neck and chest to help eliminate any obvious color difference between the face and the body.

With outdoor photography, what you see is what you get. Outdoor lighting is very unforgiving. Use little foundation and a very light hand with blush. Everything has to look great to the naked eye, and makeup has to be well blended.

For indoor photography, the amount of makeup you apply depends on lighting. Define the features and determine if the lighting will wash out the skin tone or enhance it. Extremely strong lighting requires a heavier hand and more definition. But there are many variables in determining the style you want, so you have to be open to trying varying degrees of coverage and definition.

MAKEUP FOR PHOTOGRAPHS

Keep in mind the type of photo being taken. You use different techniques for a simple portrait than for a shoot for a high-end European fashion magazine.

Portrait
Keep the look simple, and make sure the subject is comfortable with the look.

Athlete
Do what's right for the person, and stick to his or her own style.

Musician
Unless the subject asks for a change, take your cue from his or her style, and don't stray too far from it.

Actor
Always ask before you start working. Actors like to evolve and try new things.

Fashion
When working with designers, it is important to be a good observer. Look carefully at the clothes. Ask about the designer's vision for the makeup.

Magazine
This kind of work varies tremendously. It is important to understand the style of the magazine and to get the input of the photographer, editor, and stylist on the shoot. I always befriend the photo assistant. That person has the best view and lets me know when something is not quite right.

BLACK-AND-WHITE OR COLOR PHOTOGRAPHY

In general, black-and-white photography is more forgiving than color photography, but both call for careful makeup application in order to get the best results.

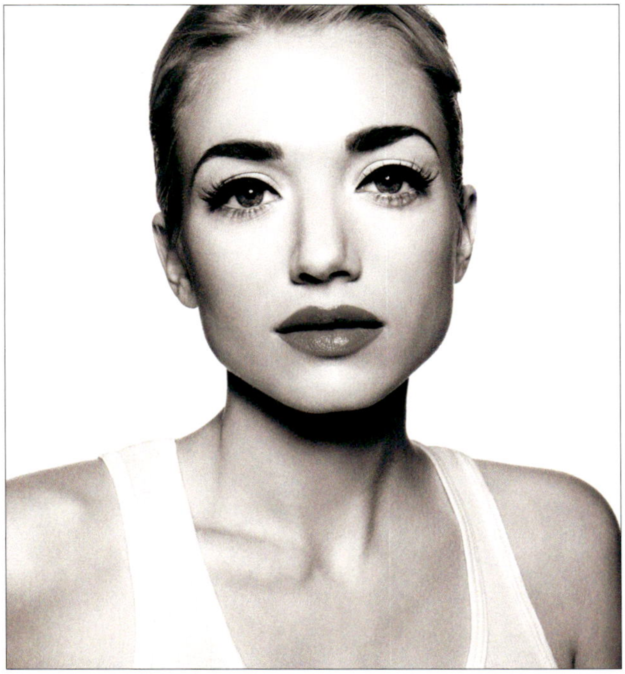

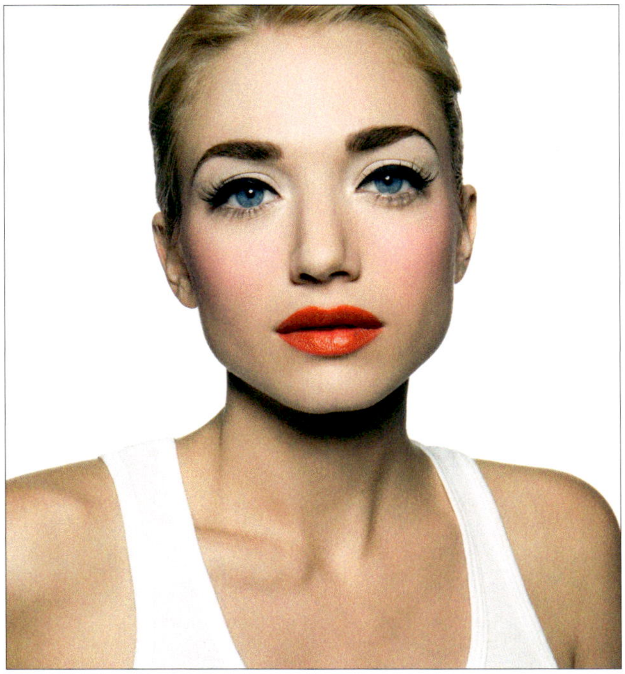

For Black-and-White Photography

Define the features. That means a precise application of eyeliner and lip liner, as well as perfectly applied blush.

Avoid using very shimmery shades on the eyes, and don't use bronzer, as it can look dirty.

Less is more. Smooth out skin and conceal any imperfections, especially under the eyes, with bright concealer that blends perfectly, but don't go overboard with too much foundation or color.

Lighting will dictate how much makeup you need.

For Color Photography

Foundation must match the skin exactly.

Never use translucent powder; it can make the face look masklike in a photograph. Instead, use warm, skin-tone-correct shades.

Don't overdo powder. Especially in close-up photography, too much powder will call attention to any peach-fuzz facial hair.

Skin needs to have even texture. Coverage depends on many variables.

Check Polaroids or digital monitor to see if any corrections have to be made.

A DYNAMIC DUO: *Gail Hadani & Paul Innis*

The photographer Gail Hadani began painting and exhibiting her work at the age of ten, but her love of singing led her to a career in opera. After years of travel and life on the road as an opera singer, she discovered her passion for photography. Paul Innis, an artist, illustrator, and makeup artist, saw her ad in *Le Book*, loved the lighting and composition, took a chance, and called her. They now work as a team almost exclusively.

My career really began when I teamed up with Gail Hadani. Gail allows me to be completely creative with no limits. Having the support of a great photographer and friend is the best tool for success in this industry…

I believe in makeup as an art form. It's wonderful to do pretty makeup, but there has to be a little art to set you apart from everyone else. You have to find that thing that is creative and beautiful. For me, it is color and three-dimensional objects. I love to glue objects to the face, making what I call beautiful art with a model's face.

"Candy Land" (photos at right) all started when Gail bought some colored sugar at Dean & DeLuca, not knowing how she could incorporate it into an interesting photograph. At the time, Gail asked me what I thought we could do with this sugar, and, at the time, I was stumped.

A year and a half later, I realized what I could do with colored sugar, and Candy Land was born. I have developed a love for using common materials to create works of art on models' faces. In this project, I started with the colored sugar, gradually adding other bright and powerful candy-inspired colors (photo at lower left). I immediately thought of Life Savers, inspiring the Life Saver–like striped lips, which became one of my pride and joys as a makeup artist (upper right photo).

I have also always been a fan of making my lashes by chopping up different types of lashes, and then combining those pieces to make different shapes. The lashes in the shot in the lower right hand corner were four pairs of lashes stacked together to create a unique shape. The lashes were custom fitted to the model's eyes, but unfortunately, they were also very heavy. So, the model was made to keep her eyes closed in between each shot.

As an artist, I believe you can use almost any products to transform a face into a work of art. Whether it is candy sprinkles, sugar, feathers, or rhinestones, it is all about thinking outside of the box to create spectacular and unique images!

—Paul Innis

Meeting Paul changed the course of my life. If it weren't for him, I would not be in this business that I have come to love with the same passion I used to have as an opera singer. We developed a distinctive style and worked so frequently together that we learned the art of making a powerful image. Both of us understand the basics of a great painting: composition, shape, light, color balance, emotion, and expression. The camera, lighting, and makeup are the paintbrushes. The set becomes a stage, where as director, I can mold the performances…

Our advice to young makeup artists: practice, practice, practice. Look, learn, create relationships, and put yourself out there.

—Gail Hadani

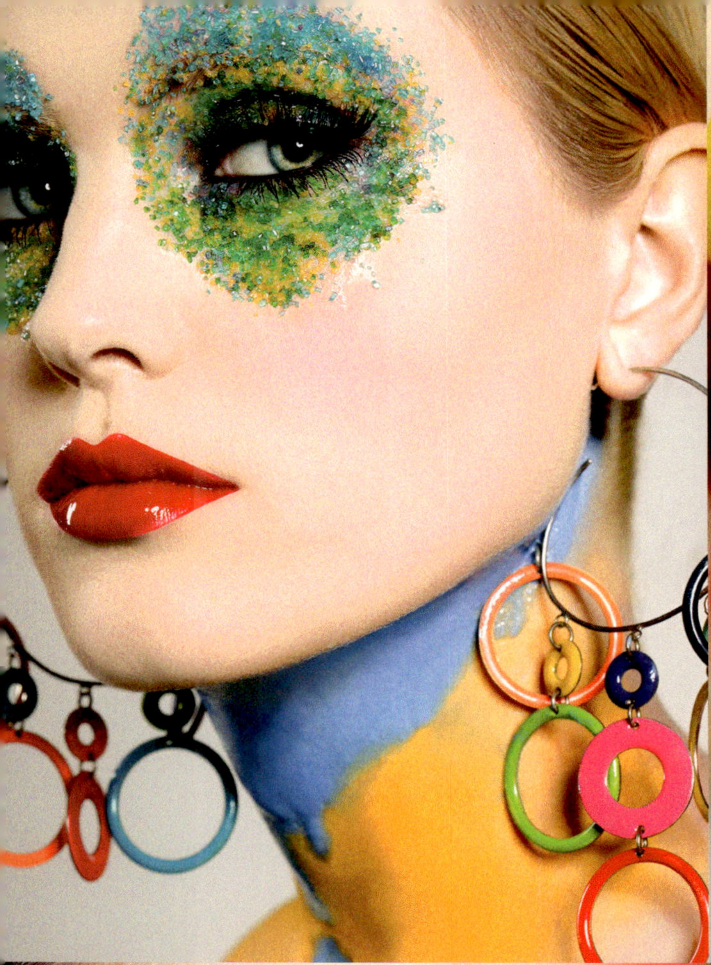
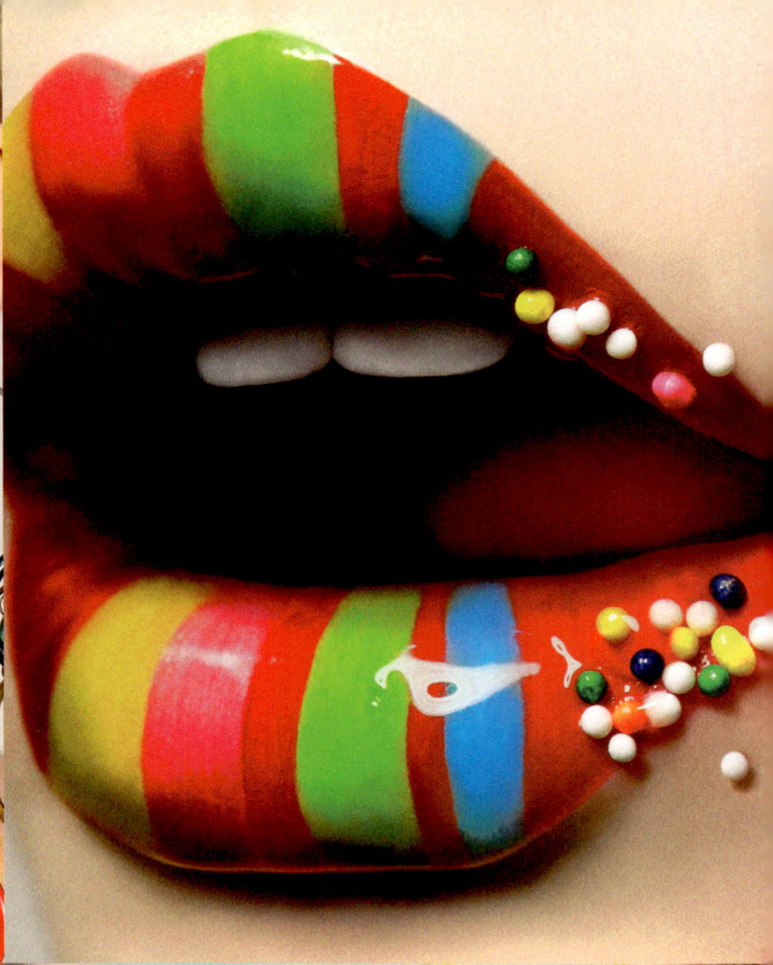
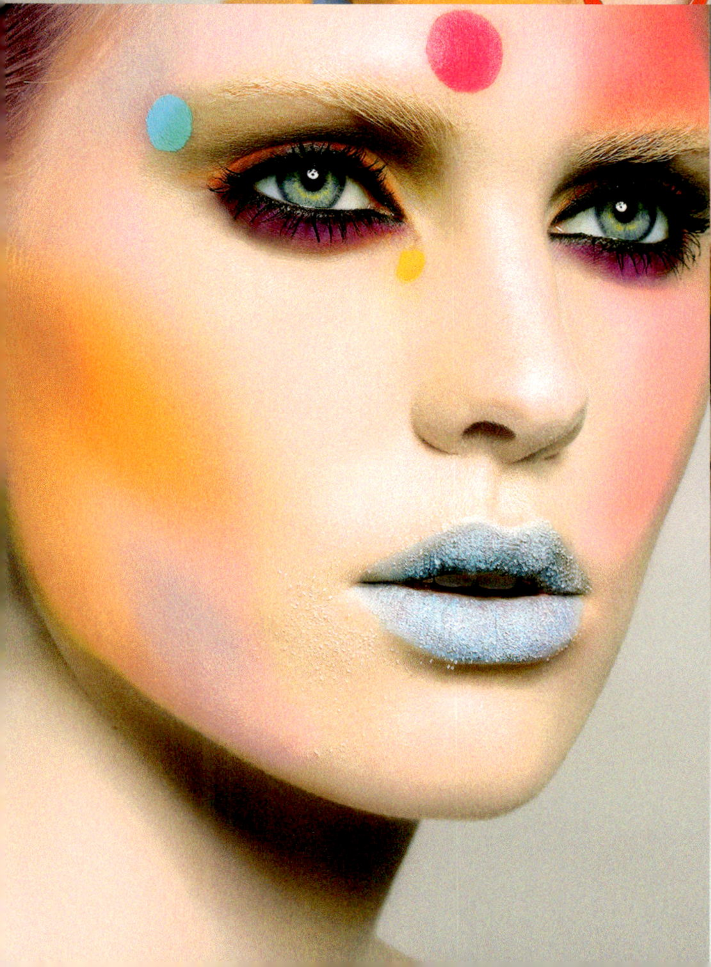
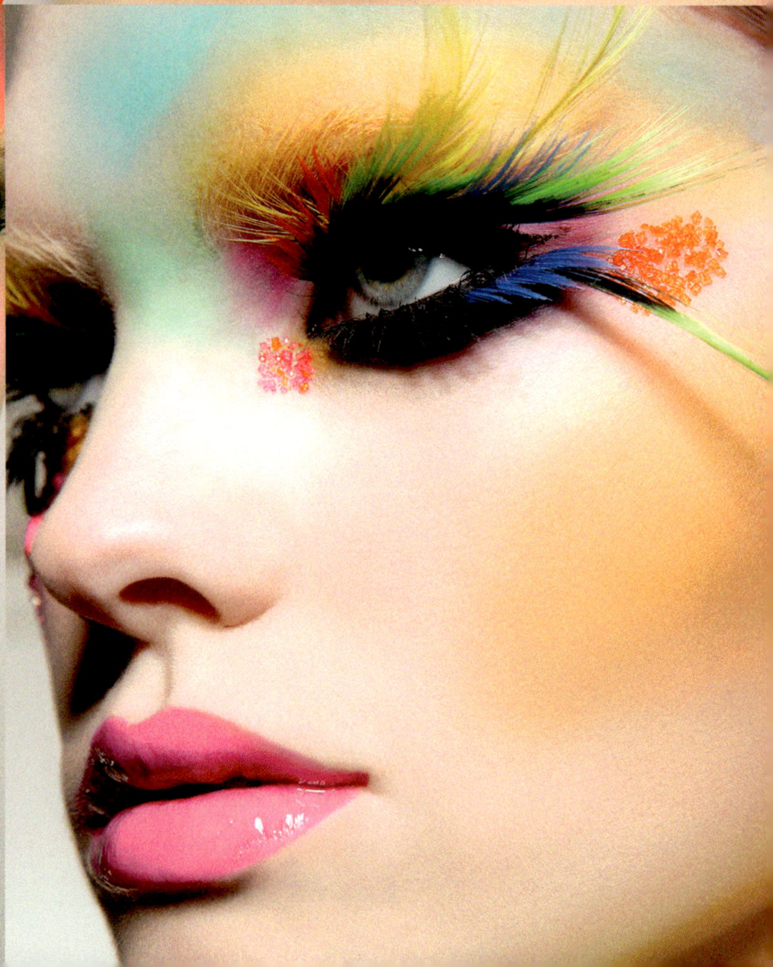

MAKEUP for MAGAZINES

The difference between doing basic makeup and doing makeup that is over the top for highly styled fashion shows or magazine work is thinking outside the box. ***Doing the unexpected*** — whether it's as simple as not putting on mascara or brows to a finished face or strengthening the brows to become a full blown experimental piece — is the difference between "basic" beauty and editorial freedom. It's all about being confident enough to experiment outside of your comfort zone.

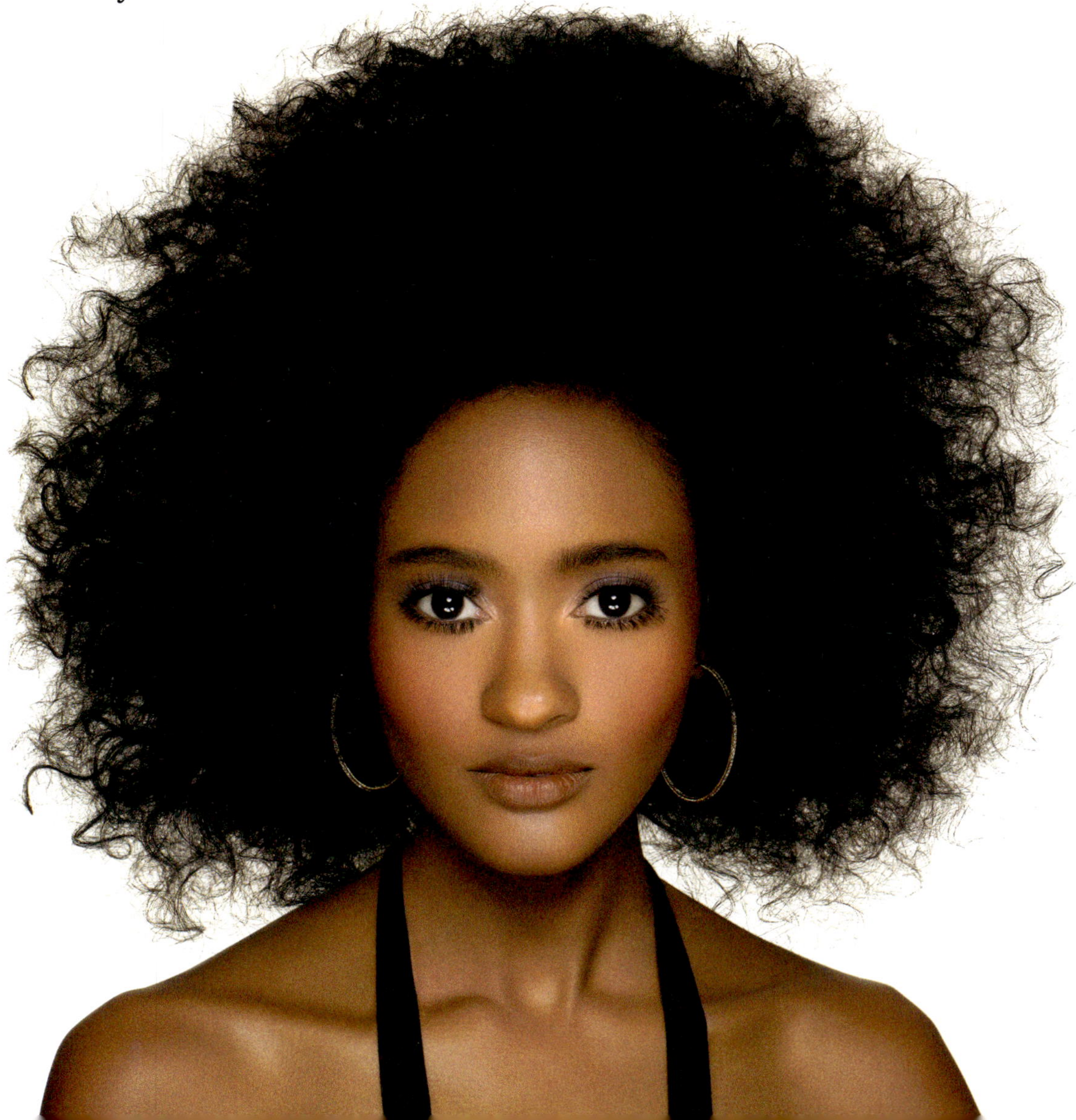

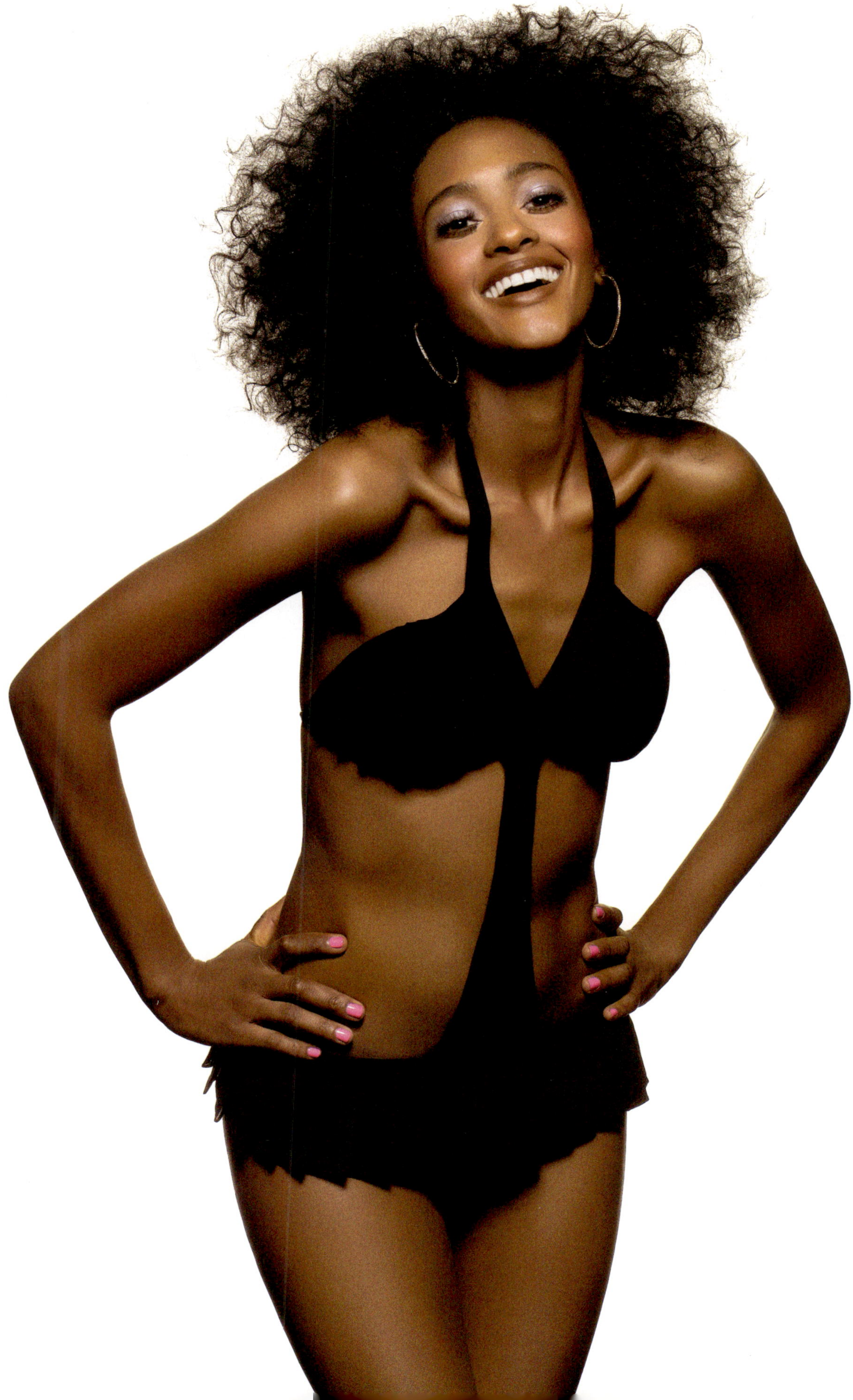

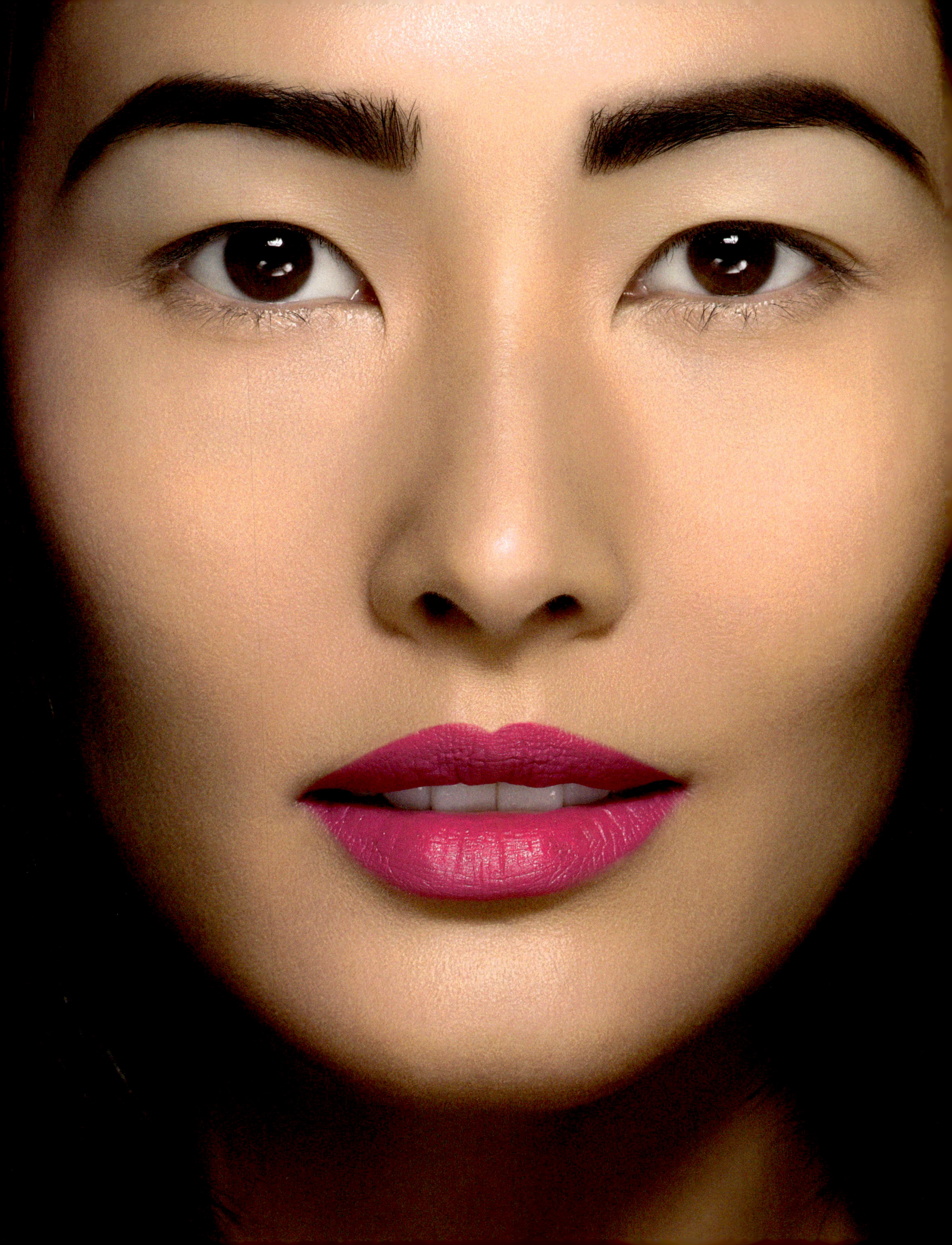

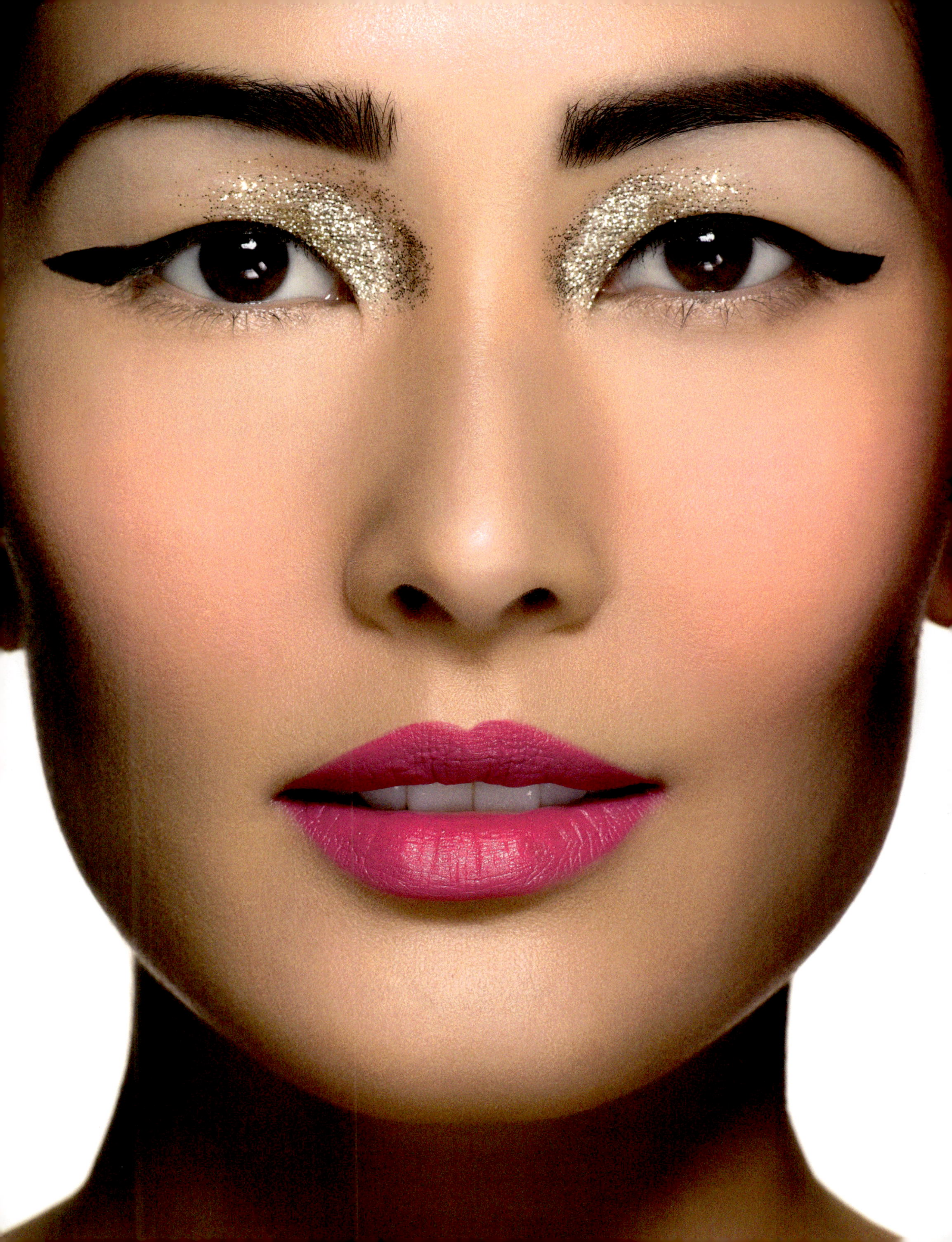

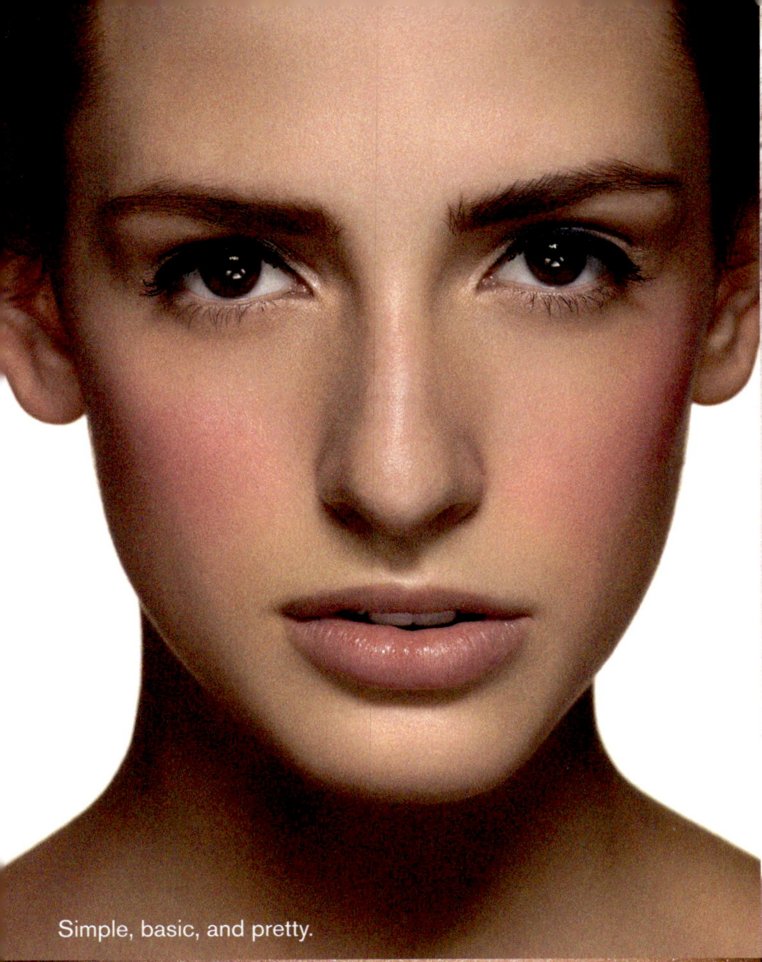

Simple, basic, and pretty.

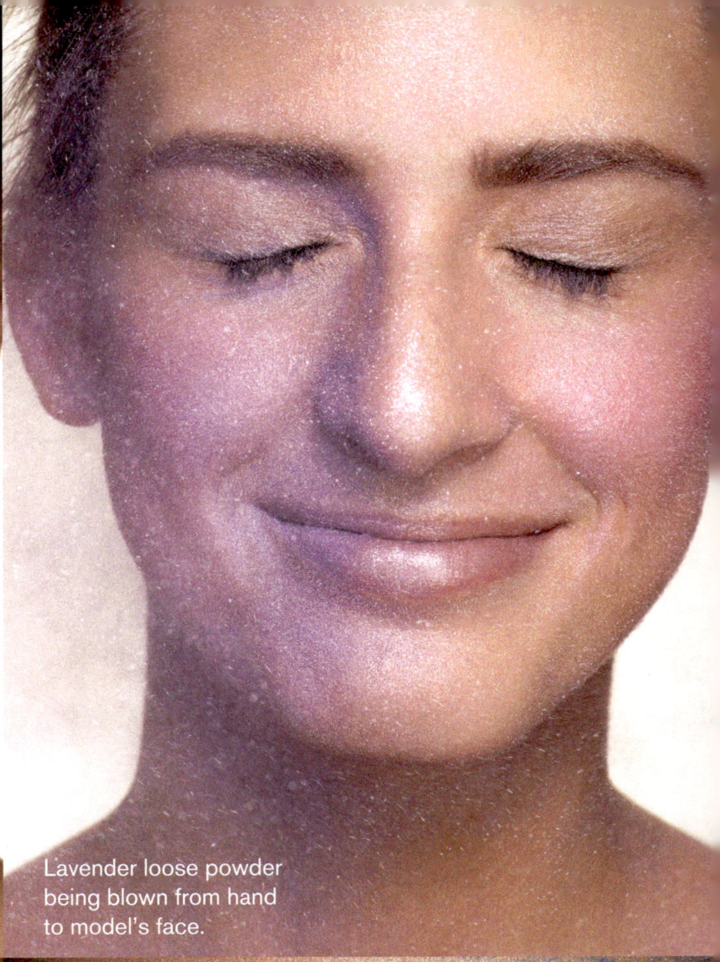

Lavender loose powder being blown from hand to model's face.

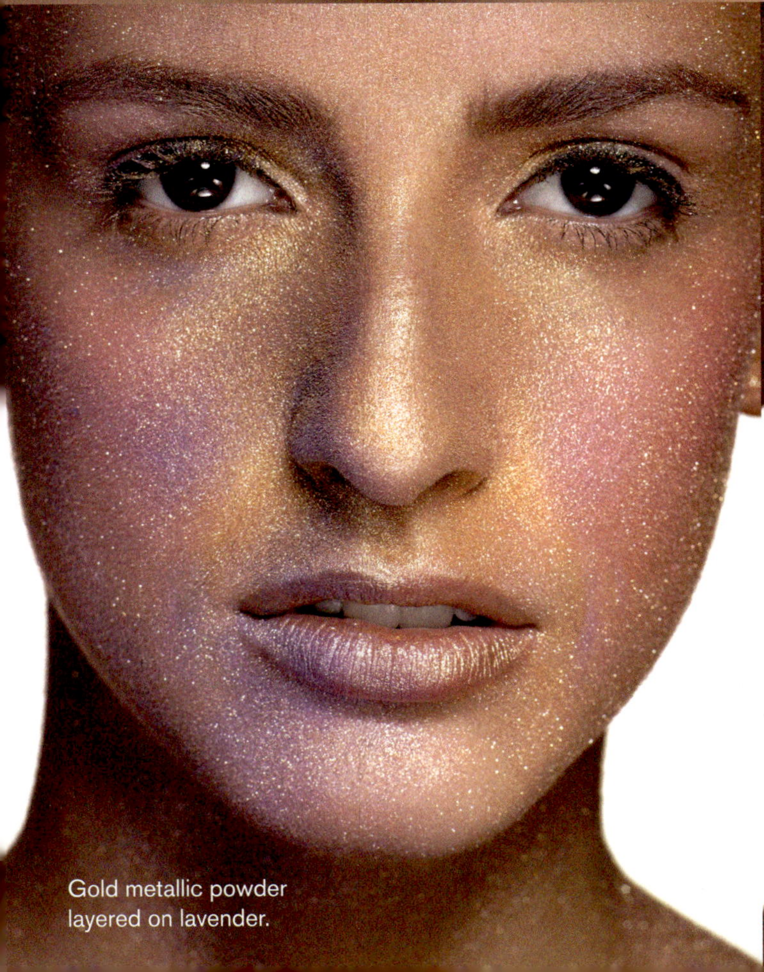

Gold metallic powder layered on lavender.

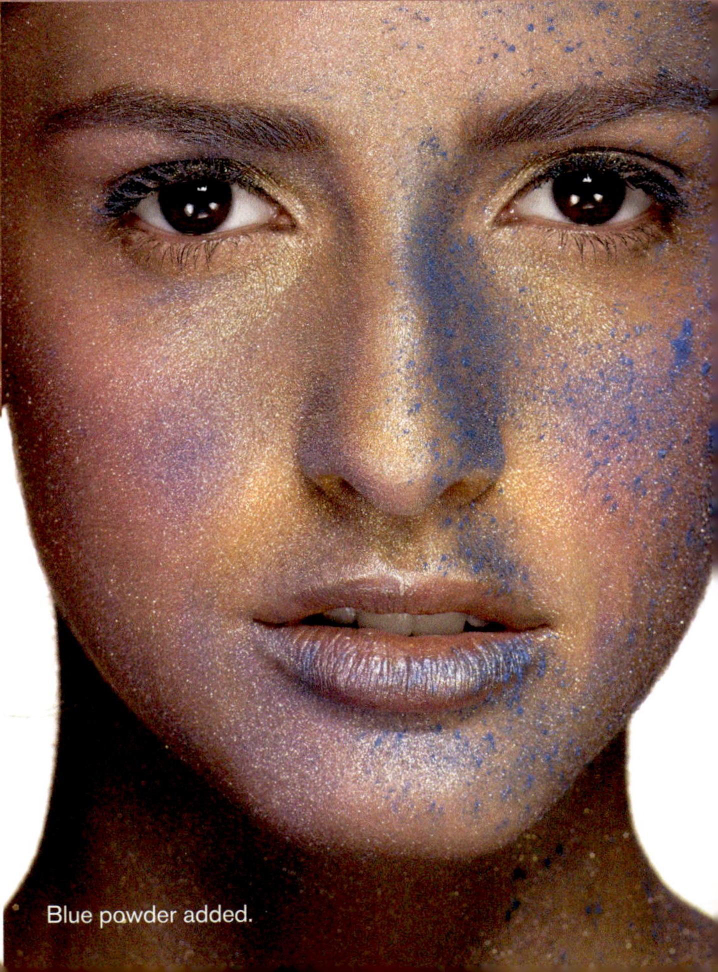

Blue powder added.

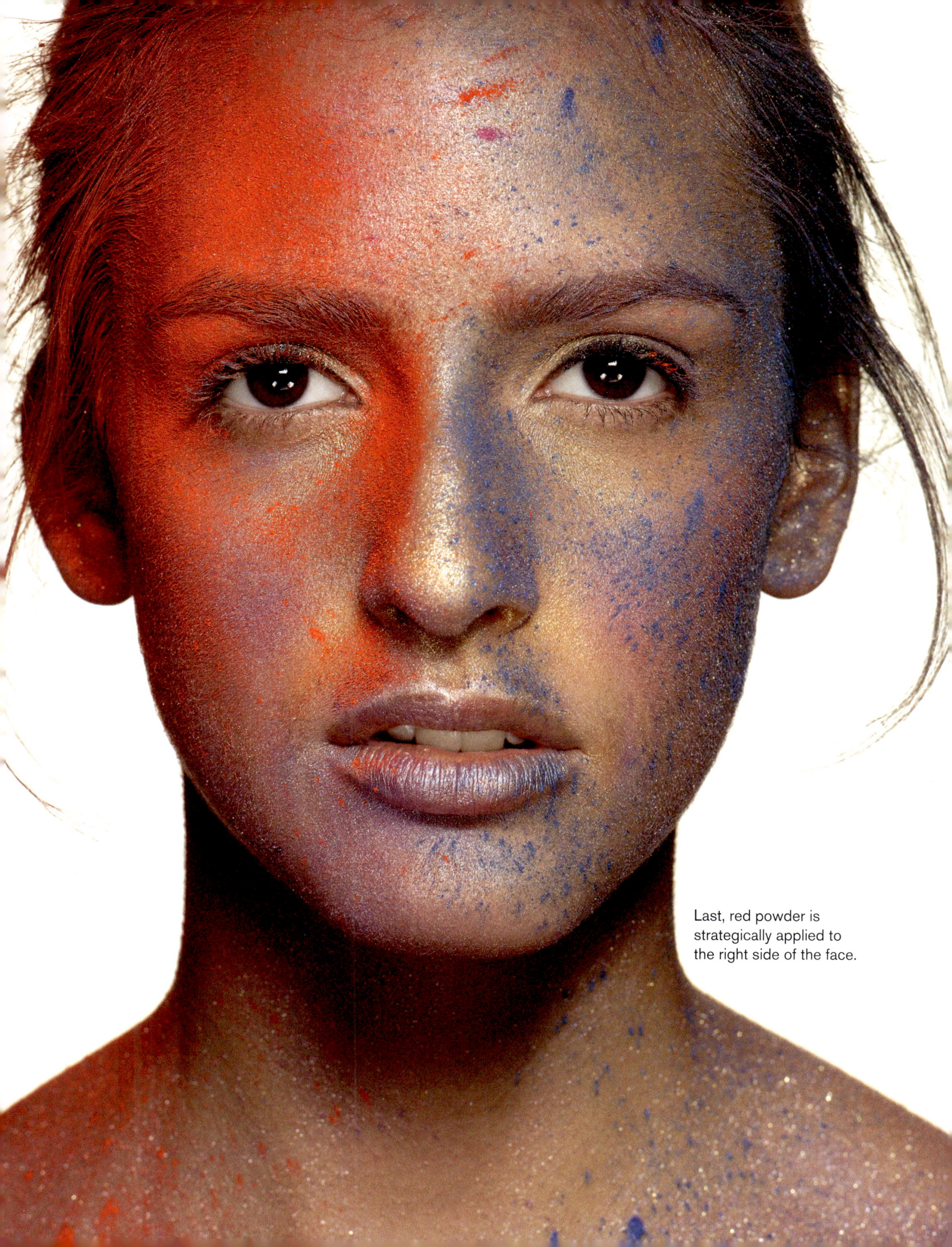

Last, red powder is strategically applied to the right side of the face.

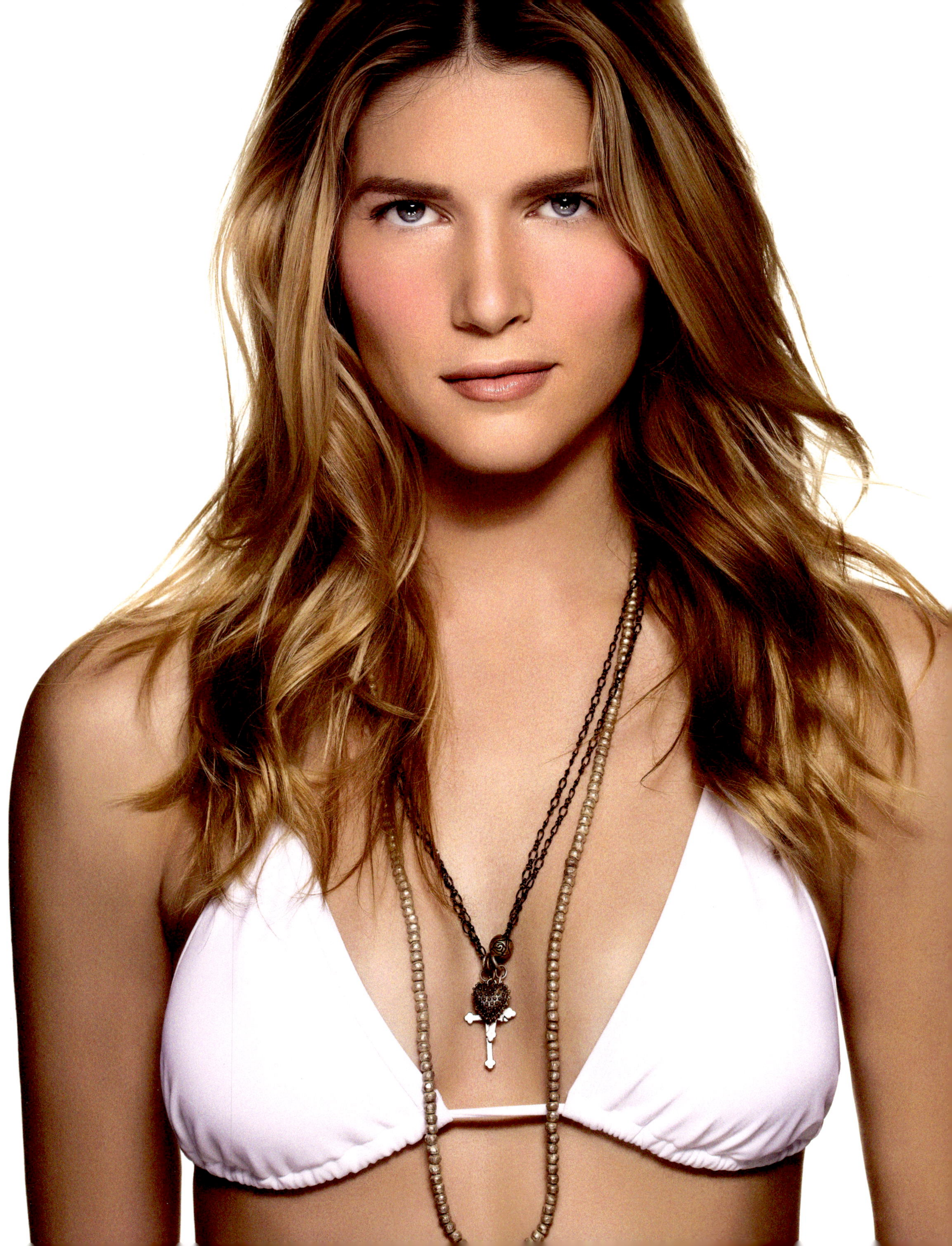

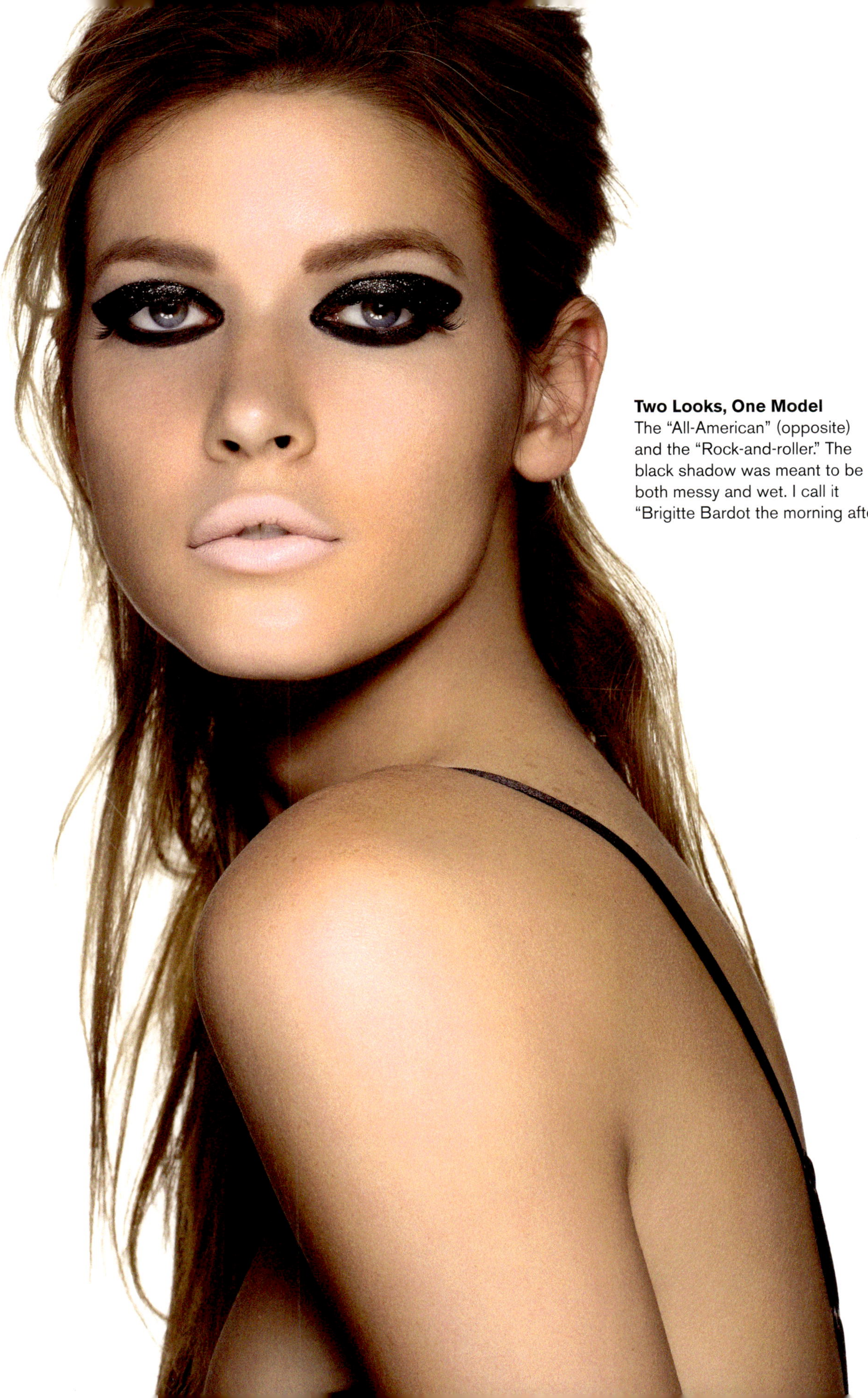

Two Looks, One Model
The "All-American" (opposite) and the "Rock-and-roller." The black shadow was meant to be both messy and wet. I call it "Brigitte Bardot the morning after."

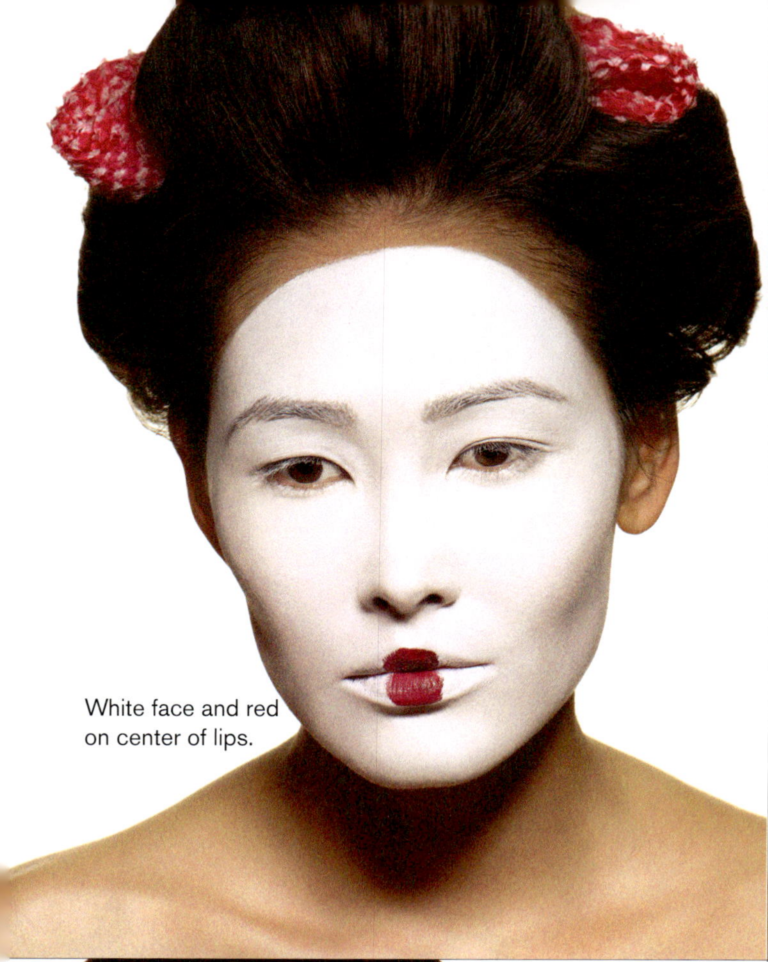
White face and red on center of lips.

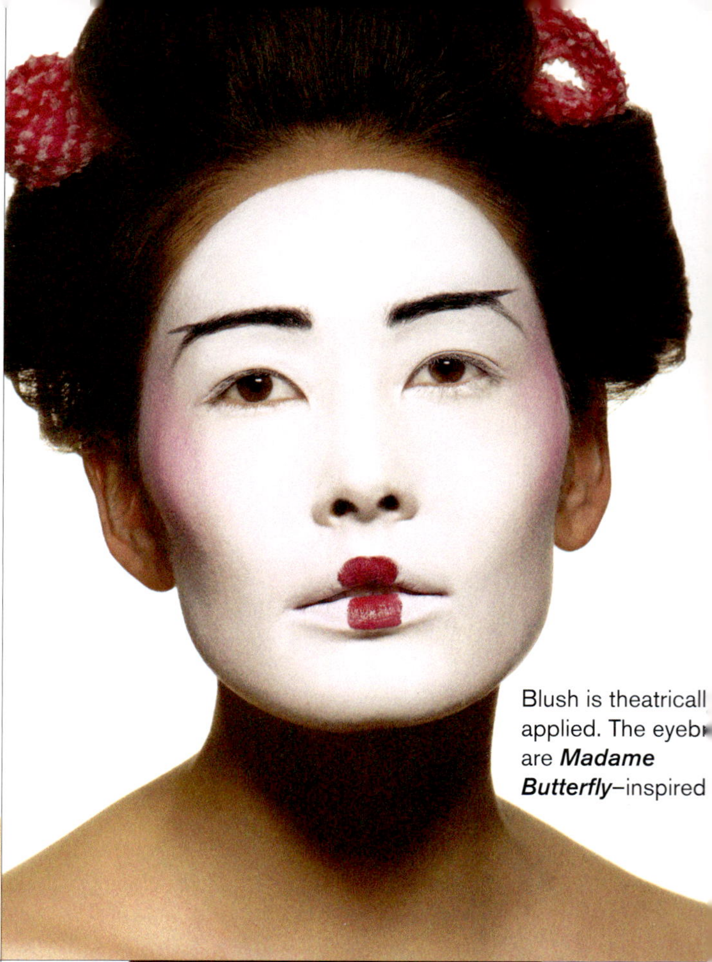
Blush is theatricall applied. The eyeb are ***Madame Butterfly***–inspired

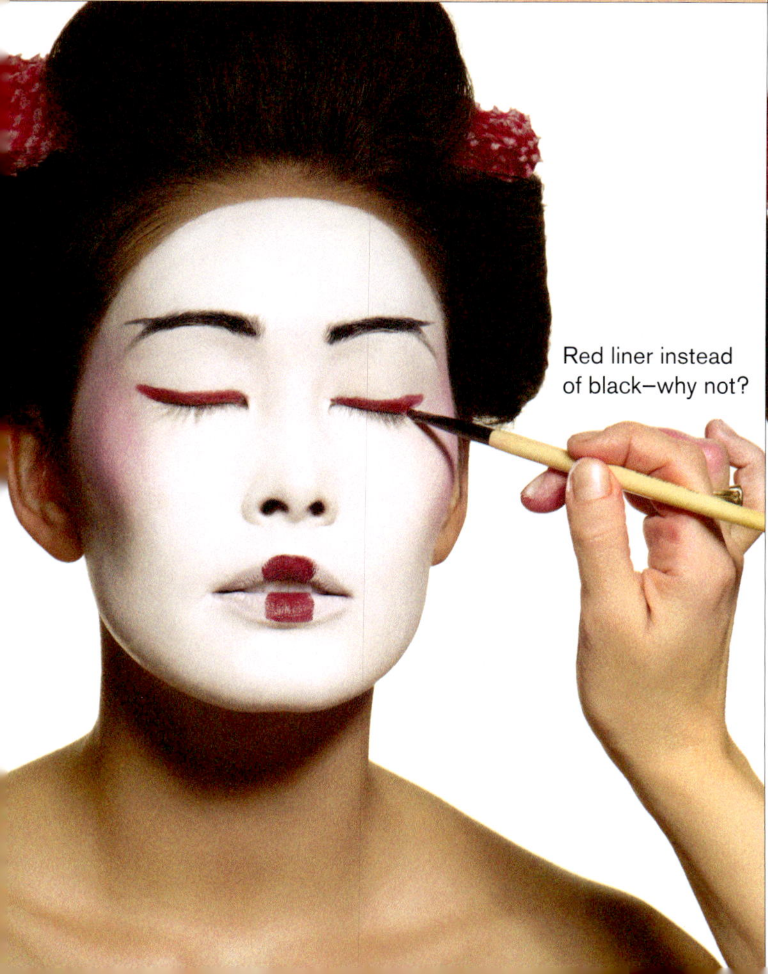
Red liner instead of black–why not?

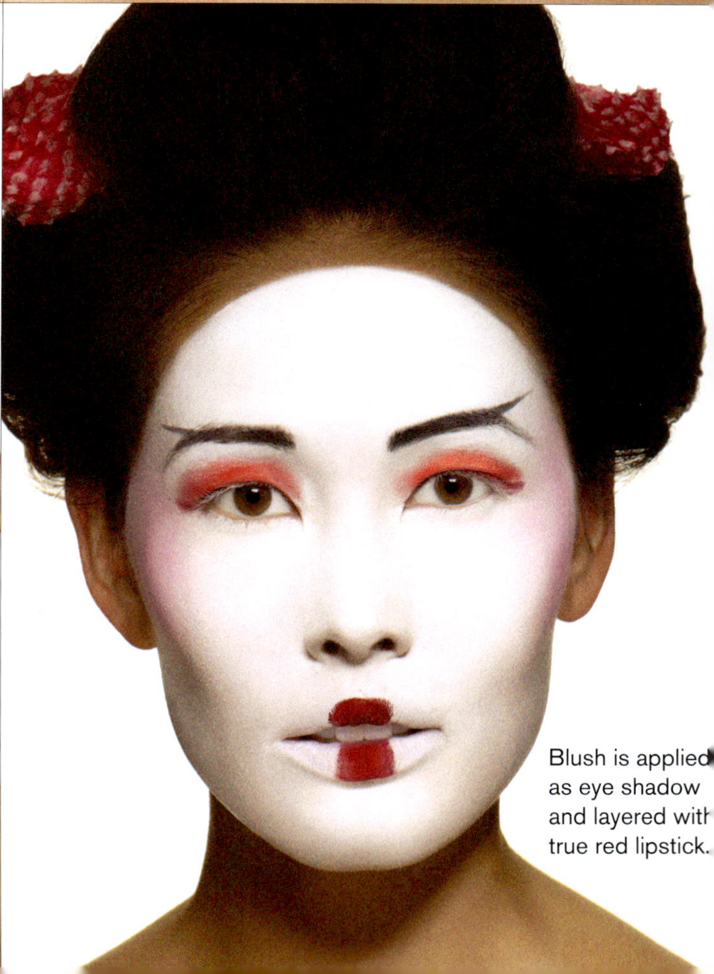
Blush is applied as eye shadow and layered wit true red lipstick.

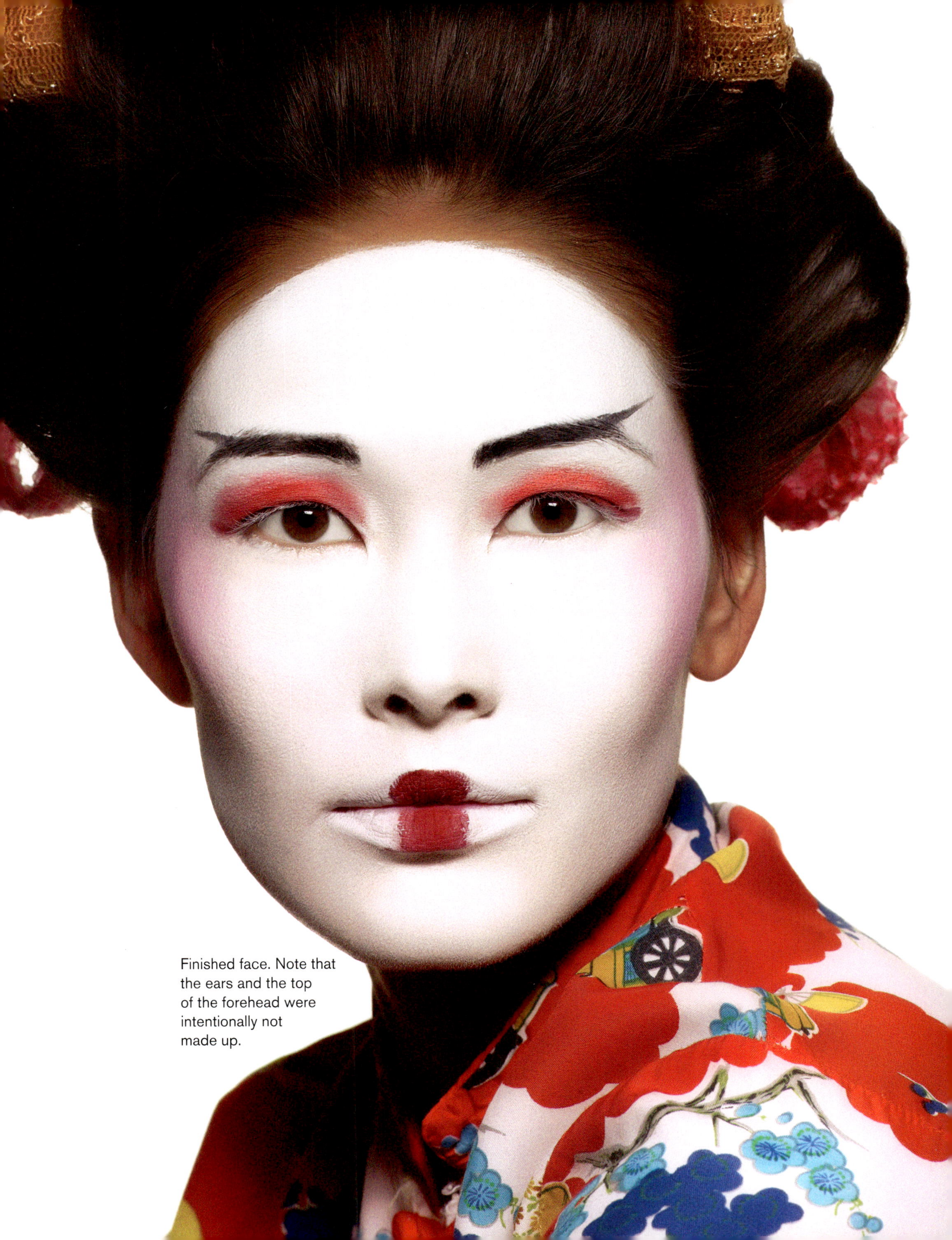

Finished face. Note that the ears and the top of the forehead were intentionally not made up.

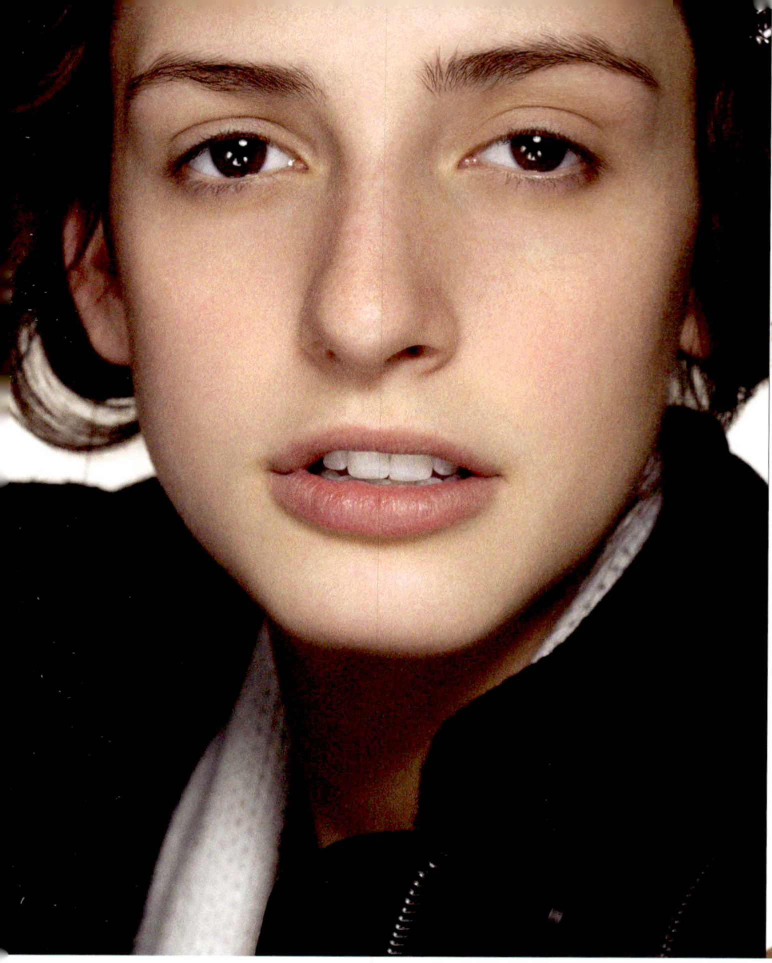

I've always loved unusual beauty. This is not a before photo. To me this face is a blank canvas.

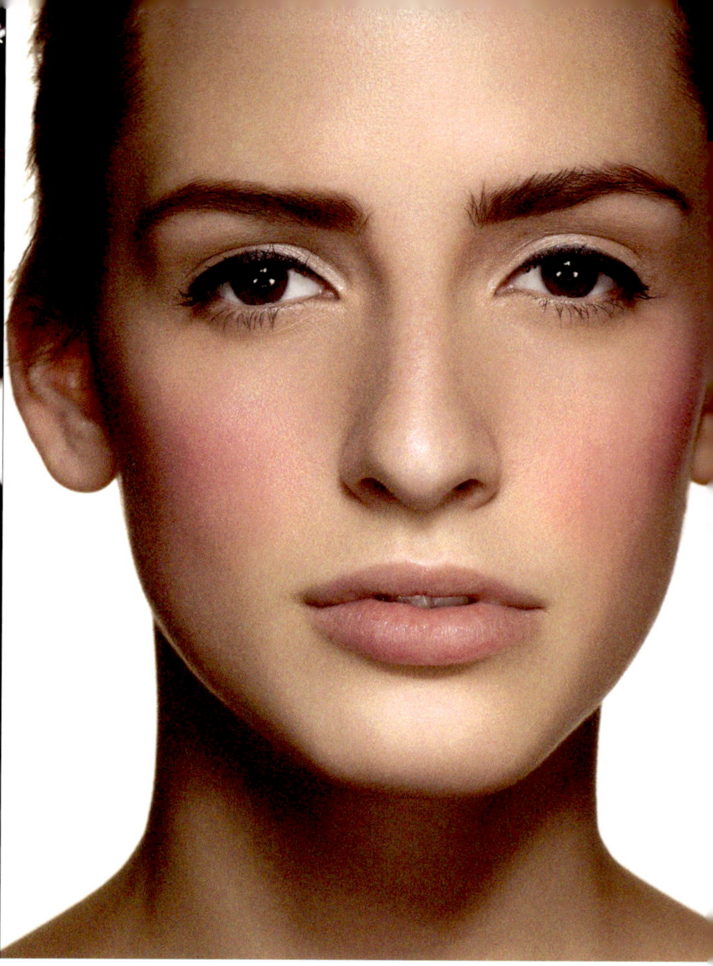

The model looks like a Joffrey Ballet dancer. Pretty, pink, and elegant.

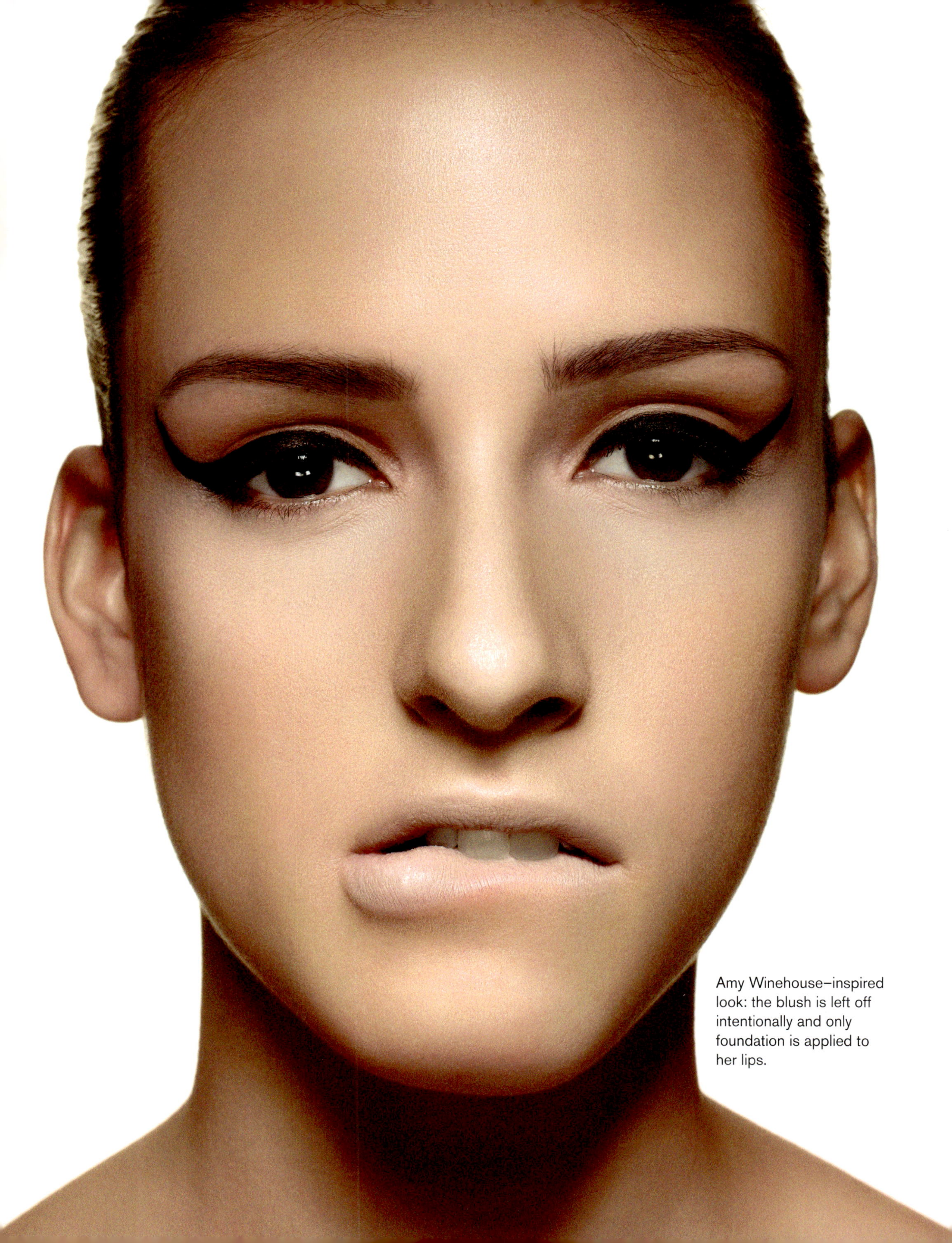

Amy Winehouse–inspired look: the blush is left off intentionally and only foundation is applied to her lips.

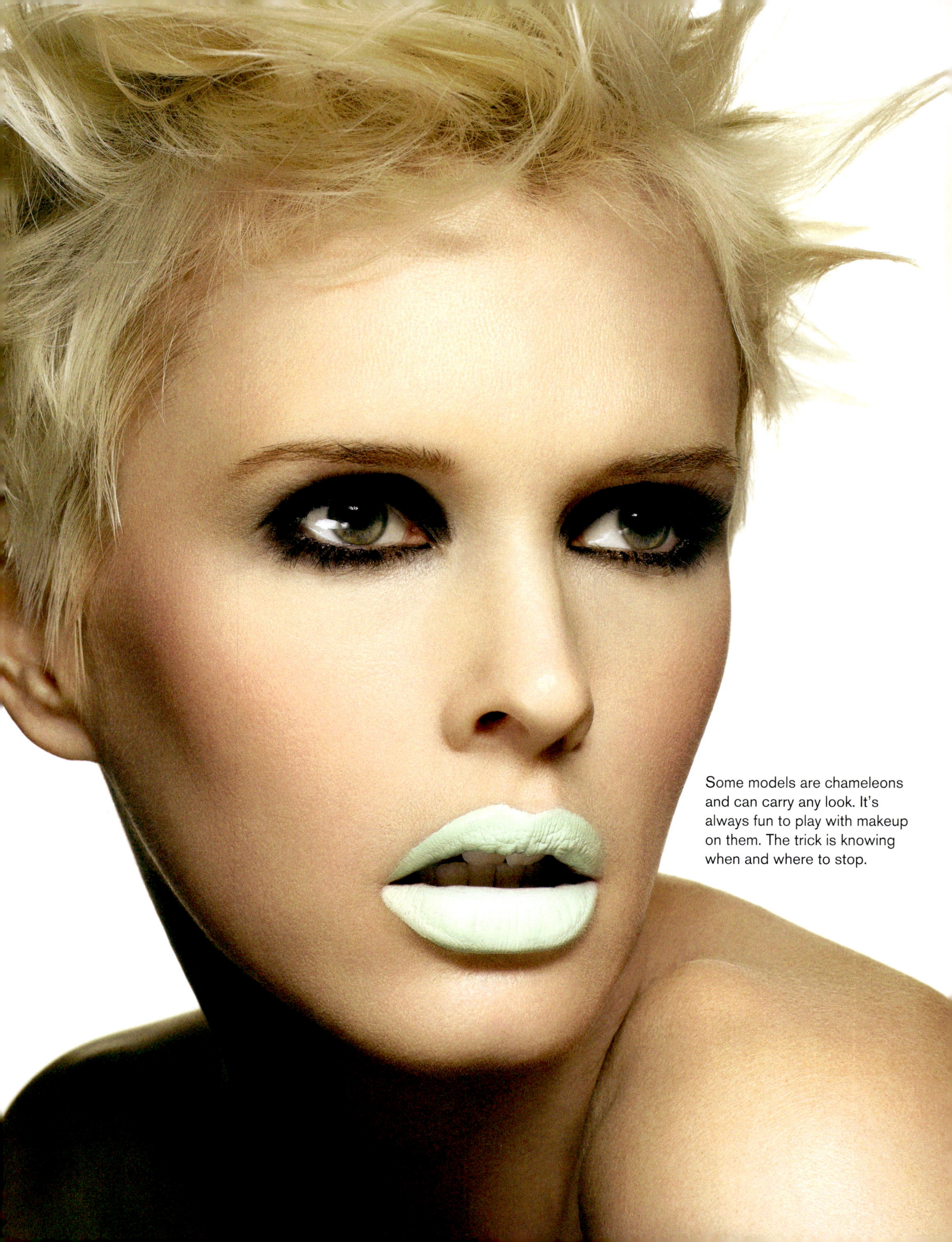

Some models are chameleons and can carry any look. It's always fun to play with makeup on them. The trick is knowing when and where to stop.

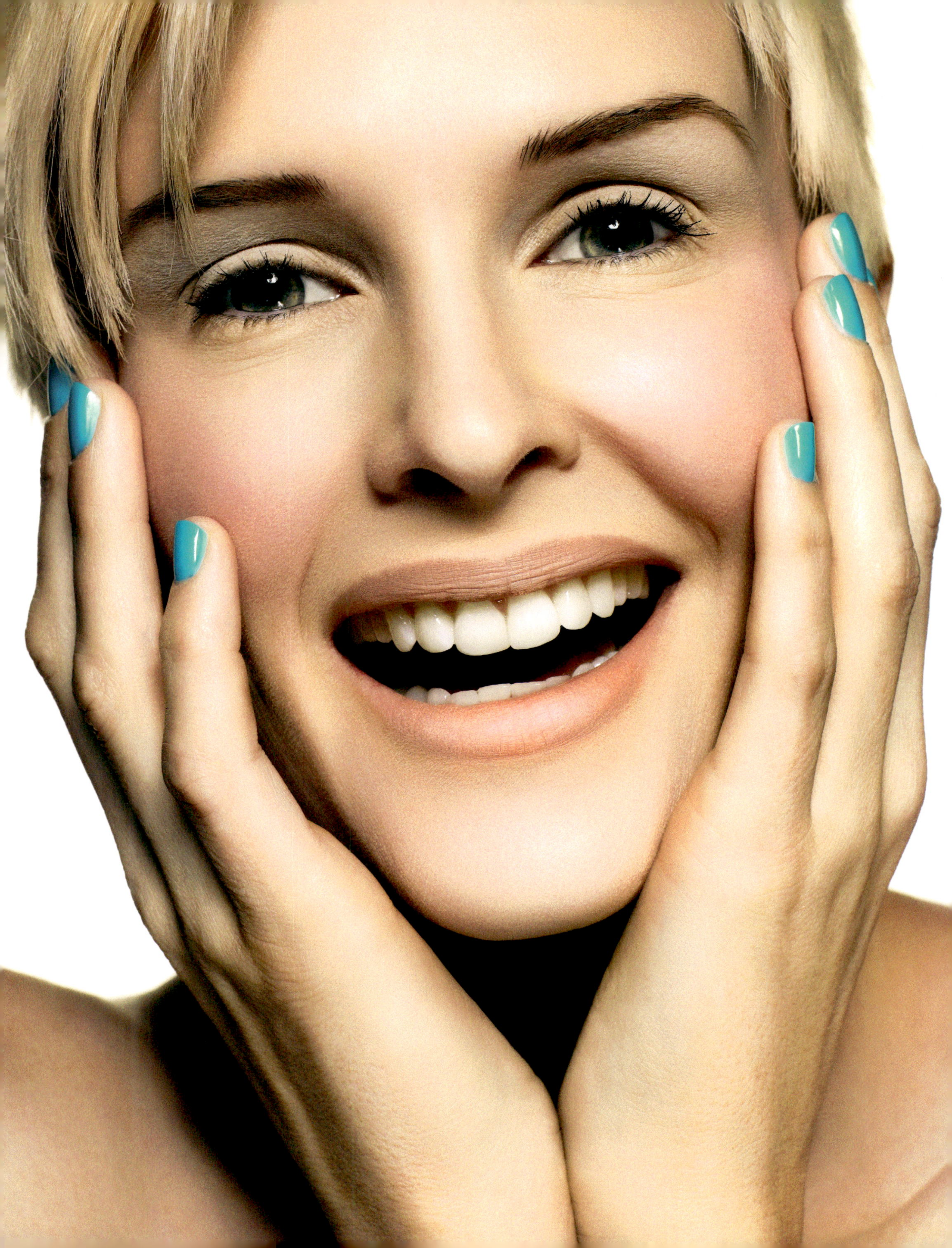

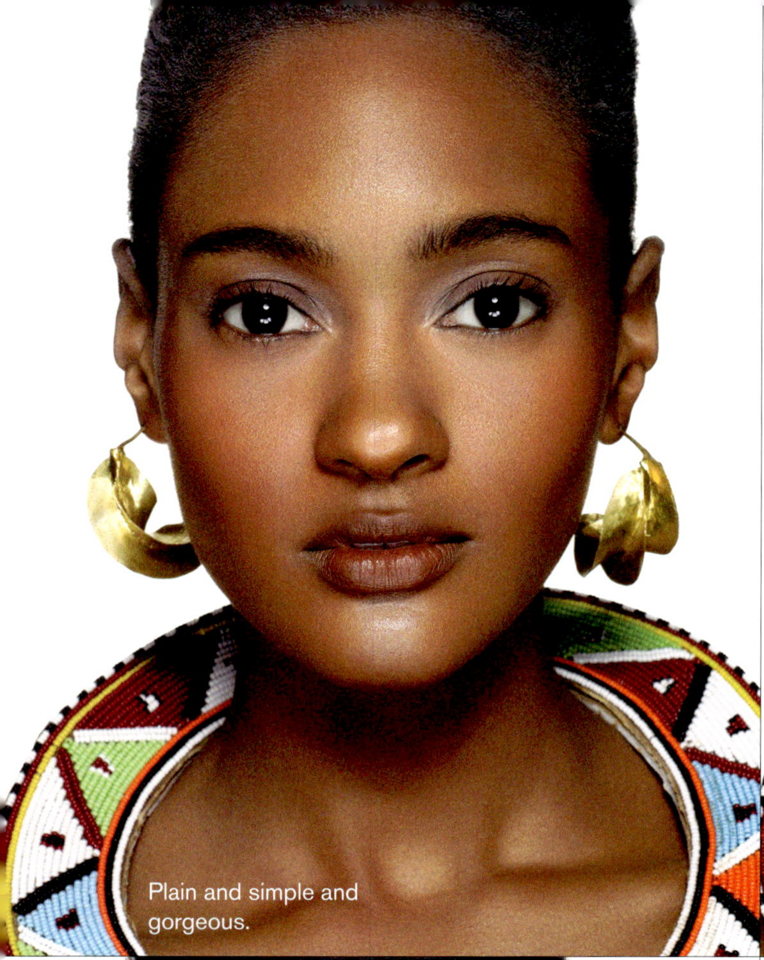
Plain and simple and gorgeous.

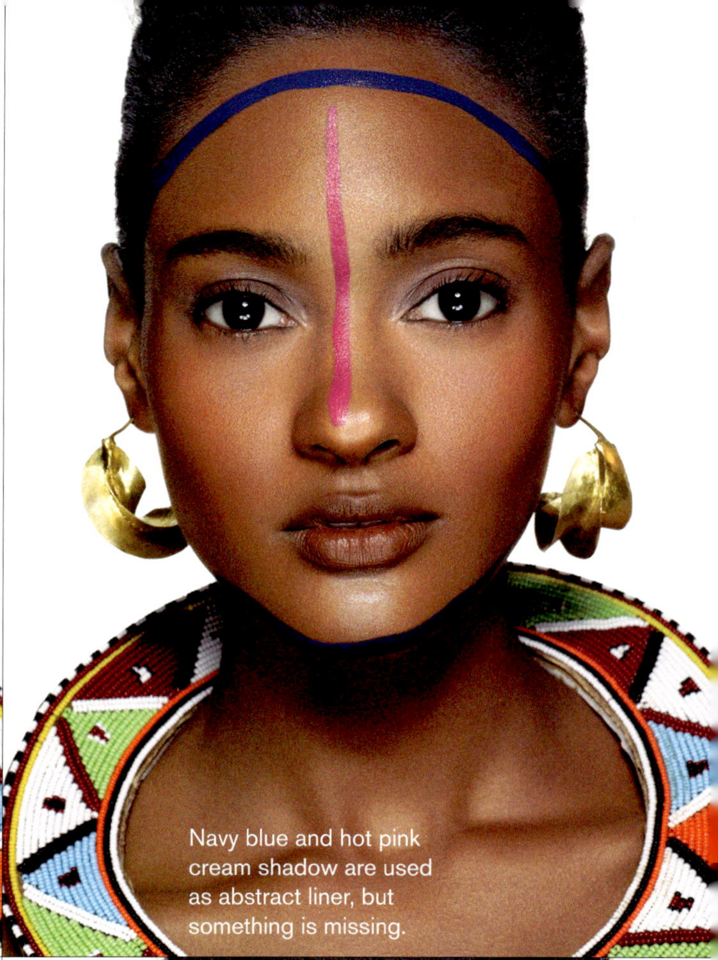
Navy blue and hot pink cream shadow are used as abstract liner, but something is missing.

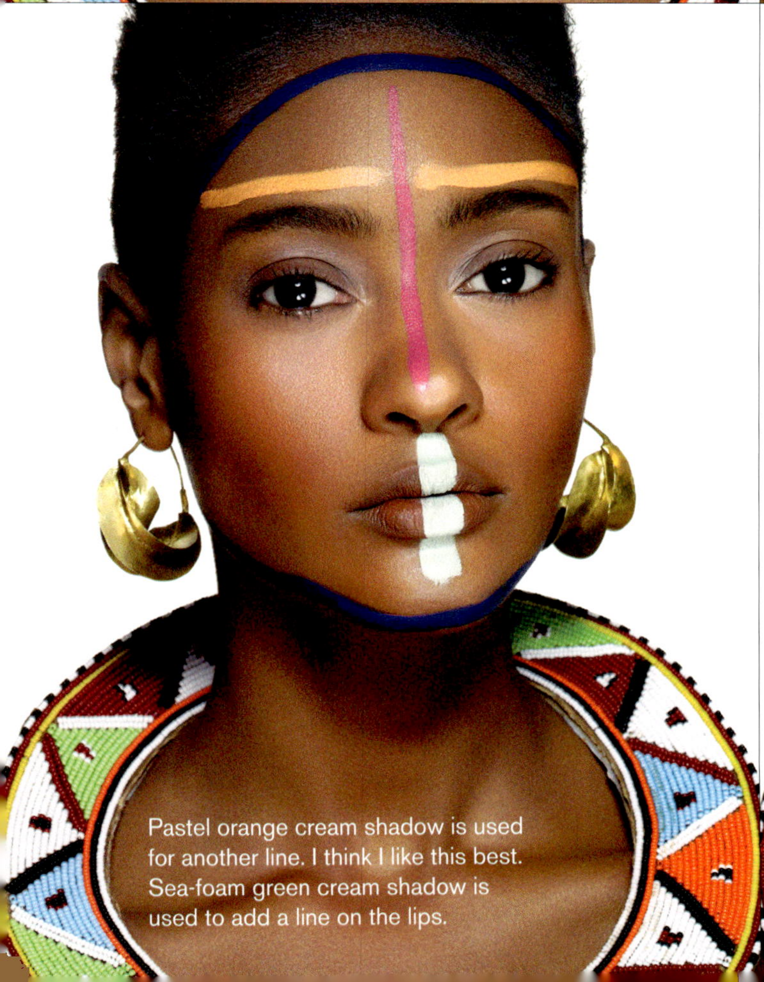
Pastel orange cream shadow is used for another line. I think I like this best. Sea-foam green cream shadow is used to add a line on the lips.

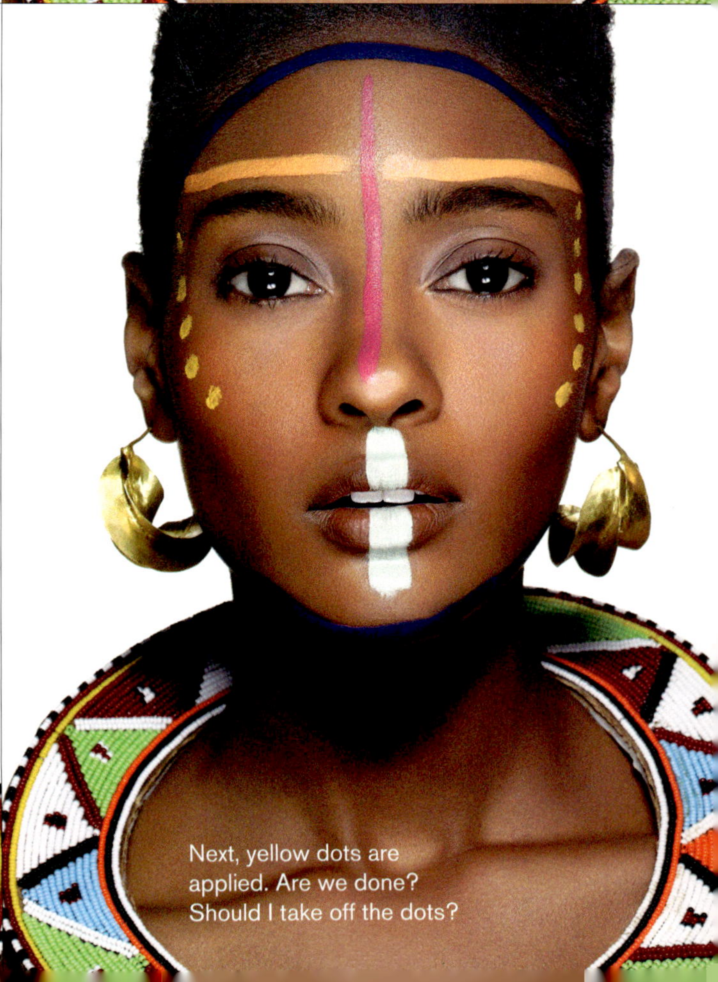
Next, yellow dots are applied. Are we done? Should I take off the dots?

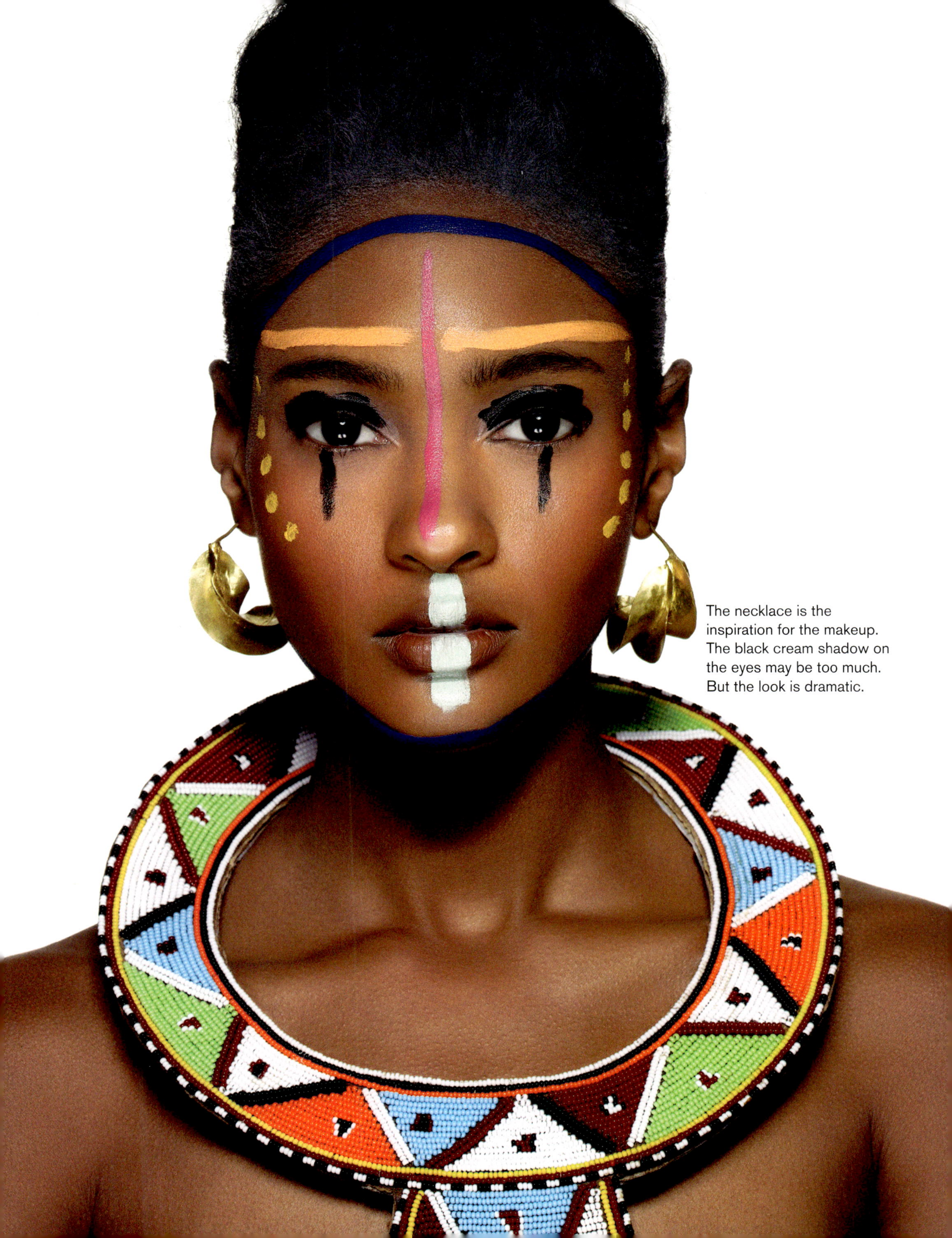

The necklace is the inspiration for the makeup. The black cream shadow on the eyes may be too much. But the look is dramatic.

MAKEUP for TELEVISION & FILM

TELEVISION

There is a misconception that makeup done for television has to be heavy. That is not the case. The bright lights of television studios can wash out makeup colors, but don't overcompensate with too heavy a hand. Use the same products you would use for day. Just make sure they are pumped up a notch, and perfectly blended.

Brighten the under-eye area by layering pink-toned corrector under yellow-toned concealer. Then set it with loose powder applied with a powder brush or puff. This step is an absolute necessity as television lights increase shine.

Use full-coverage foundation followed by powder to keep it matte. Sheer tints are too subtle for television.

Even if a glow is desired, it needs to be added to the cheeks at the end of the makeup application.

Color tends to wash out, so always use two shades of blush—one natural shade followed by a brighter pop of color. Correct blending is a must.

Avoid lip colors that are too light unless the subject's lips are so full that you want to downplay them. Television tends to wash out natural tones.

Define lips with pencil.

Make sure hands, arms, neck, and ears all match the face.

Bronzer is a great help, especially on the neck.

High-Definition Television

High-definition television is extremely unforgiving. (It definitely wasn't invented by a woman over twenty years old.) It conveys very sharp contrast with great detail. The makeup you apply has to be both fluid and perfectly blended. Foundation that is not correctly applied will look like it's melting off the face. Remember two words: *coverage* and *blending*.

Always check makeup in the monitor to see how it reads with lighting.

Blemishes need to be expertly covered.

FILM

Directors, lighting, and scripts dictate what style of makeup needs to be done. Communicate with everyone involved, ask lots of questions, and do lots of testing. The real makeup challenge, when working on films, is maintaining continuity. Scenes are often shot out of sequence, and part of a makeup artist's job is to make sure the character looks the same in each scene. It can be a slow process, so always have a digital camera and a notebook handy to keep track of the shots. Lighting and style dictate what the makeup should look like.

NINE MEMORABLE WOMEN

These women are all icons and their looks have inspired many makeup artists to recreate them either in movies or editorial work. Whether it's a direct period piece or just an element—these are the looks that inspire editors and photographers.

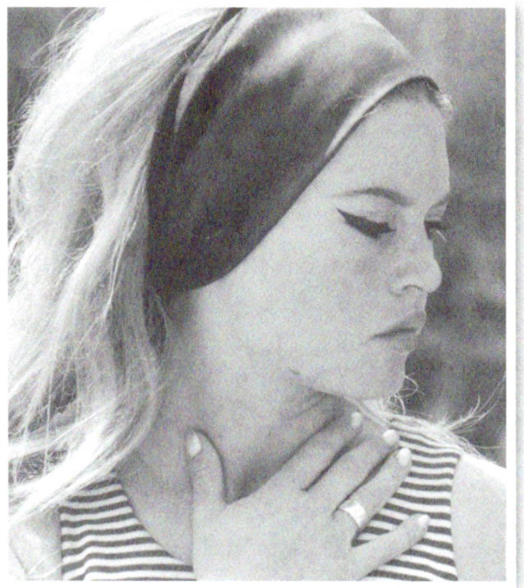

Brigitte Bardot
Light foundation and blush, extra pale lips, and classic medium-thick eyeliner.

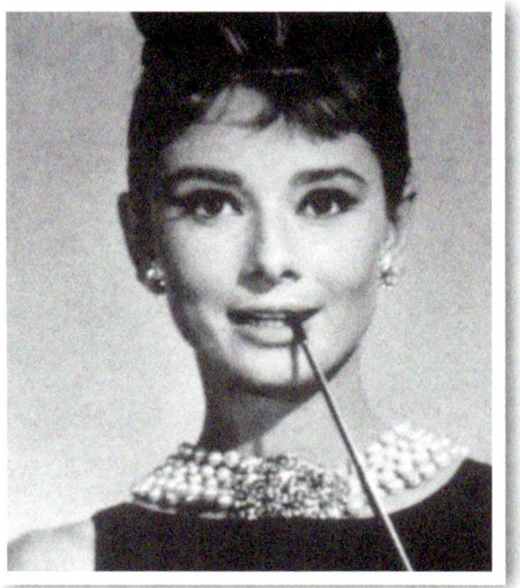

Audrey Hepburn
Her look was all about the strong squared-off brow, a matte powdery face, and natural colors.

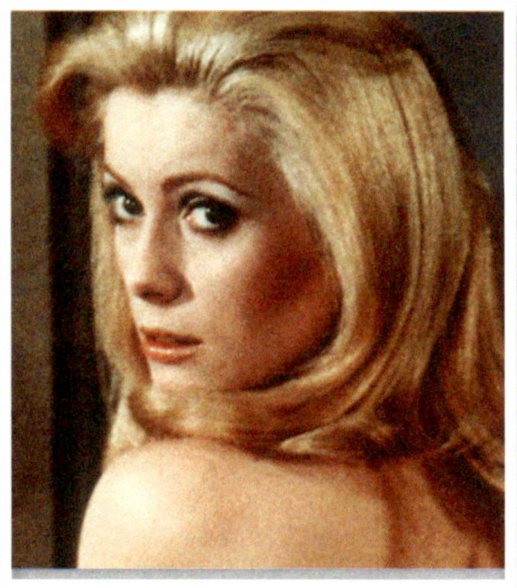

Catherine Deneuve
Sexy kitten, smoky eyes, and medium lips.

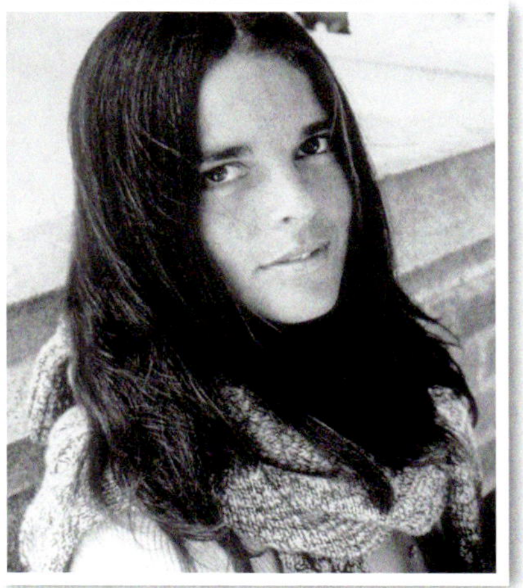

Ali McGraw
The icon of the natural American look. Brown eyeshadow, simple dark brown liner, naturally strong brow, clean skin, tawny cheek, and nude lip.

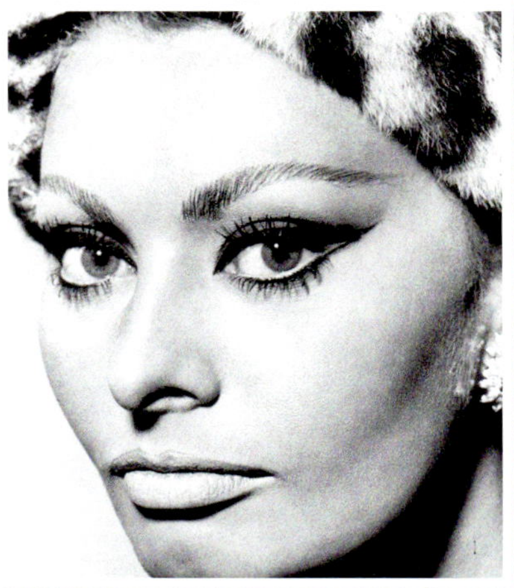

Sophia Loren
Classic Italian, sexy yet understated. Her strong features don't need a lot. Strong brows, medium lips, clean black eyeliner, and a little blush.

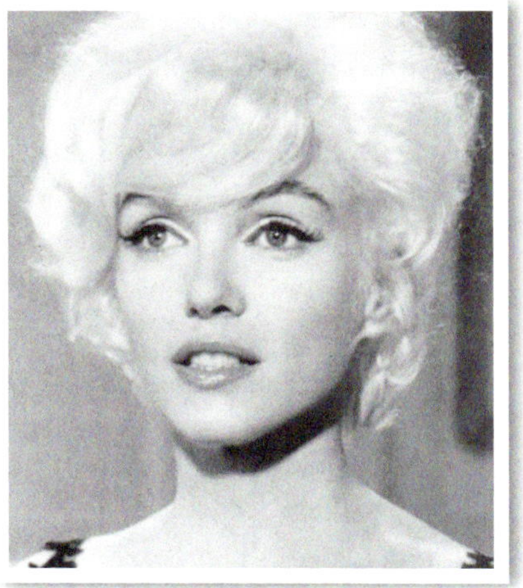

Marilyn Monroe
Her makeup was all about a sexy face. Strong brows, white eyelids, smoky contour, false eyelashes, and strong eyeliner, often with a red lip—classic 50s.

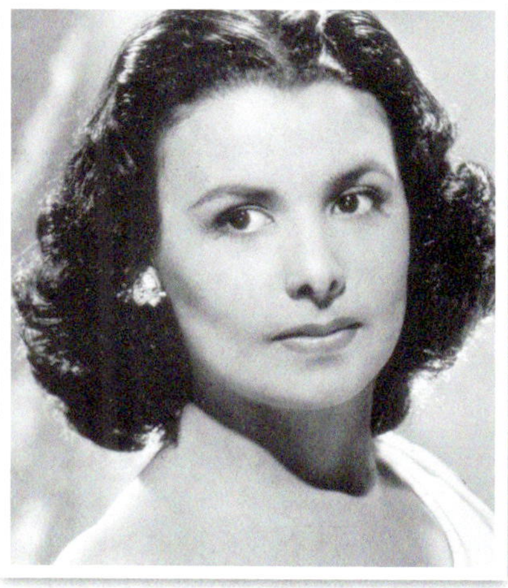

Lena Horne
40s glamour—burgundy lips, eyes lined on top, shadow artfully applied, strong brow, and visible black false eyelashes.

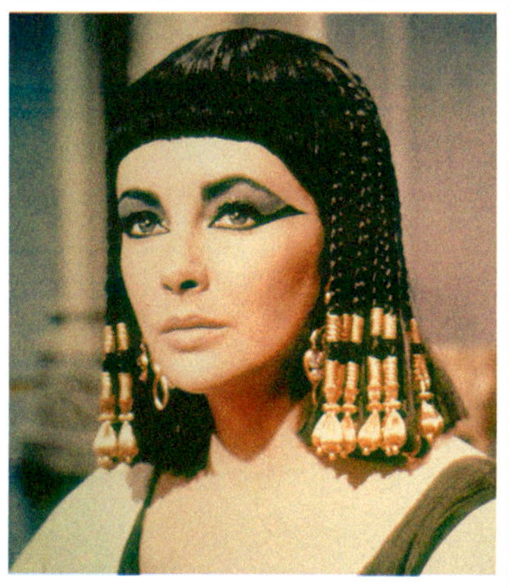

Elizabeth Taylor
Whether playing the title role in *Cleopatra* or Martha in *Who's Afraid of Virginia Woolf*, she always had her violet eyes rimmed with black shadow, eyeliner, and lashes.

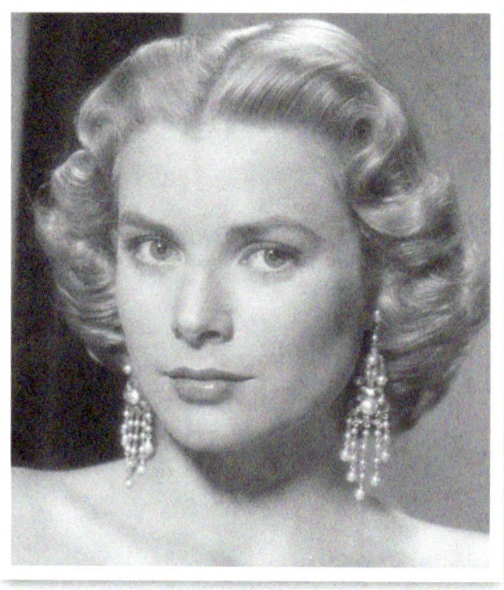

Grace Kelly
A Hollywood princess: classic blonde and "Ralph Laurenesque" at a black-tie ball.

MAKEUP for FASHION SHOWS

Working as a makeup artist at a fashion show is similar in many ways to doing the makeup for a theatrical production. Just as theatrical makeup has to represent the vision of the director or the playwright, ***the final look you see on the runway is a collaboration between the designer, the makeup artist, the hairstylist, and the model.*** As fashion shows have increasingly become a media circus, with television cameras and photographers recording every aspect of the event both on the runway and backstage, the makeup artist's role has become even more important. It is not enough to make a model look beautiful; a makeup artist must be able to speak about the designer's vision and the current style trends.

Working with models is like working with a blank canvas. You can experiment and try things that would probably look horrible on a real woman but look great on the runway or in a photo. I do believe that if the model likes her look, the shoot will go better. I have had to apologize for creating a severe look that the model hates but is required by the designer or photographer. ***All of these situations take confidence, patience, communication, and a willingness to take risks.***

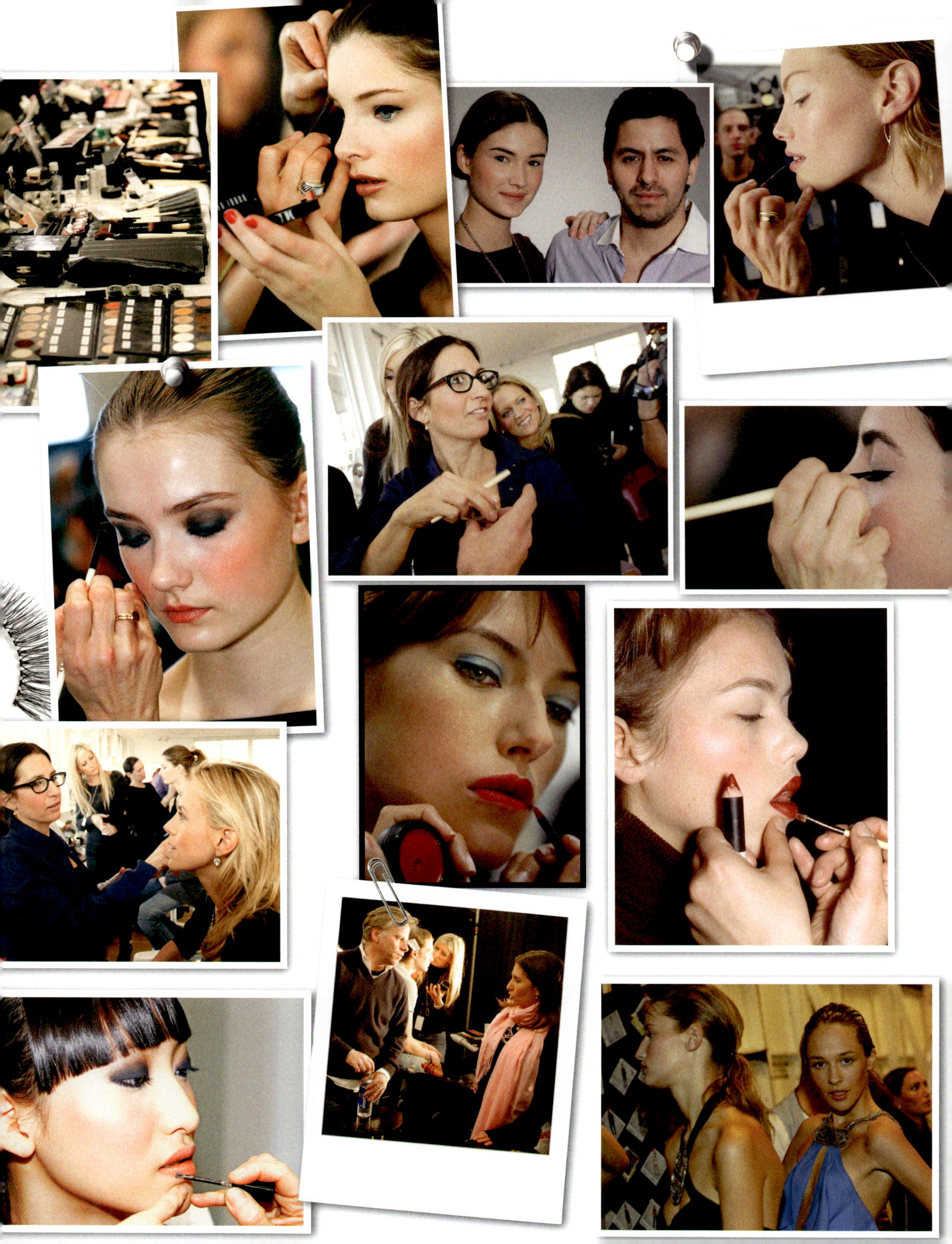

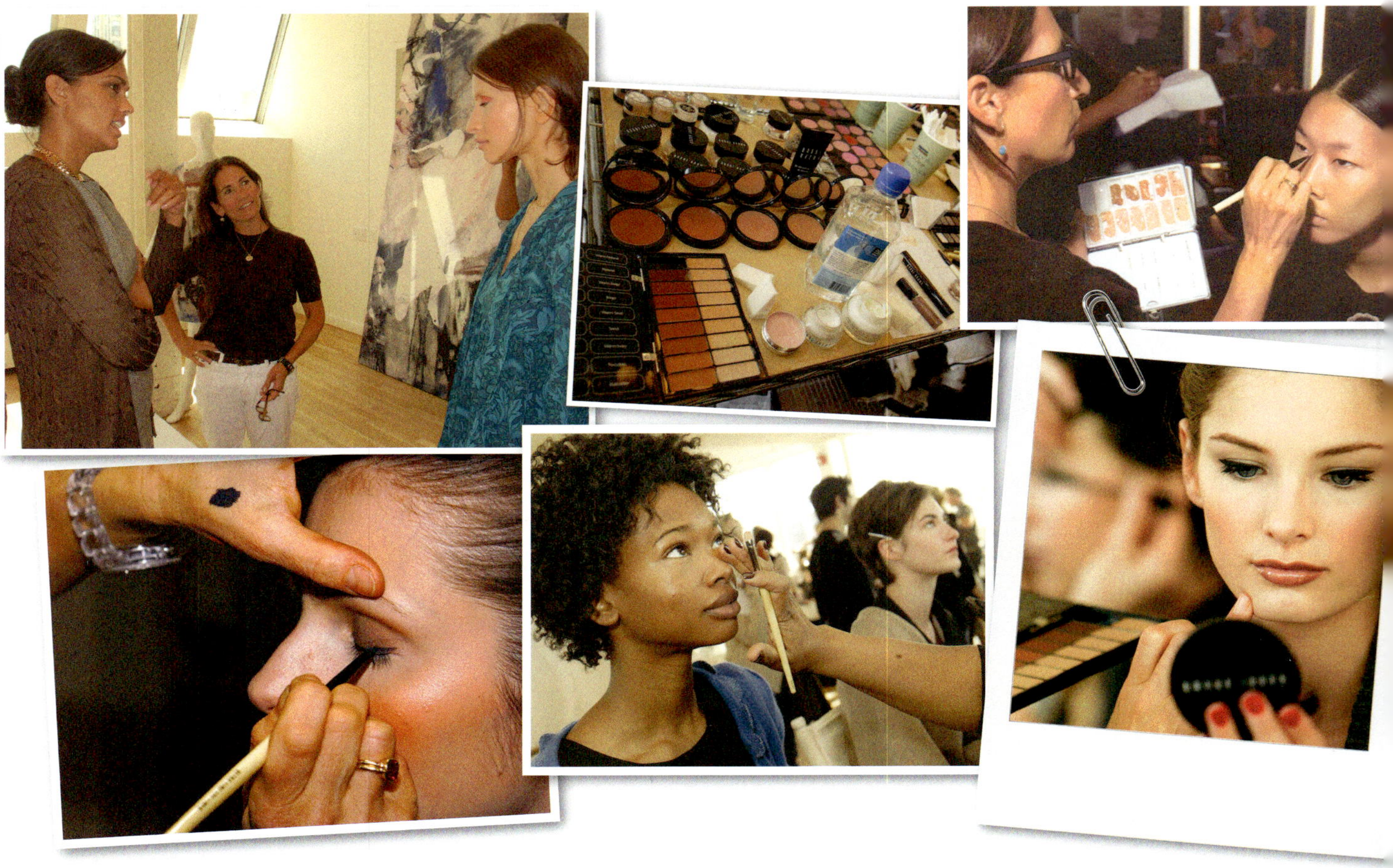

WHAT HAPPENS BEFORE THE SHOW

The Makeup Test

If it's the first time you've worked with a designer, research his or her design style and history. This will give you an idea of the aesthetics of past shows.

About a week before the fashion show, the makeup artist and designer meet to discuss the look. After viewing the clothes, the designer will give you his or her vision for the collection. Designers are very visual, but aren't always able to communicate what they want. Your role is to interpret their vision. Most designers have photos of inspirational objects to help you with the interpretation. Ask a *lot* of questions. If the designer mentions he wants a strong eye, ask if he's thinking Sophia Loren in the 60s or the modern Gucci eye. Keep asking until you feel confident that you have the right vision in your head.

Next, do some trials and experiment with some options to show the designer and stylist your interpretations of the look. You may get the right look quickly, or it can take quite a long time. Sometimes makeup is done on a pretty assistant, but show makeup works best on a model. There is a reason models are models: they showcase makeup better than other people.

Once the final look is approved, sketch it. Purchase anything you think you will need that is not already in your kit, and complete a face chart that includes all of the products, with color identification, location on the face, and any special information needed to complete the look. You will need a makeup team. Find out how many models will be walking and hire one artist for every two to three models.

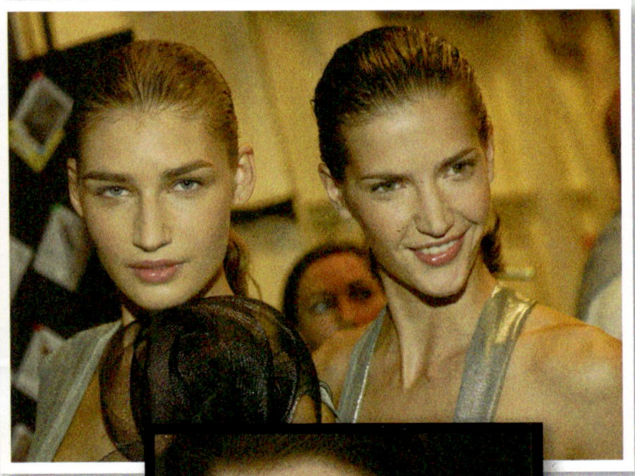
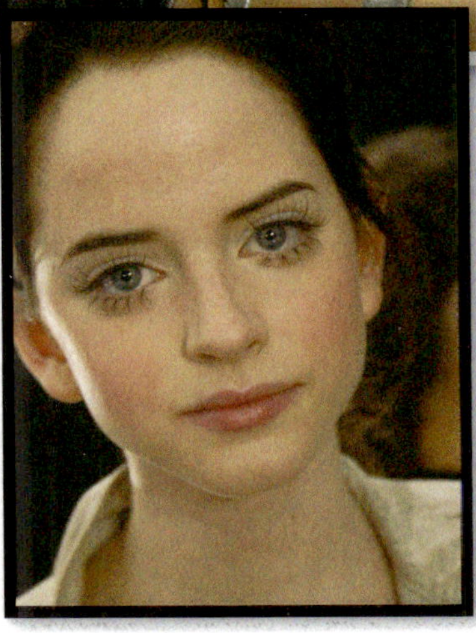
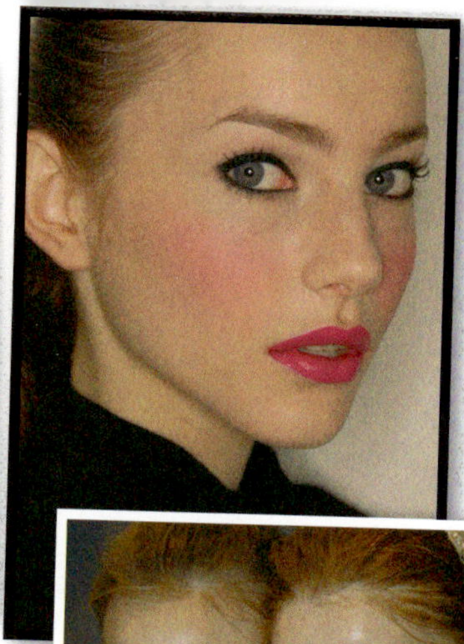
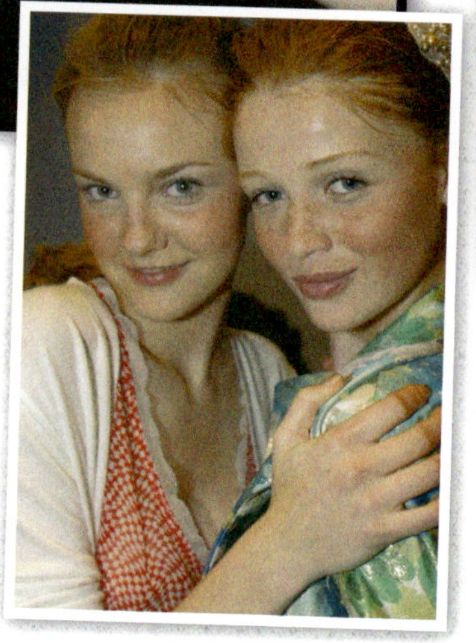
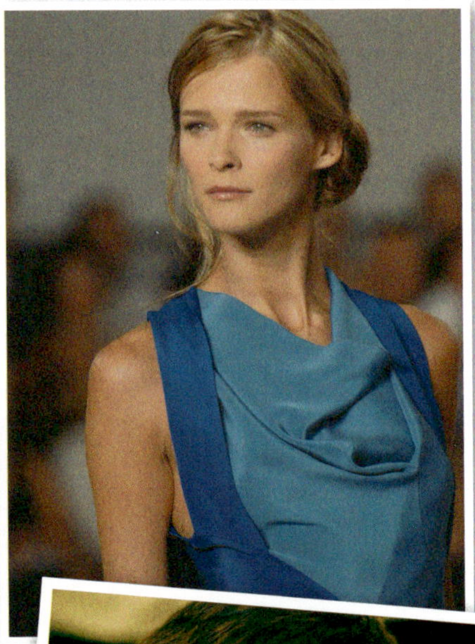
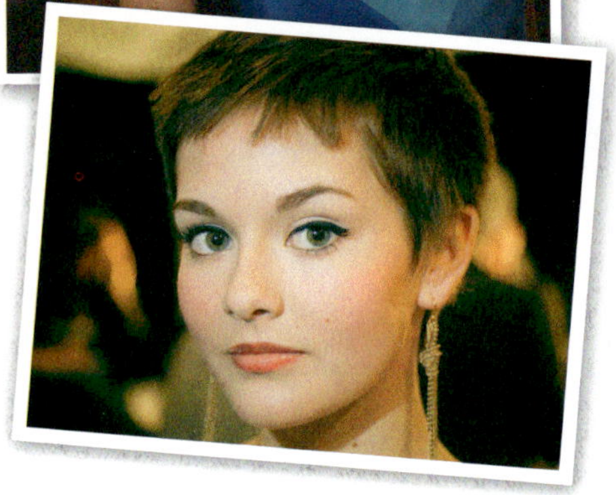

WHAT HAPPENS DURING THE SHOW

Stay calm. This is the key to working on a fashion show. There will be plenty of chaos, lots of distractions, and last-minute emergencies. You also have to be flexible; sometimes makeup is completely changed thirty minutes before the show.

On the day of the fashion show, you need to arrive two to four hours before the show is scheduled to begin.

Start by using one of the models to do a trial run of the makeup. When her face is done, bring her out onto the runway so you and the designer can check the results under the lights. If you have assistants working with you, bring them out as well so they hear what you and the designer decide.

Once the look gets approved, the team begins to work. Adjust the colors for each model's skin tone. Even if the designer says he wants pastel pink on everyone's cheeks, remember that the exact same color won't work on different skin tones.

Many of the models will arrive backstage from another show. They will already have a full face of makeup on, and you will have only minutes to change their look completely. To save time, hand the model a tissue covered in non-oily makeup remover, and instruct her to wipe off her lipstick and eye shadow. You can have her leave the foundation and mascara on, but you must check it carefully to determine whether it will work with the look you're trying to create. No matter how little time you have, if the foundation isn't right, you must take it all off and start from scratch.

Right before the show begins, you need to check the models for refreshing or additional powder to combat shine.

Even after the models start heading down the runway, your job is not done. As the models change clothes, they might mess up their lips, or they might need a touch-up with powder. Your job is to continue standing by, ready to fix whatever might need fixing.

WORKING with CELEBRITIES

Working with celebrities is fun and challenging. Just like every woman, they want to find a look that is right for them while looking beautiful. ***Whether you are doing their makeup for an early-morning television appearance, a movie premiere, a photo shoot, or the Oscars, you have to adapt the look to suit the clothes, lighting, and occasion.*** And as with any relationship, if it's your first time working with a certain celebrity, go slowly, ask a lot of questions, and hand her the mirror frequently to avoid getting big surprises at the end of the application. If it is a celebrity you've worked with regularly, just ask a few quick questions about what she's going to be wearing and the look she wants.

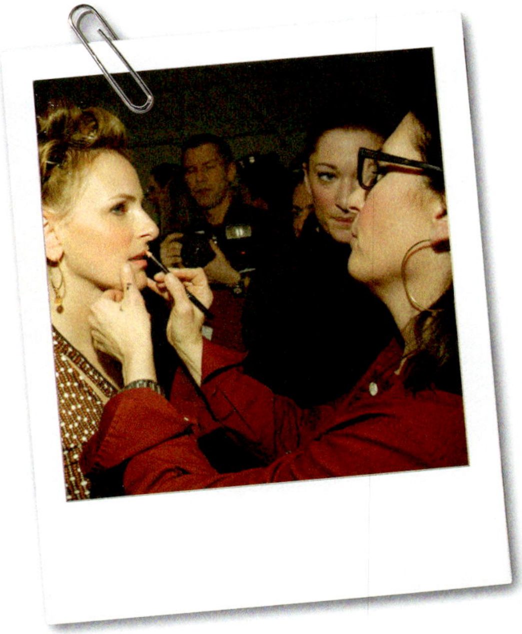

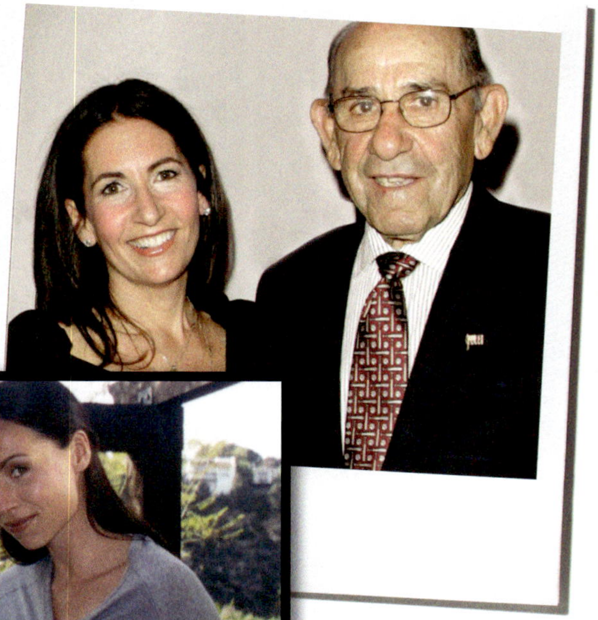

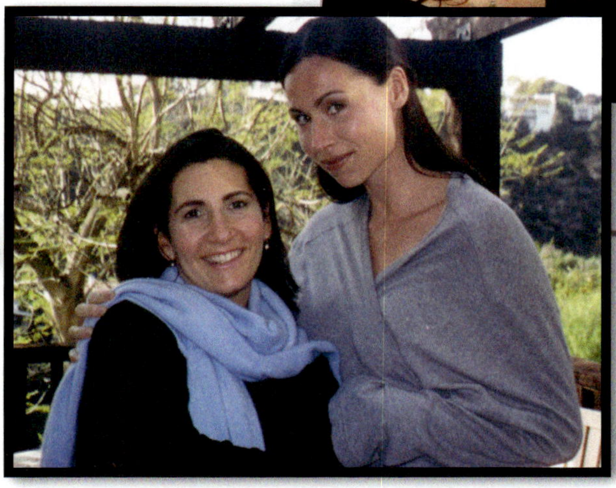

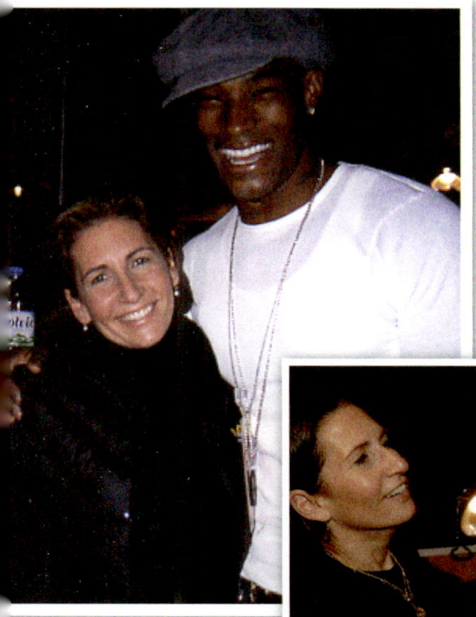
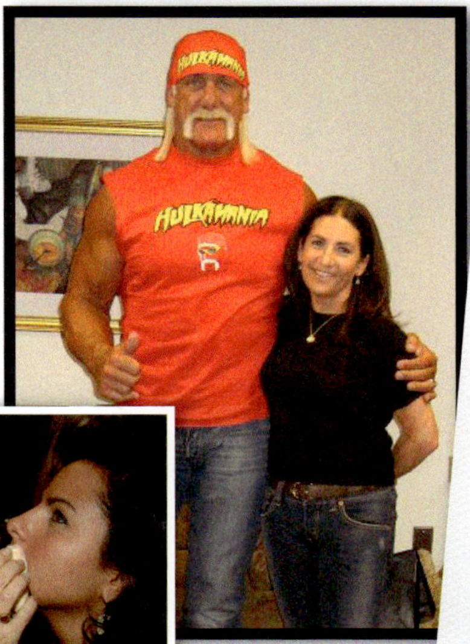
HULKAMANIA
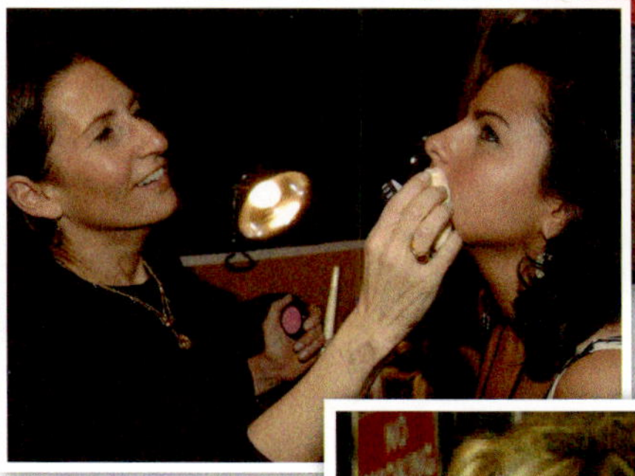
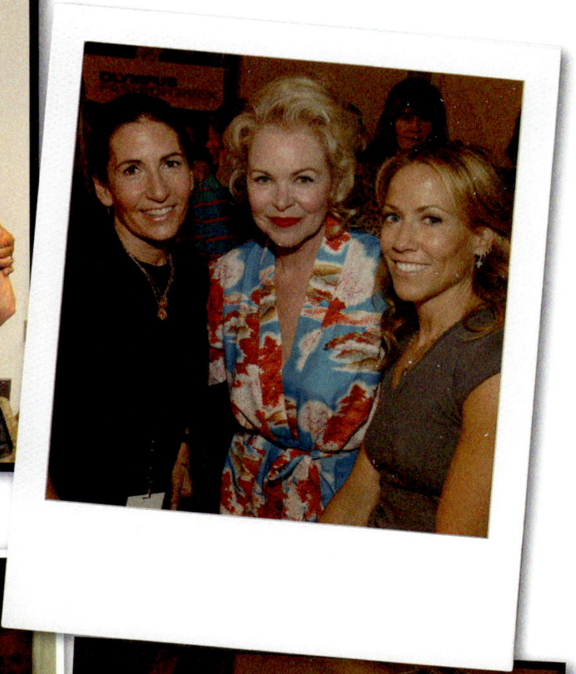
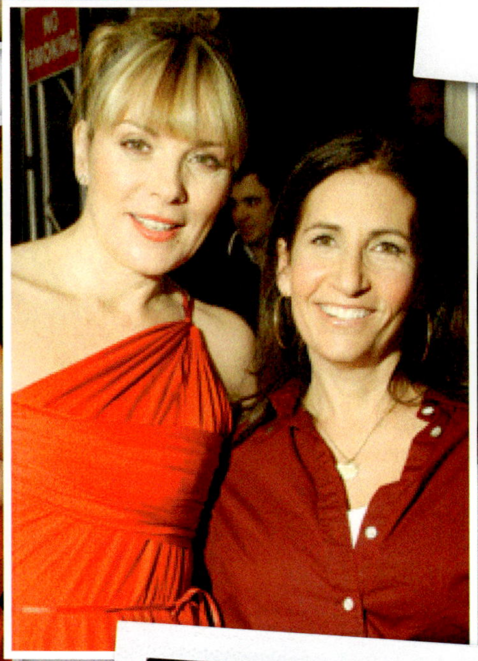
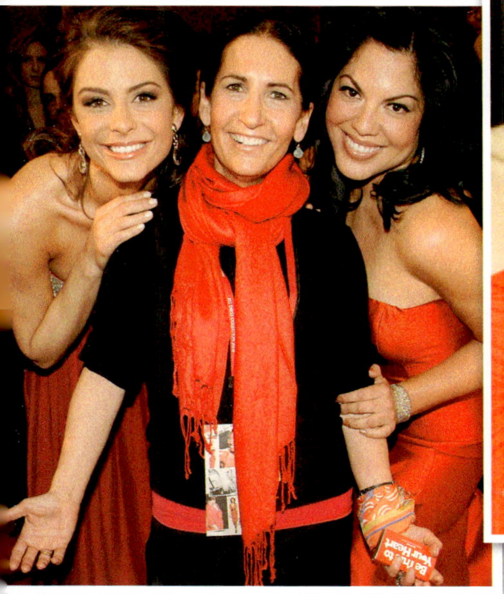
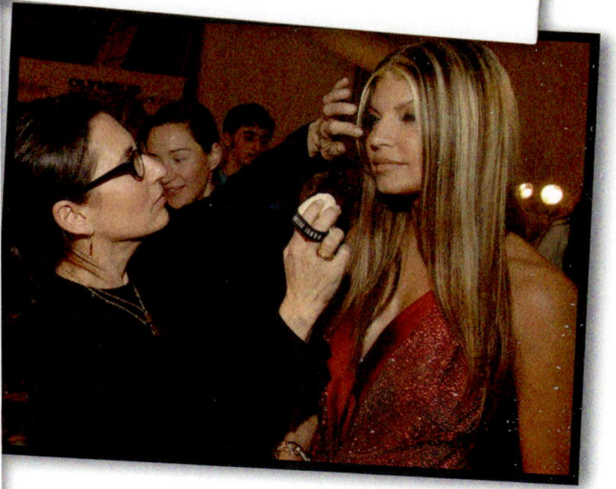
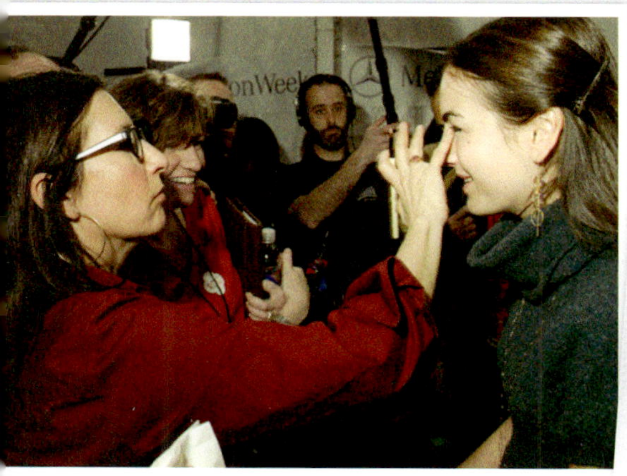
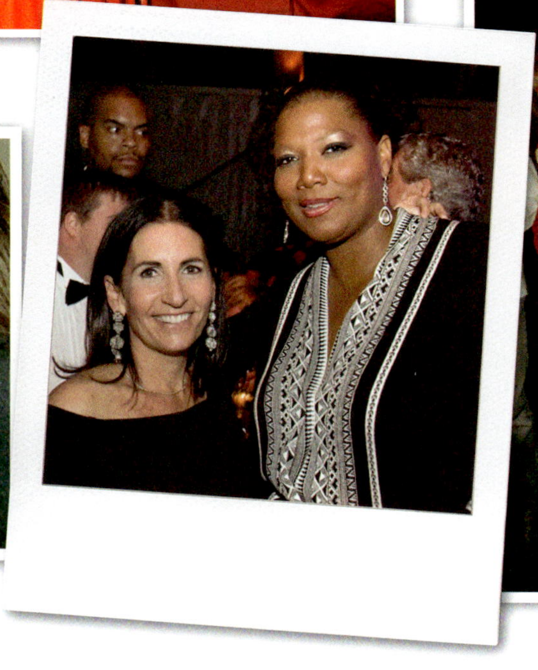
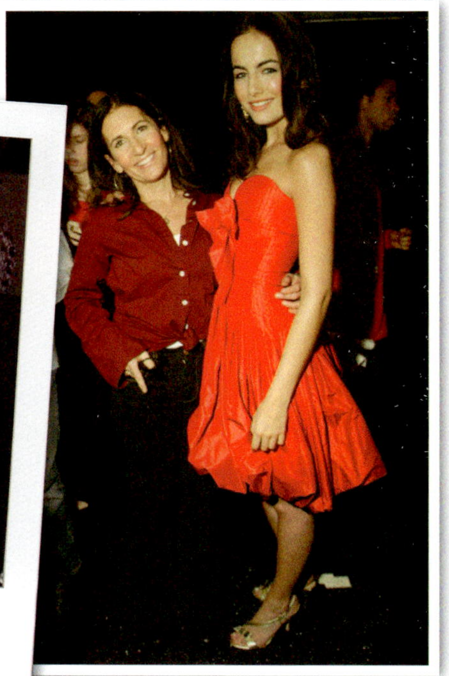

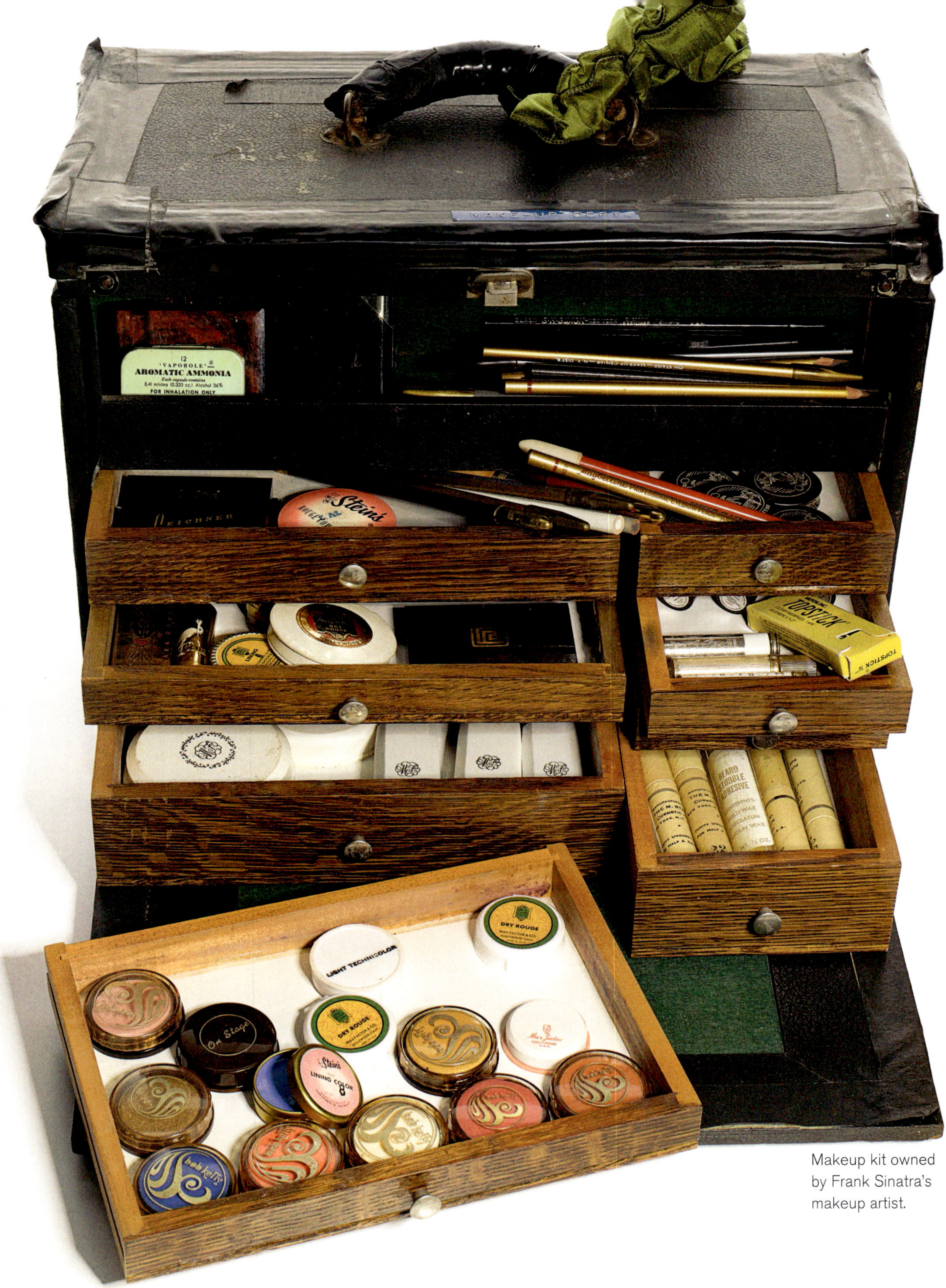

Makeup kit owned by Frank Sinatra's makeup artist.

Chapter 12

MEMORABLE MAKEUP MOMENTS & LEGENDS

the HISTORY of MAKEUP

c. 500,000 B.C.E. Cave dwellers in Africa and South America cover their bodies with mud applied in decorative patterns. The mud also functions as an insect repellent.

c. 3000 B.C.E. Egyptians use more than thirty different types of cosmetic balms and ointments made from ingredients such as beeswax, vegetable oil, and animal fat. Moisturizers are considered so essential, they are routinely distributed to workers and farmers.

Egyptian women have elaborate makeup chests, equipment, and products. They give themselves egg white facials, use complexion cream, and apply perfumed oils. Women paint their faces with a (deadly) powder made from lead carbonate and water. Nails are painted with henna, and lipsticks are available in several orange-based shades. The use of red is banned, as it is considered magical. To outline the eyes, they use either powdered kohl or crushed ant's eggs. Eye shadows in red or green are created using plant stems. Other makeup tools include stone pestles for grinding, bronze or silver mirrors, ivory or alabaster spoons, bronze jars for holding face cream, linen, razors, ivory combs, and pumice.

c. 2000 B.C.E. An Egyptian papyrus includes formulas for removing wrinkles, pimples, age spots, and other blemishes. One mixture includes bullock's bile. Egyptians who want to get rid of wrinkles are told to apply a mixture of incense, olive oil, crushed cyperus, and wax to the face and to leave it on for six days.

Overseers stop all work on the pyramids until makeup supplies (kohl, green malachite, and galena) that help to protect the eyes of workers from the sun are delivered.

c. 2500 B.C.E. Sumerians invent the first tweezers to get rid of unwanted hair and use a flat bone to push back cuticles.

c. 1800 B.C.E. Gold dust is used by Babylonian men to powder their hair.

c. 1500 B.C.E. Egyptian women use body oils scented with frankincense and myrrh to moisturize and protect their skin from the dry, dusty climate.

Mesopotamian soldiers are paid in bottles of oil and perfume, which are more highly valued than cash.

c. 1200 B.C.E. Egyptians of this era are wearing a full face of cosmetics. They create eye shadows out of malachite, a copper ore that has a greenish tone, to line their bottom lids. Eyelashes and upper lids are darkened with powder made from lead ore.

c. 600 B.C.E. Makeup and lavish clothing is worn by all Babylonians of rank. An ambitious warrior named Parsondes was said to have complained to King Nebuchadnezzar about the governor Nanarus's focus on beauty rather than on government. When word got back to the governor, Nanarus ordered that the warrior shave all his hair and wear makeup and perfumed oils.

c. 400 B.C.E. Women from various cultures use powders made from crushed minerals, such as ocher, hematite, and white lead, to color their skin.

FIRST CENTURY B.C.E. Roman women use saffron or wood ash as eye shadow and antimony to darken their lids, lashes, and brows. Fucus, a purple pigment, is mixed with saliva and used for rouge and lip color. Blue paint is used to outline veins, which are seen as a sign of beauty. Nails are buffed with sheep's fat. Pumice is used to whiten teeth.

SECOND CENTURY A.D. Women in Palestine apply a mixture of starch, white lead, and crimson dye to their faces as an early form of blush.

THIRD CENTURY A.D. Talmudic law forbids Jewish women from applying makeup on the Sabbath.

636 The first glass mirror is invented. Women hang them, placed in elaborate cases, on a chain from their girdles, and men keep theirs under their hats.

1370 Charles V of France receives a gift of Hungary water, a body rub made of an alcohol base with rosemary, cedar, and turpentine. Soap is a luxury, but the use of these waters sweetens the smell of the body.

c. 1400 Cosmetics, including a white paste made of flour to cover the face, become increasingly popular among the French aristocracy. Women pluck their hairlines and even remove their eyebrows in the name of beauty.

c. 1500 Renaissance women use a mixture of honey and egg whites to condition their skin. White lead is applied to reduce the appearance of wrinkles. Mercuric sulphide is used for rouge. To keep complexions clear, some wash their faces in urine or a mixture of rose water and wine. To reduce ruddiness, raw veal soaked in warm milk for several hours is placed on the affected area.

c. 1550 Catherine de Médicis uses a skin tonic made from crushed peach blossoms mixed with almond oil.

1597 *Gerard's Herbal* is published. This is one of the first printed publications to include recipes for various skin creams, including one for acne.

c. 1600 To soothe chapped lips, it is recommended that sweat from behind the ears be applied to the affected area.

1603 Queen Elizabeth I dies and is rumored to have an inch and a half of makeup on her face at the time of her passing. This is not uncommon in an era when no one washes their faces, and makeup is used to cover the horrible scars left by smallpox.

LATE 1600s A doll-like look with a pure white face and scarlet cheeks is all the rage. A foundation of white ceruse, which contains lead, is mixed on a palette with water or egg white and applied to the skin. Rouge is commonly applied by rubbing a piece of Spanish felt or wool that has been dyed scarlet onto dampened cheeks.

LATE 1600s TO 1700s Silk taffeta or thin leather patches in shapes like flowers, stars, and moons become a popular product to temporarily conceal smallpox scars on the face. More than just cover-ups, however, the patches signal a woman's availability if placed near the lips. Engaged women wear them on the left cheek and switch to the right after marriage. Some even carry small patch boxes with them to social events to replace any that fall off. Small scenes are sometimes pasted over an eyebrow, and profiles of family members are sometimes worn on the face.

c. 1830 Women put a few drops of belladonna into their eyes to dilate the pupils, creating a dreamy look. Belladonna is a plant extract used since ancient times as a poison.

1846 Pond's Extract, a commercial cold cream, is introduced.

1867 The department store B. Altman and Company opens a "making up" department to teach women to apply rouge, powder, and eyebrow pencil.

1886 Avon, the door-to-door cosmetics line, is founded by David Hall McConnell, a former door-to-door book salesman.

c. 1900 Guerlain introduces the first lip colors to come in stick form.

1891 Polish-born Helena Rubinstein opens the world's first modern beauty salon, in Australia. She sells a simple face cream inspired by her mother's beauty cream. The product is an instant hit among Autralian women. In 1902 Helena expands her business to London, followed by Paris in 1906 and New York in 1912.

1908 Actresses are the only people who know much about makeup, as it is used exclusively for the stage. No woman dares to go out in public with more than the lightest dusting of rice powder. Rice powder makes the face appear lighter but also swells up in the pores of the skin, enlarging them. Helena Rubinstein starts to produce a tinted face powder that is more natural looking, does not have harmful side effects, and has a broad appeal.

1909 Rubinstein's lifelong rival, Elizabeth Arden, opens her Fifth Avenue salon.

1909 The Russian immigrant Max Factor opens his first makeup studio in Hollywood.

1909 Eugène Schueller, a French chemist, opens the French Harmless Hair Dye Company, selling the first safe commercial hair dye product. A year later, he renames his product L'Oréal.

c. 1910 The first pressed compact powders—complete with mirrors and puffs—are introduced.

1910 *The Daily Mirror Beauty Book* is published. The makeup hints and recipes for homemade lotions reflect the fact that cosmetics have become publicly accepted for the first time in almost one hundred years. The little booklet includes references to a device that curls lashes, a homemade eyebrow darkener, and astringent lotion, and it suggests using a pencil line to elongate the eyes.

1910 Tattoos are extremely popular in Britain. George Burchett, a famous tattooist, practices his art on men and women alike. His card indicates that he can tint and shade complexions and remove moles, blemishes, and other marks.

1914 After seeing his sister Maybel apply petroleum jelly to her lashes, T. L. Williams formulates the first mascara. He forms a company, named Maybelline after his sister, to manufacture the new product.

c. 1920 Coco Chanel makes tans chic, calling a suntan an important "fashion accessory."

1920s The flapper Clara Bow is everyone's favorite "it" girl. Her look includes heavy eyeliner and ultrathin eyebrows.

The opening of chain stores, in which products and prices can be examined by all, make inexpensive cosmetics available to everyone.

1922 Elizabeth Arden opens a salon on Bond Street in London.

1930 When she finds that her new cream can heal and improve the skin in a matter of hours, Elizabeth Arden names the product Eight Hour Cream. It remains a best seller to this day.

1932 Revlon launches its first nail enamel.

1939–1945 World War II restricts the manufacture of cosmetics. Petroleum and alcohol, two principal ingredients used in makeup, are needed for war supplies.

1940s Joan Crawford's heavily penciled-in, arched eyebrows become the trademark look for the 1940s career woman.

1943 Estée Lauder launches her company with a line of six products.

1952 Revlon's Fire and Ice, an all-out sexy red lipstick color, is launched and becomes an instant success.

1960 The Color Additive Amendment requires that coloring ingredients in cosmetics be tested for safety and approved by the FDA.

1967 Estée Lauder launches a new line called Clinique, which emphasizes scientific skincare and cosmetics.

1967 The supermodel Twiggy popularizes a dramatic eye look; she draws lashes around the eye with a pencil and applies numerous false lashes, creating a doe-eyed effect.

1970s Natural makeup is all the rage.

Models to know: Veruschka, Marissa Berenson, Lauren Hutton, Margaux and Mariel Hemingway, Cheryl Tiegs, Christie Brinkley, Beverly Johnson.

Beauty icons: Jacqueline Kennedy Onassis, Bo Derek, Farrah Fawcett, whose poster was the top-selling poster in history.

1972 Ilana Harkavi, a former professional dancer, launches Il Makiage. The line is positioned as "the makeup artist's makeup."

1974 Lauren Hutton becomes the first model to sign an exclusive cosmetics contract. Revlon signs her for $100,000.

1975 Trish McEvoy launches a line of makeup brushes to fill the demand for high-quality makeup tools.

1977 Calvin Klein launches a line of cosmetics, which relaunches in 2005.

1980s Makeup is strong and exaggerated. Color trends are bold—lots of blues and fuchsias. Avon and Mary Kay create palettes to take the guesswork out of choosing a color scheme.

Models to know: Rosemary McGrath, Pat Cleveland, Esme, Lisa Taylor, Jerry Hall.

Beauty icons: Madonna, Grace Jones, Jane Fonda, Pat Benatar.

1984 Canadians Frank Toskan, a makeup artist and photographer, and Frank Angelo, a hair salon owner, launch Make-up Art Cosmetics, or MAC. Their line, which is originally designed for use in fashion photography, wins a wide following with its socially conscious motto: "All ages, all races, all sexes."

Make Up For Ever is launched by Dany Sanz and Jacques Waneph to meet the unique needs of the stage and fashion industries.

1985 Paulina Porizkova signs on as the face of Estée Lauder for six million dollars.

1990 Hollywood makeup artist Carol Shaw launches LORAC, a line featuring oil and fragrance-free foundations.

1988 Ultima II relaunches the Naked Collection.

1990s Makeup is all about looking natural.

Models to know: Linda Evangelista, Christy Turlington, Naomi Campbell, Cindy Crawford, Tatjana Patitz.

Beauty icons: Jennifer Aniston, Jennifer Lopez.

1991 New York makeup artist Bobbi Brown launches Bobbi Brown *essentials* with ten brown-based lipsticks at Bergdorf Goodman.

1994 Kate Moss appears on Calvin Klein Obsession perfume ads and billboards

Jeanine Lobell launches Stila cosmetics.

Fashion model Iman launches IMAN, a line of cosmetics for women of color.

François Nars launches NARS with twelve lipsticks at Barneys New York. In 1996 he shoots his first advertising campaign for his brand, and continues to do so today.

1995 Frustrated by the lack of bold, vibrant colors, Vincent Longo launches his own line.

1996 Crème de la Mer, a potent cream developed by aerospace physicist Max Huber, is relaunched.

Laura Mercier launches her line of cosmetics.

1999 Sonia Kashuk launches the Sonia Kashuk Professional Makeup collection for Target. This marks the first partnership between a high-profile makeup artist and mass-market retailer.

2000s–Present Fake tans, sun beds, and tanning products are all the rage, mineral-based makeup enters the marketplace, and makeup brands explode.

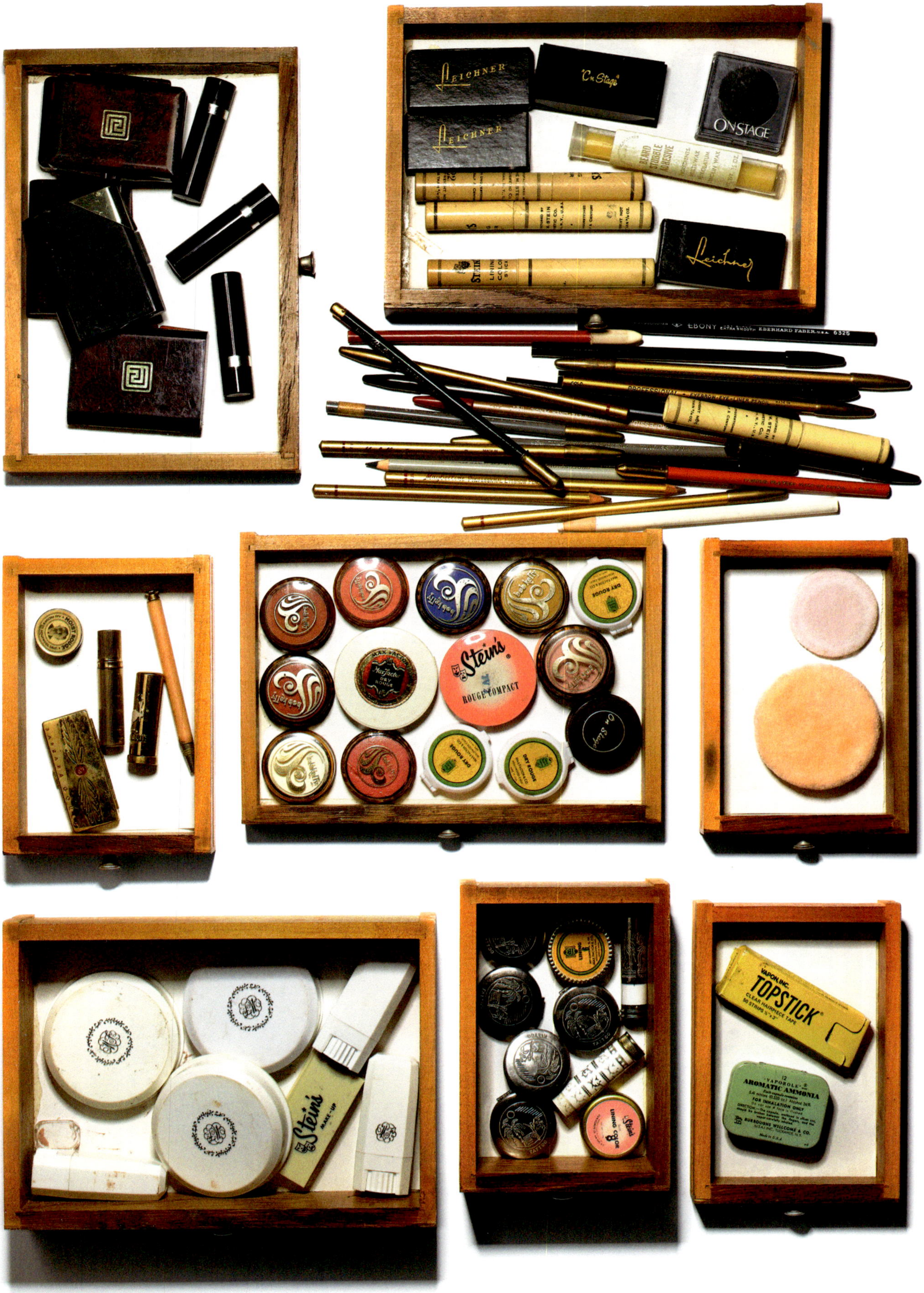

LEICHNER
"On Stage"
ONSTAGE
LEICHNER
Leichner
EBONY
EBERHARD FABER
Stein's
ROUGE COMPACT
DRY ROUGE
Stein's
MAKE-UP
VAPON INC.
TOPSTICK
CLEAR HAIRPIECE TAPE
AROMATIC AMMONIA
FOR INHALATION ONLY
BURROUGHS WELLCOME & CO.

WHO'S WHO in MAKEUP

These are the pioneers ***who helped shape the beauty industry*** and also greatly influenced me as an artist.

Helena Rubinstein

(1870–1965)

Born in Poland, she was the eldest of eight daughters. After immigrating to Australia, she opened the world's first modern beauty salon. She later relocated to the United States, opened a salon in New York City, and became a lifelong rival of Elizabeth Arden. In 1962, Rubinstein's salon was the first to introduce the concept of a "day of beauty." It consisted of an exercise class, massage, lunch, facial, shampoo, hairstyling, manicure, pedicure, and makeup session and cost $35.

Max Factor

(1877–1938)

Born in Poland as Max Faktor, his name morphed into Factor in 1904, when he went through Ellis Island on his way to becoming an American. In Los Angeles, he began selling his lotions and makeup, and soon he had developed a new type of makeup formulated specifically for the movies. It was called "flexible greasepaint" because, unlike standard film makeup, it didn't crack. In 1920, Factor introduced his cosmetics to the public, giving the average woman a chance to buy a little bit of Hollywood glamour at her local drugstore.

Coco Chanel

(1883–1971)

Although primarily remembered as a fashion designer, Chanel also created some of the world's most memorable perfumes. In 1922, she introduced Chanel No. 5, which to this day is a worldwide best seller.

Elizabeth Arden

(1884–1966)

Born in Ontario, Canada, as Florence Nightingale Graham, she moved to New York in 1908, where she worked as a bookkeeper at E. R. Squibb Pharmaceuticals Company. Whenever possible, Graham spent time in the company's lab, learning the skills she would later use to create her own skincare lotions. She jumped at an opportunity to go to work for a "beauty culturist" doing skin treatments. There she met Elizabeth Hubbard and, in 1909, the two opened their own Fifth Avenue salon. When the partnership ended, Graham retained her partner's first name, Elizabeth, and chose the last name Arden, from the Tennyson poem "Enoch Arden." Thus, Elizabeth Arden was born. She quickly expanded her repertoire from giving skincare treatments to creating makeup colors. She worked tirelessly for her self-made company into her eighties.

Charles Revson

(1906–1975)

In 1932, Revson went into business with his brother and a chemist named Charles Lachman. They founded a company called Revlon and launched it with the introduction of a nail polish. Revlon became known for nail polishes in a wide variety of colors. Eventually, they marketed matching lipsticks, including the legendary Fire and Ice shade of bold red.

Estée Lauder

(1908–2004)

As an enterprising young woman, Lauder began selling the skin creams created by her uncle, a chemist. In 1948, she convinced the managers at Saks Fifth Avenue to give her counter space to sell her line. She is credited with pioneering the concept of "gift with purchase," giving away free samples to her customers. In 1953, she introduced her first fragrance, Youth Dew, a bath oil meant to be lavishly splashed over the entire body. By 1984, annual sales of that product had reached $150 million.

Mary Kay Ash

(1918–2001)

Born in Hot Wells, Texas, Mary Kay Ash worked in direct sales until 1963, when she retired to write a book to assist women in business. The book turned into a business plan and by September 1963, with only five thousand dollars, she founded Mary Kay Cosmetics with her son, Richard Rogers. They developed a line of skincare products and color cosmetics, initially sold out of a storefront in Dallas, Texas. With the Golden Rule as the founding principle of her company, she insisted that her employees keep their lives in balance. She authored a total of three books, all of which became best sellers. Her book on people management, has been included as a text at the Harvard Business School. At the time of Ash's death, Mary Kay Cosmetics had over 800,000 representatives in 37 countries, with total annual sales of more than $2 billion at retail.

Shu Uemura

(1928–2007)

The founder of shu uemura cosmetics, he was the first to merge makeup and art through makeup performances on stage and his seasonal Mode Makeup collections. His career began in Hollywood in 1955 and it took off when he was called to substitute for Shirley MacLaine's makeup artist. His first product, Unmask Cleansing Oil, came out in 1960. His first makeup school opened in Tokyo shortly thereafter. His first open workshop/concept cosmetics boutique opened in 1983. The Tokyo Lash Bar, with a huge variety of false-lash concepts, was launched in 2007.

Way Bandy

(1941–1986)

Bandy was one of the best-known freelance makeup artists of the 70s and 80s. He created Calvin Klein's first cosmetics collection, which featured burgundy packaging. His best-selling books are a great source of information and inspiration to makeup artists today.

George Newell

(1954–1992)

George Newell began his career as a model and makeup artist in Houston. He moved to New York in 1977 to work as a freelance makeup artist, and became famous for a Halston layout he did for *Vogue* in 1979, where he served as both a fashion model and a makeup artist. In the early 1980s he established George Newell, Inc., a management and talent agency in Los Angeles, representing photographers, stylists, makeup artists, and hair stylists. During his career he designed many *Vanity Fair* and *Vogue* covers.

Frank Toskan & Frank Angelo

(1948–1997)

In 1985, these two Canadians joined creative forces to form MAC (Make-up Art Cosmetics). Toskan was a makeup artist and photographer, and

Angelo operated a chain of beauty salons. Toskan was frustrated with the available cosmetic offerings, all of which had glossy finishes that he thought reflected too much light in photographs. The company marketed an expanded color line (to suit more skin tones) and products with matte finishes. Today, MAC is known as much for its ethical policies and good works as it is for its products.

Kevyn Aucoin

(1962–2002)

As a child growing up in Louisiana, Aucoin studied fashion magazines and tried to duplicate the looks he saw on his younger sister, Carla. After attending beauty school, he moved to New York in 1983. His big break came when a beauty editor at *Vogue* asked to see his book. In 1986, he did his first *Vogue* cover shoot with the photographer Richard Avedon. During his career, he worked with countless A-list celebrities and showcased his work in three books: *The Art of Makeup*, *Making Faces*, and *Face Forward*.

Ariella

Ariella is best known for her longtime collaboration with the photographer Richard Avedon. She did the makeup for countless American *Vogue* covers as well as the iconic photo in 1981 featuring Natassja Kinski entwined with a boa constrictor.

Serge Lutens

Serge Lutens is a French photographer, filmmaker, hair stylist, perfumer, and fashion designer. In 1962, he moved to Paris, where *Vogue* magazine hired him to create makeup, hair, and jewelry looks. During the 60s he worked with photographer greats such as Richard Avedon, Bob Richardson, and Irving Penn. He created a makeup line for Christian Dior in 1967. In 1980, he was hired by Shiseido to develop its image internationally and to create the fragrance Nombre Noir. Both the fragrance and its packaging were considered ahead of their time. In the early 90s he designed Les Salons du Palais Royal, a perfume boutique, and in 2000, launched his own brand.

Alberto Fava

Alberto Fava began his career as a makeup artist in Rome in 1970, assisting Gil Cagne. In the 1970s he collaborated with fashion magazines, started to design makeup for fashion shows, and worked with several prominent photographers. As beauty editor for *Mirabella* magazine, he helped envision and plan the style and content of beauty stories.

Sandy Linter

Sandy Linter is a legendary makeup artist in New York City. Linter has spent the past thirty years working with celebrities and models. She is recognized throughout the beauty community for her age-defying techniques, which have been known to take off more years than cosmetic surgery. A frequent contributor to the country's leading fashion and beauty magazines, Linter's work has appeared in *Vogue*, *Harper's Bazaar*, and *Vanity Fair*.

Linda Mason

Linda Mason reinvented the role of makeup on the runway in the late 70s. Her artistry was an integral part of signature looks for designers such as Gaultier and Mugler and for the label Comme des Garçons. In 1987, she started Linda Mason Elements, Inc.

Mary Quant

Working as a fashion designer in London in the 50s, Mary Quant was on a mission to make youthful fashion affordable. Her King's Road boutique became a Mecca for girls in search of the mod look and Quant's famous miniskirts. In the 60s she expanded her line to include paintbox makeup—a collection of bold, fun colors in a compact container.

Bonnie Maller

New York–based freelance makeup artist Bonnie Maller is best known for introducing the natural makeup look in the late 70s. She created looks for Ralph Lauren, Perry Ellis, and Calvin Klein, and her work was showcased in magazines around the world. She collaborated frequently with the photographer Bruce Weber.

Stéphane Marais

Stéphane Marais is a French makeup artist and entrepreneur whose quirky imagery has earned him global attention. He is widely known for his collaboration with Peter Lindbergh, his consulting work for Shiseido, and his ability to be understated and dramatic at the same time. He opened a flagship store in Paris in 2002.

Linda Cantello

Linda Cantello's career began in the early 80s, and since then she has worked in high-luxury advertising campaigns, collaborated with top photographers, and worked with some of the best fashion and beauty publications. She was commissioned by MAC and Kanebo to recast their color lines and recently launched her signature makeup and skincare line.

Mary Greenwell

Mary Greenwell began her career in the 80s in Paris. She has since worked with every big-name photographer, and trained many of today's makeup artists. Her eye for detail and color led to a contract with Shiseido, where she created new colors, taking the collection in a new direction. She is a regular artist at fashion shows and has a large celebrity clientele. Her work has been seen in all the leading magazines, in editorial, and in ad campaigns for Yohji Yamamoto, Valentino, DKNY, Estée Lauder, Guerlain, L'Oréal, Max Factor, and Comme des Garçons.

Barbara Daly

British makeup artist Barbara Daly began working in the 1960s and is popularly known for her work on the 1971 Stanley Kubrick film, *A Clockwork Orange*. She was called on by Diana, Princess of Wales, to do her wedding day makeup. And she is the creator of a makeup line available at the UK retailer Tesco.

François Nars

Born in the South of France, François Nars attended the Carita makeup school in Paris. In 1984, he began working with fashion's top publications, collaborated with top designers, including Dolce & Gabbana, Marc Jacobs, and Karl Lagerfeld, and with legendary photographers, such as Richard Avedon, Patrick Demarchelier, Steven Meisel, Helmut Newton, Irving Penn, and Bruce Weber. Frustrated with the cosmetics lines available, Nars developed and successfully launched NARS, a cosmetics and skincare company, in 1994. He is also a professional photographer and the author of *X-Ray* (1999) and coauthor of *Makeup Your Mind* (2002).

Joey Mills

Joey Mills was widely known in the 70s and 80s for his classic American style. His work appeared in countless magazine covers, editorials, and advertising campaigns.

Reggie Wells

A veteran in the makeup industry, Reggie Wells has worked with countless actresses, painting his iconic, glamorous sculpted faces. Reggie is also widely known for his work with Oprah Winfrey as both a guest and behind-the-scenes makeup artist. He is an Emmy Award winner and author of *Face Painting*.

Tom Pecheux

Tom Pecheux lives and works in Paris. He is a beauty designer and key makeup artist for some of the top makeup brands, including Shiseido and MAC. His work on fashion shows for Prada, Karl Lagerfeld, and Alberta Ferretti, among others, has won him a loyal following in the fashion industry. He's also worked with countless musicians including Madonna and Avril Lavigne on music videos, collaborating with the top fashion designers in the business.

Dick Page

This British makeup artist has a reputation as an industry leader. He is known for his editorial, advertising, and runway work. Since 1997, he has worked with Shiseido in Japan on its premier domestic line of cosmetics, and in 2001, he was made artistic director of the makeup line. He redesigned and relaunched the line in August 2002 as Inoui ID. In March 2007, he was named artistic director of Shiseido The Makeup. Page frequently contributes to *Allure* with his own insider's page of tips and ideas entitled "The Makeup Guy." He currently acts as the key makeup artist for the runway shows of Michael Kors, Narciso Rodriguez, Marc Jacobs, Marc by Marc Jacobs, and United Bamboo.

Pat McGrath

Pat McGrath is a British makeup artist known for her wide range and inventive use of materials: her makeup is often handmade, and she works mainly with her fingers rather than with brushes. McGrath's big break came while working with Edward Enninful at *i-D* magazine in the early 90s. She became known for her dramatic, stylized designs, including bodies drenched in paint and petals glued to faces. She designed Armani's cosmetics line in 1999 and in 2004 was named global creative-design director for Procter and Gamble, where she is in charge of Max Factor and Cover Girl cosmetics, among other brands.

Laura Mercier

Raised in Provence, Laura Mercier trained at the Carita school, where she specialized in makeup application. In her early career, she began working closely with Thibault Vabre, a well-known French makeup artist. In 1985, Mercier moved to New York to join the team to launch American *Elle*. She soon began working for advertising campaigns for major corporations, editorial spreads for magazines, and multiple cosmetics and clothing companies, and worked with Madonna to create looks for print, television, and film. She then contracted with Elizabeth Arden to design the makeup looks for advertising campaigns and worked on Chanel's advertising campaigns in France. In 1996, Mercier developed her own line, which is now in four hundred stores in twenty-one countries.

Sam Fine

Sam Fine began his education in makeup behind the cosmetics counters of department stores. He studied art in New York while continuing to work in the cosmetics department of a large specialty store. His transition to freelance artist occurred when Naomi Campbell's makeup artist was unavailable for a show and she called Sam. He is known especially for his work with African American women and as the author of *Fine Beauty*.

Joanne Gair

Joanne Gair is an artist and image maker who has emerged as the premiere makeup artist/body painter in the world. From New Zealand, Gair has an interest in art photography. Her work as a makeup artist and body painter has appeared in editorial covers, layouts, fashion campaigns, advertising, music videos, commercials, and motion pictures.

Heidi Morawetz

Heidi Morawetz was the creative director of Chanel's makeup

studio in Paris for over thirty years. Morawetz created the "face" of each season for the runway shows. She developed Chanel's famous Rouge Noir nail polish (Vamp) in 1994; the blood red shade is still Chanel's best-selling nail polish color. She began as a freelance makeup artist and stylist until Dominique Moncourtois discovered her work and brought her into Chanel. Together with Moncourtois, Morawetz built the Chanel makeup business into the success it is today.

Dominique Moncourtois

Dominique Moncourtois spent thirty-six years as the director of Chanel's Makeup Creation. As a child, he spent holidays in Paris with his great aunt, a former model who introduced him to the art of makeup. From 1963 to 1967 he worked as a makeup artist and wigmaker in the film industry, and in 1968, he joined Chanel. He continues to create and develop new looks and technology for makeup.

Fulvia Farolfi

Fulvia Farolfi's work appears in *Vogue*, *Harper's Bazaar*, and *W* magazines, to name a few, and she works regularly with top photographers including Irving Penn, Bruce Weber, and Raymond Meier. She's a fixture at the runway shows in New York and Europe and has developed makeup lines for Emporio Armani and Shiseido.

Charlie Green

Charlie Green began her career in London, working on music videos for talents like Kylie Minogue and Bryan Ferry, then headed to Paris where she made her name collaborating with photographers David LaChapelle and Michael Thompson, and designers like Vivienne Westwood and Chloé. Now based in the United States, Green is a celebrity and editorial favorite.

Paul Starr

Paul Starr is a Los Angeles–based celebrity-makeup artist whose clients include Jennifer Garner, Salma Hayek, Michelle Pfeiffer, Angelina Jolie, and countless others. He has worked with photographers such as Patrick Demarchelier, David LaChappelle, and Annie Leibovitz. Starr has worked over twenty years in film, music videos, and print, and he has also worked with Estée Lauder on a makeup collection.

Gucci Westman

Gucci Westman studied makeup in Paris, then headed to Los Angeles, where she focused on special-effects makeup. She was "discovered" when photographer Annie Leibovitz called on her for a 1996 *Vanity Fair* cover shoot. In addition to working regularly with the beauty and fashion industry's top magazines and designers, Gucci has lent her expertise to the cosmetics company Lancôme.

Scott Barnes

Scott Barnes came to New York City at the age of seventeen to begin a career as a painter. A graduate of Detroit's Center for Creative Studies, and New York's Parsons School for Design, he began to find work on fashion photography shoots. Scott used his painting skills to model faces for fashion and soon secured an agent for his work. His work is known for its sexiness with a global sensibility and has been published by *Vogue*, *InStyle*, *Elle*, *Vanity Fair*, *Rolling Stone*, and *Premiere*. He works regularly with celebrated photographers such as Herb Ritts, Patrick Demarchelier, Annie Leibovitz, and Matthew Rolston, as well as many A-list celebrities.

Joe Blasco

Joe Blasco began his study of the art of makeup at the early age of seven. He was awarded a scholarship to cosmetology school, and after graduating in 1964 at the age of eighteen, he arrived in Hollywood to work for the Max Factor cosmetics company. In 1967 he set out to pursue a career in Hollywood as a makeup artist. He took a job as an instructor with a small makeup school and recognized the need for a course that taught motion picture and television makeup artistry. He became known for his work in special makeup effects. In 1976 he opened the first of two renowned makeup training centers.

Diane Kendal

Diane Kendal's signature look—one that's rock and roll but gorgeous and approachable—has made her an industry favorite. She collaborates regularly with Catherine Malandrino, Jean Paul Gaultier, Balenciaga, Carolina Herrera, and Calvin Klein. Her work appears frequently in *W*, *Vogue*, and *Vanity Fair*. Additionally, she regularly represents MAC at Fashion Week and designed Calvin Klein's cosmetic line from 2002 to 2003.

RESOURCE GUIDE

Theatrical Makeup Stores

ALCONE 235 West 19th Street, New York, NY 10019; alconeco.com; 212-633-0551,

BALL BEAUTY SUPPLY 416 North Fairfax Avenue, Los Angeles, CA 90036; 323-655-2330

CINEMA SECRETS 4400 Riverside Drive, Burbank, CA 91505; 818-846-0579

FREND'S BEAUTY SUPPLY 5270 Laurel Canyon Boulevard, North Hollywood, CA 91607; 818-769-3834

THE MAKEUP SHOP 131 West 21st Street, New York, NY 10011; 212-807-0447

NAIMIE'S BEAUTY CENTER 12640 Riverside Drive, Valley Village, CA 91607; www.naimies.com; 818-655-9933

RAY BEAUTY SUPPLY 721 8th Avenue, New York, NY 10036; 800-253-0993

RICKY'S 590 Broadway New York, NY 10012; 212-226-5552 / 1574 Third Avenue, New York, NY 10079; 212-996-7030 / 107 Montague Street, Brooklyn, NY 11201; 718-522-5011

SALLY BEAUTY SUPPLY Locations nationwide; sallybeauty.com; 800-ASK-SALLY

Makeup Artist Agencies

NEW YORK AGENCIES

THE ARTIST LOFT 580 Broadway, Suite 606, New York, NY 10012; www.aartistloft.com; 212-274-0961; Attn: Sara Mouzianni

ARTISTS BY TIMOTHY PRIANO 131 Varick Street, Suite 905, New York, NY 10013; 212-929-7771; Attn: David Kelley

ART + COMMERCE 755 Washington Street, New York, NY 10014; www.artandcommerce.com; 212-206-0730; Attn: Joshua Hiller

BRIAN BANTRY AGENCY 4 West 58th Street, Penthouse, New York, NY 10019; 212-935-0200

JED ROOT 61A Walker Street, New York, NY 10013; www.jedroot.com; 212-226-6600; Attn: Kelly Obaski Hass

MAGNET: 270 Lafayette Street, Suite 901, New York, NY 10012; www.magnetla.com; 212-941-7441

MAREK 508 West 26th Street, New York, NY 10001; 212-924-6760

NEW YORK OFFICE 15 West 26th Street, New York, NY 10010; www.nyoffice.net; Attn: Julianne Hausler

OLIVER PIRO 128 West 26th Street, 3rd Floor, New York, NY 10001; www.oliverpiro.com; 212-925-2112; Attn: Massu Nedjat

R. J. BENNETT REPRESENTS 530 East 20th Street, Suite 2B, New York, NY 10009; www.rjbennettrepresents.com; 212-673-5509; Attn: Rose Bennett

CALIFORNIA AGENCIES

ARTISTS BY TIMOTHY PRIANO 8447 Wilshire Boulevard, Beverly Hills, CA 90211; 323-782-0021; Attn: Jared Franco

ARTIST UNTIED www.artistuntied.com; 323-933-0200

ATELIER MANAGEMENT 543 South Spring Street, Los

Angeles, CA 90013; 323-933-2983; Attn: Brian

CELESTINE 1548 16th Street, Santa Monica, CA 90404; www.celestine.com; 310-998-1977; Attn: Frank Moore

CLOUTIER 1026 Montana Avenue, Santa Monica, CA 90403; www.cloutieragency.com; 310-394-8813; Attn: Imari McDermott

LUXE 6442 Santa Monica Boulevard, Los Angeles, CA 90035; 323-856-8540; Attn: Nadia

TRACEY MATTINGLY LLC/AVANT GROUPE 1617 Cosmo Street, Loft 402, Los Angeles, CA 90028; 323-467-0000; Attn: Tracey Mattingly, Cale Harrison, or Jessica Johnson

ZENOBIA 130 South Highland Avenue, Los Angeles, CA 90036; www.zenobia.com; 323-937-1010; Attn: Keith or Heidi

Creative Directories

ASSOCIATION OF FILM COMMISSIONERS INTERNATIONAL www.afci.org. Published annually. This directory has listings for film and television productions globally.

THE BLACK BOOK www.blackbook.com. Published annually in December. It is a directory of advertising photography—an excellent resource for finding photographers to send your work.

LA 411 www.la411.com. Published annually in January. It lists the names and contact information of professionals in the television, video, and film industries in Los Angeles. The book includes rate tables and information on union rules.

LE BOOK www.lebook.com. Published annually. It is an international guide to the fashion world. It includes contact information for designers, modeling agencies, catalog companies, and photographers.

MIAMI PRODUCTION GUIDE www.filmflorida.com. Published annually in December. It lists film and television production resources in Miami.

SELECT www.select-magazine.com. Published six times a year. Issues focus on different cities and provide information including clubs, agencies, and more. It is a good source for finding catalog and entertainment photographers.

THE WORKBOOK www.workbook.com. Published annually, in January. It is a resource for the graphic arts industry and is great for finding photographers, stylists, makeup artists, costumers, etc., who work in advertising. Select a target group for a mailing. The Workbook will give you a count, and for a small fee will send you labels for your promotional mailing.

Suggested Reading

Designing Your Face by Way Bandy (Random House, 1984)

Face Forward by Kevyn Aucoin (Little, Brown & Co., 2001)

Making Faces by Kevyn Aucoin (Little, Brown & Co., 1997)

Make-up Artist magazine http://makeupmag.com

Stage Makeup by Richard Corson (Prentice Hall, Inc., 1990)

Other Books by Bobbi Brown:

Bobbi Brown Beauty (Harper Style, 1997)

Bobbi Brown Beauty Evolution (Harper Resource, 2002)

Bobbi Brown Living Beauty (Springboard Press, 2007)

Bobbi Brown Teenage Beauty (Cliff Street Books, 2000)

ACKNOWLEDGMENTS

This book was a labor of love and could not have been done without the talented and hardworking team that made it possible. First I want to thank Jill Cohen, who managed this intricate process and worked with me every step of the way. A special thank-you to my editor, Karen Murgolo, whose hard work and patience were invaluable—and to the rest of the publishing team at Hachette Book Group, including Jamie Raab, Matthew Ballast, Tom Hardej, Dorothea Halliday, Pamela Schechter, Melissa Bullock, Nicole Bond, and Peggy Boelke.

I'm grateful to my creative director, Ruba Abu-Nimah, who always surprises me with her aesthetic. Thanks also to designer Eleanor Rogers, and everyone else who brought this book to life: writers Debra Bergsma Otte and Sally Wadyka, Matthias Gaggl, John Cassidy, Jason Nakleh, Billy Jim, Daymion Mardel, Kellie Kulton, Gail Hadani, Nicolai Grosell, Maxine Tall, Brian Hagiwara, Bret Baughman, Sydney Wicks, John Eaton, Guy Aroch, Joy Glenn, and Rosanne Guararra. Thank you to Henry Leutwyler for the stunning photos, to Lise Varrette for the beautiful and perfect step-by-step shots, and to Ben Ritter for the behind-the-scenes reportage. Thanks to the photographers who contributed advice, including Patrick Demarchelier, Walter Chin, and Troy Word. My heartfelt appreciation goes to my makeup artists who worked on this book, including Kimberly Christine Soane, Elizabeth Keiser, Sarah Sugarman, Tanya Cropsey, Ellice Schwab, and Waltaya Culmer. And thank you to hair stylist Yannick d'Is and his assistant, Mako, to hair stylist Mario Diab, and to manicurist Roza Israel.

Thanks to everyone at Bobbi Brown Cosmetics. A shout-out to my support team, including Matthew Riopelle, Joe Pinto, Kristen Boscaino, and Ron Hill. And big thanks to my incredibly fun and tireless PR team, including Veronika Ullmer, Gretchen Berra, Jay Squire, Ashley Badger-Wakefield, Elizabeth Just, Samantha Bailye, and the HL Group. Thank you also to the creative team, including Dorothy Mancuso, Marie Clare Katigbak, Nicole Kirkitsos, and Sarah Honeth, and to the product development team, including Sarah Robbins, Sotiria Cherpelis, and Gabrielle Nevin. And as always, my deep appreciation to Maureen Case, president of Bobbi Brown Cosmetics, my friend, biggest supporter, and all around great human being (breathe!).

PHOTO CREDITS

Guy Aroch: 89; **Walter Chin**: 175 (top right); **Patrick Demarchelier**: 175 (bottom right); **Nicolai Grosell**: 2; **Gail Hadani**: 179; **Brian Hagiwara**: 8, 11, 12, 13, 14, 18, 19, 37, 66, 68 (compact), 84 (lip pencil), 90 (brush), 91 (brush), 93, 98 (makeup), 99 (brush), 112 (brush), 133, 166 (jar, bottle), 167, 168 (nail polish); **Henry Leutwyler**: endpapers, ii, vii, viii, 6, 9, 10, 16, 17, 21, 22, 24, 25, 26, 27, 28, 29, 31, 35, 40 (cigarettes), 42, 44, 46, 48, 49, 51, 53 (Darker Peach), 54 (brush cleaning), 57 (makeup), 58, 61, 63, 65, 67, 69, 70, 71, 73, 74, 75, 76 (makeup), 77 (makeup), 78, 81, 82, 83 (lipsticks), 85 (makeup), 86, 95 (eye shadow), 97 (makeup), 100, 101, 104, 105, 110, 111, 114, 116, 124, 126, 131, 135, 137, 139, 142, 149, 157 (Bobbi with feet on desk), 162, 165, 166 (blush), 168 (tools), 169, 170, 175 (top left), 180, 181, 182, 183, 184, 185, 186, 187, 188, 189, 190, 191, 192, 193, 194, 195, 204, 210, 222, 223, 224; **Patrick McMullan**: v, 202 (Bobbi with Yogi Berra); **Ben Ritter**: 144, 147, 173; **Lise Varrette**: 40 (model), 52, 53 (Corrector Application for Asian Eyes), 54 (model), 55, 57 (three models), 59, 68 (model), 72, 76 (model), 77 (model), 83 (model), 84 (model), 85 (model), 90 (model), 91 (model), 92, 95 (model), 96, 97 (model), 98 (model), 99 (model), 102, 103, 106, 107, 108, 109, 112 (model), 113, 115, 118, 119, 120, 121, 122, 123, 177; **Troy Word**: 175 (bottom left).

Face Chart (125): Illustrated by **Tobie Giddio**.

Nine Memorable Women (197): Brigitte Bardot: MPTV.net; Catherine Deneuve: MPTV.net; Audrey Hepburn: MPTV.net; Lena Horne: © 1978 **Maurice Seymour** / MPTV.net; Grace Kelly: Photo by **Bert Six** / MPTV.net; Sophia Loren: MPTV.net; Ali MacGraw: © 1978 **Ken Whitmore** / MPTV.net; Marilyn Monroe: MPTV.net; Elizabeth Taylor: MPTV.net.

Fashion week and special event photography courtesy of: **Berit Bizjak**, **Dan Lecca**, **Patrick McMullan**, **WireImage**: 128, 129, 153, 199, 200, 201, 202, 203.

Other photography from Bobbi Brown's personal collection: 5, 157, 159, 161, 202, 203.

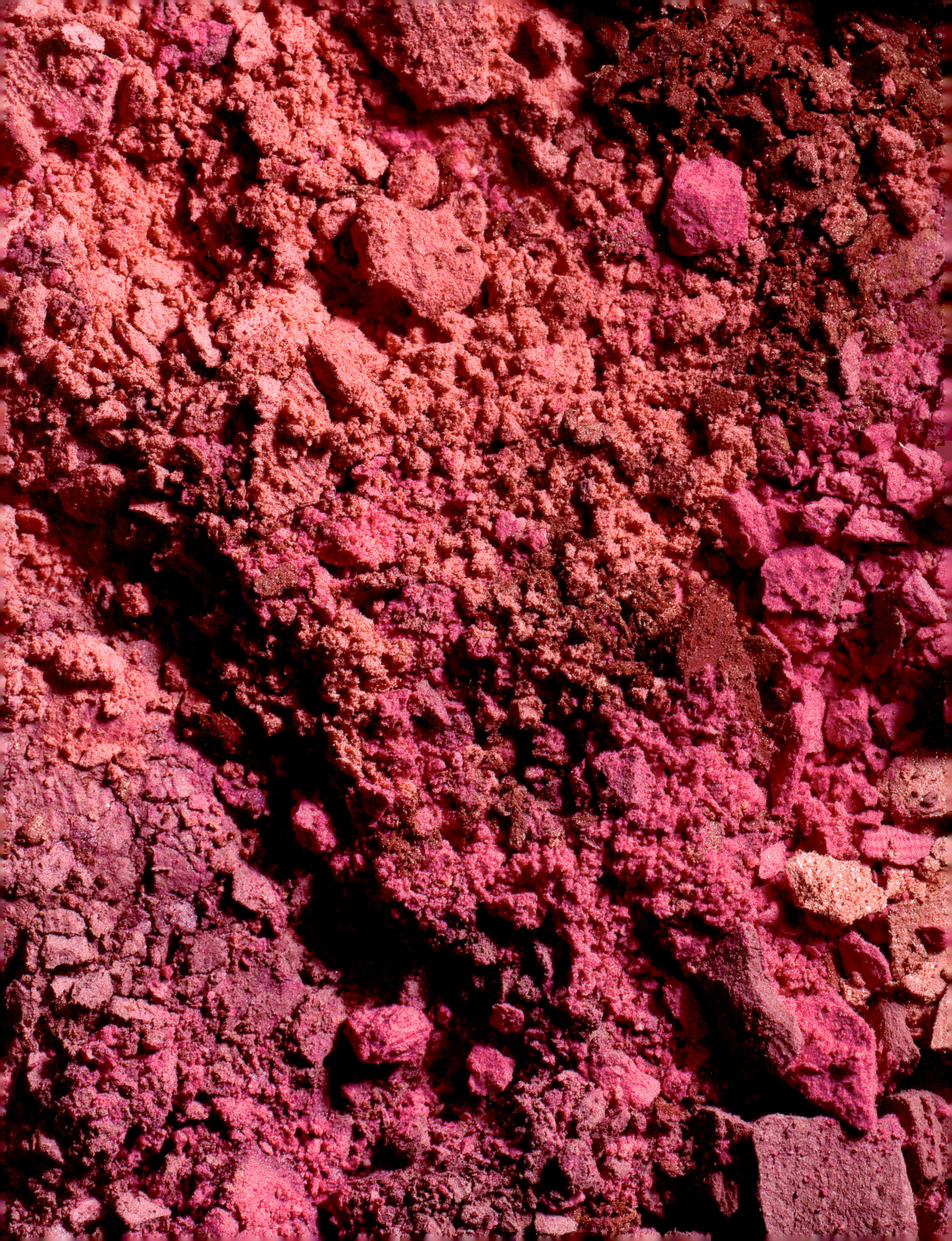

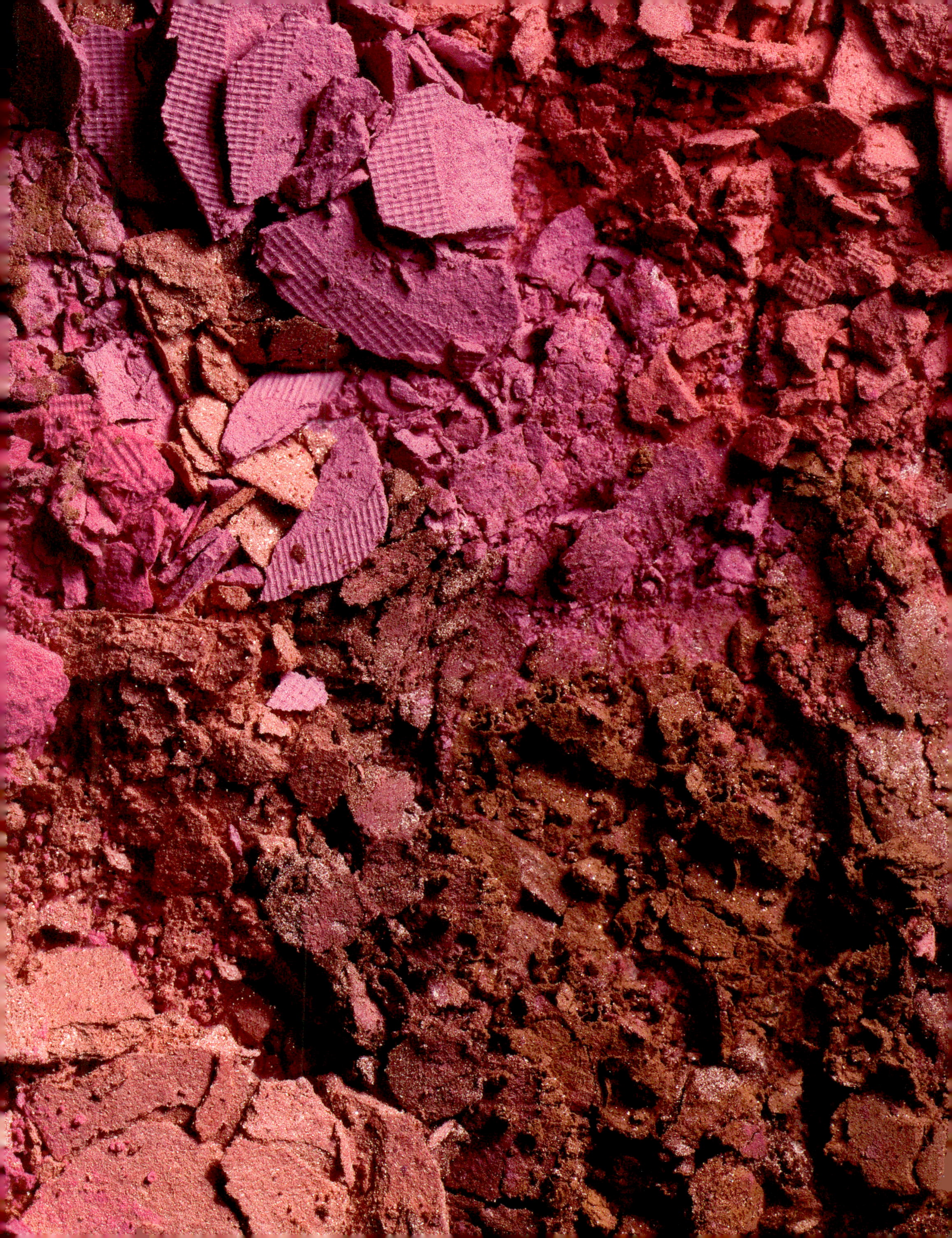

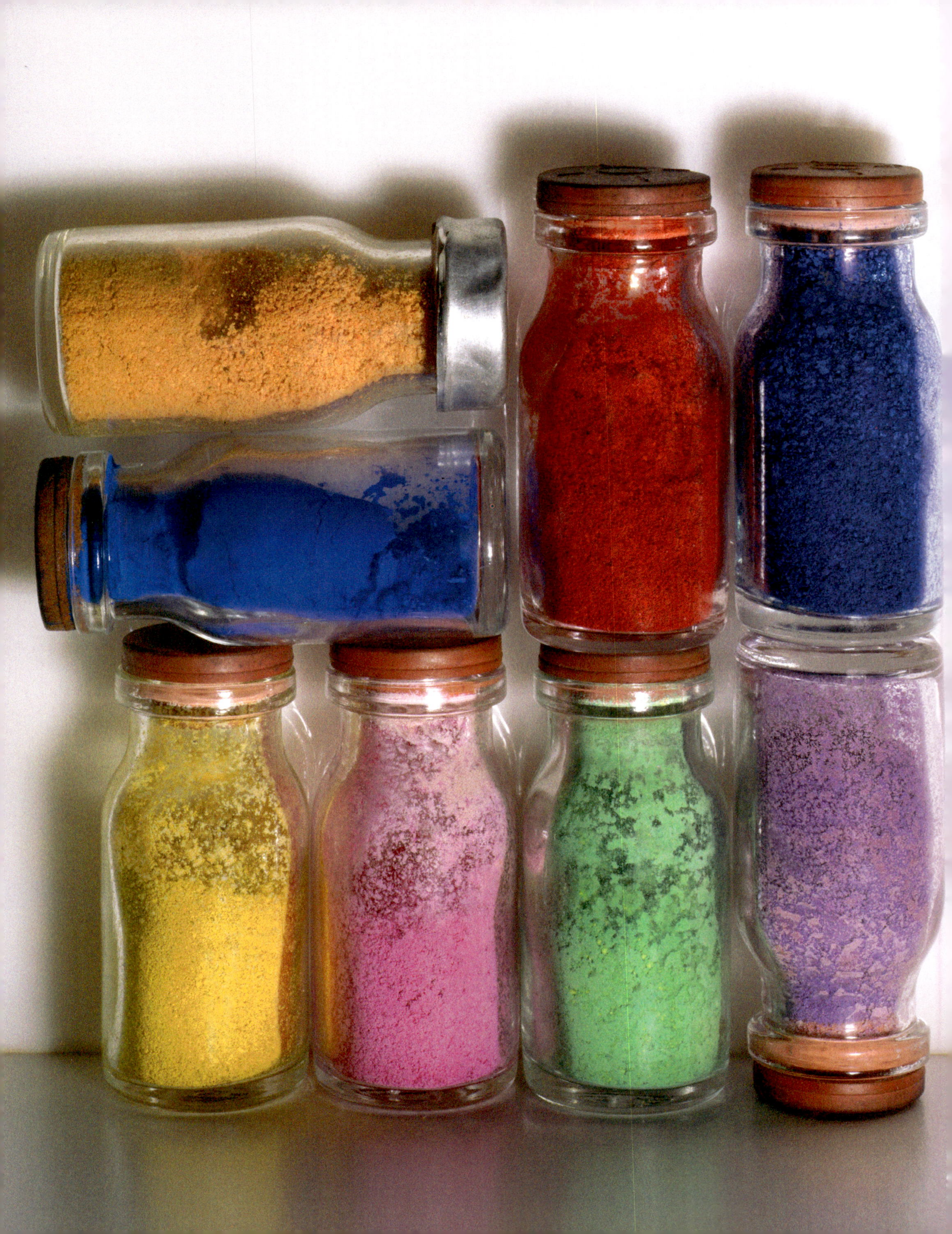

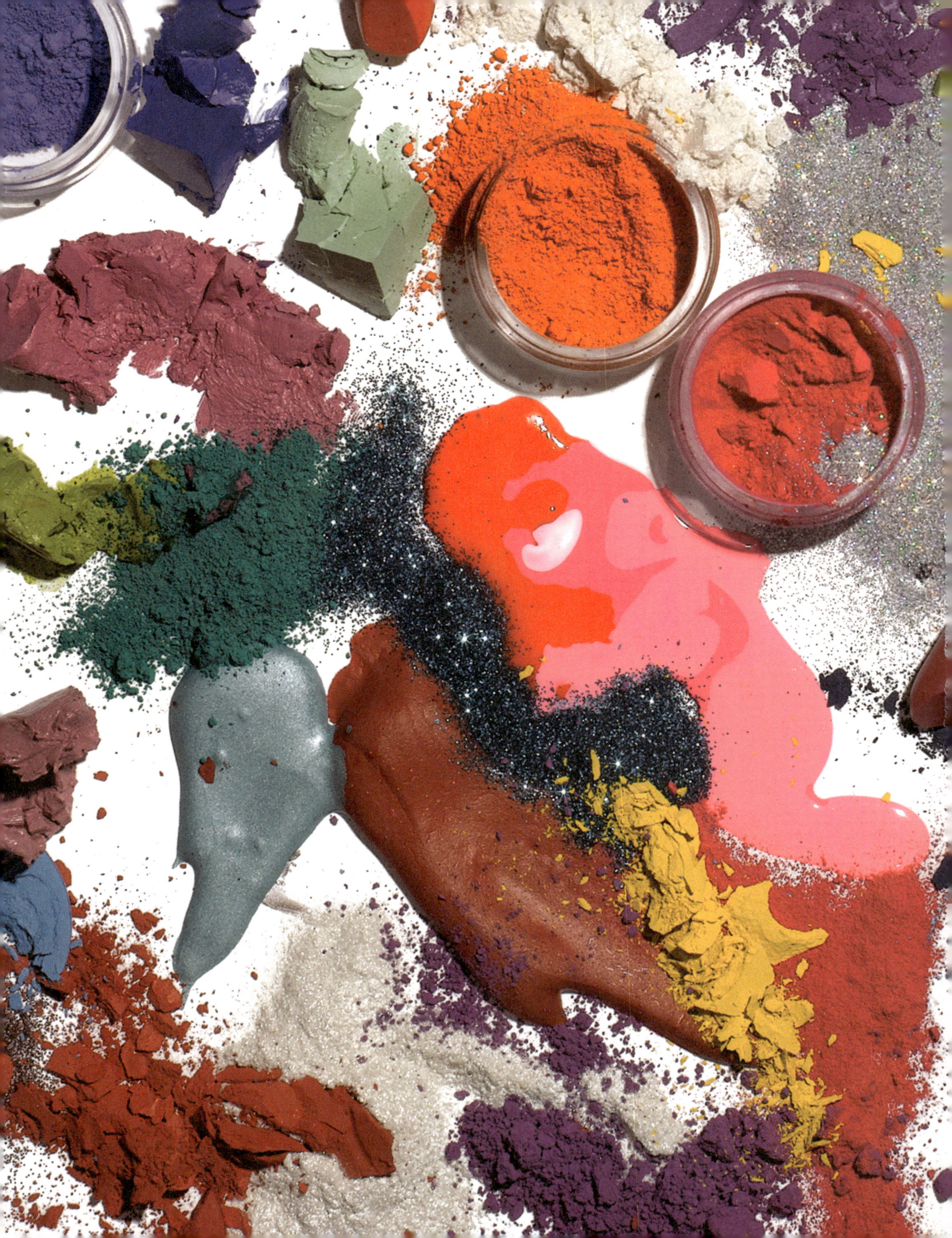